I0044380

Computed Tomography: Principles, Techniques and Clinical Applications

Computed Tomography: Principles, Techniques and Clinical Applications

Edited by Robert Meyer

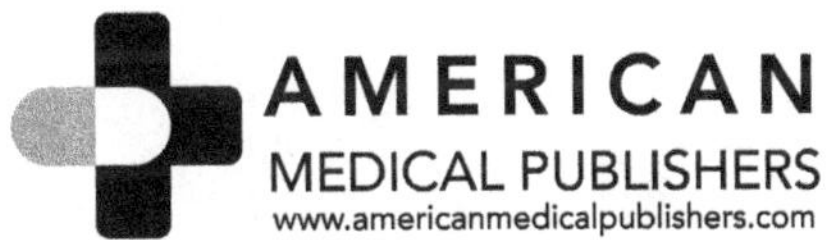

American Medical Publishers,
41 Flatbush Avenue,
1st Floor, New York,
NY 11217, USA

Visit us on the World Wide Web at:
www.americanmedicalpublishers.com

ISBN: 978-1-63927-068-2

Cataloging-in-Publication Data

Computed tomography : principles, techniques and clinical applications / edited by Robert Meyer.
p. cm.
Includes bibliographical references and index.
ISBN 978-1-63927-068-2
1. Tomography. 2. Tomography--Technological innovations. 3. Radiography, Medical.
4. Imaging systems in medicine. 5. Diagnostic imaging. I. Meyer, Robert.
RC78.7.T6 C66 2022
616.075 7--dc23

Table of Contents

Preface

I am honored to present to you this unique book which encompasses the most up-to-date data in the field. I was extremely pleased to get this opportunity of editing the work of experts from across the globe. I have also written papers in this field and researched the various aspects revolving around the progress of the discipline. I have tried to unify my knowledge along with that of stalwarts from every corner of the world, to produce a text which not only benefits the readers but also facilitates the growth of the field.

Computed tomography is an imaging procedure that makes use of computer-processed combinations of many X-ray measurements. The X-ray measurements are taken from different angles to produce cross-sectional images of particular areas of a scanned object. This helps in seeing inside the object without cutting. Computed tomography is an important tool in medical imaging which supplements medical ultrasonography and X-rays. It is primarily used for preventive medicine or screening for disease, such as CT scanning of head, lungs, angiography, etc. CT scanning of the head is used to detect medical conditions such as bone trauma, tumors, infarction and calcifications. CT scanning of lungs is used for detecting both acute and chronic changes in the lungs parenchyma. In angiography, it is used to visualize arterial and venous vessels throughout the body. In cardiac imaging, it is performed to gain knowledge about cardiac and coronary anatomy. This book unravels the recent studies in the field of computed tomography. The topics covered herein deal with the core aspects of this field. This book will prove to be immensely beneficial to students and researchers in medical imaging.

Finally, I would like to thank all the contributing authors for their valuable time and contributions. This book would not have been possible without their efforts. I would also like to thank my friends and family for their constant support.

Editor

1

Use of fuzzy edge single-photon emission computed tomography analysis in definite Alzheimer's disease

Robert Rusina[1*], Jaromír Kukal[2], Tomáš Bělíček[2], Marie Buncová[3], Radoslav Matěj[4]

Abstract

Background: Definite Alzheimer's disease (AD) requires neuropathological confirmation. Single-photon emission computed tomography (SPECT) may enhance diagnostic accuracy, but due to restricted sensitivity and specificity, the role of SPECT is largely limited with regard to this purpose.

Methods: We propose a new method of SPECT data analysis. The method is based on a combination of parietal lobe selection (as regions-of-interest (ROI)), 3D fuzzy edge detection, and 3D watershed transformation. We applied the algorithm to three-dimensional SPECT images of human brains and compared the number of watershed regions inside the ROI between AD patients and controls. The Student's two-sample t-test was used for testing domain number equity in both groups.

Results: AD patients had a significantly reduced number of watershed regions compared to controls ($p < 0.01$). A sensitivity of 94.1% and specificity of 80% was obtained with a threshold value of 57.11 for the watershed domain number. The narrowing of the SPECT analysis to parietal regions leads to a substantial increase in both sensitivity and specificity.

Conclusions: Our non-invasive, relatively low-cost, and easy method can contribute to a more precise diagnosis of AD.

Background

Alzheimer's disease (AD) is the most common neurodegenerative dementia. Diagnostic criteria are based mainly on clinically altered cognition. Early diagnosis of AD is crucial for maximizing treatment benefits. Neuroimaging may be helpful in increasing diagnostic precision, but correlations between localized atrophy, mainly in the temporal regions, on MRIs, and AD pathology are still controversial, and promising new techniques like PET amyloid imaging are not in routine use. Low beta-amyloid and elevated tau protein levels in cerebrospinal fluid have been correlated with AD at a sensitivity of 85-94% and a specificity of 83-100% [1]. However, other studies have not been able to confirm these results and widespread consensus is lacking regarding its utility in everyday practice [2].

* Correspondence: robert.rusina@ftn.cz
[1]Department of Neurology, Thomayer Teaching Hospital and Institute for Postgraduate Education in Medicine, Prague, Czech Republic
Full list of author information is available at the end of the article

Single photon emission computerized tomography (SPECT) is a widely used diagnostic method based on analysis of regional cerebral blood flow (rCBF); with restricted rCBF considered to reflect hypometabolism and consequently hypofunction. Typical SPECT AD patterns show reduced rCBF in both temporal and parietal regions, and, in a recent review, were capable of distinguishing AD from healthy controls (sensitivity = 65% - 71%; specificity = 79%) [3]. SPECT studies with autopsy-confirmed diagnoses reported sensitivities of 86 to 95% and specificities of 42 to 73% [4,5]. Since "raw" data needs further treatment, final results from SPECT investigations are, at least partly, operator-dependent and both specificity and sensitivity vary among centers. Because of its low sensitivity and specificity, routine use of SPECT is not recommended for diagnostic purposes [6].

Currently, new methods for signal processing and supervised learning have demonstrated the potential of computer aided diagnostic systems [7,8].

Computer based analysis of SPECT data is of increasing interest in the field. The superiority of 3-dimensional stereotactic surface projection analysis (3D-SSP) over visual inspection for differentiating patients with very early AD from control subjects using brain perfusion SPECT has been reported [9]. The authors found that 3D-SSP had an accuracy of 86.2% for differentiating patients with AD from control subjects when analyzing the posterior cingulate gyri and precunei. In contrast, visual inspection only had an accuracy of about 74.0%. Voxel-based analysis (using specific voxel-based Z score maps) may be helpful in differentiating AD from vascular dementia and non-demented patients using a method which is not influenced by inter-observer differences among radiologists [10]. These procedures, however, necessitate special software applications and are not routinely used in many countries.

Nevertheless, reasonable financial costs and the possibility of using SPECT repetitively for monitoring disease progression, offer arguments for routine use of SPECT, assuming that specificity and sensitivity can be increased through improved data processing.

The aim of our study was to develop a procedure with at least comparable accuracy to the results of visual inspection in differentiating AD patients from controls and at the same time avoid the need for special additional equipment.

Methods

Our study is based on a post hoc (retrospective) analysis of raw SPECT data, acquired between 2003 and 2005. The data were analyzed with respect for patient privacy and the protocol was approved by the local Ethics Committee.

We enrolled SPECT data from 17 adult patients with definite Alzheimer's disease confirmed by autopsy, as defined by NIA-Reagan Institute criteria as well as the Consortium to Establish a Registry for Alzheimer's disease criteria.

We routinely perform SPECT in patients with cognitive impairment as a routine diagnostic procedure. Therefore, in our setting, the data from SPECT scans and the confirmation of clinical diagnosis of AD were very timely (within a few weeks). All patients included in the study were diagnosed with mild to moderate AD (later confirmed by autopsy) according to NINCDS-ADRDA and DSM-IV criteria; additionally all patients were diagnosed with dementia.

Control cases included 10 patients with amyotrophic lateral sclerosis (ALS), without signs or complaints of cognitive dysfunction, who underwent SPECT and a detailed cognitive evaluation as part of a previously published research protocol [11].

SPECT studies were performed using a standardized protocol, which started 40 minutes after injection with 740 MBq 99mTcHMPAO (hexamethylpropyleneamine-oxime labeled with 99mTechnetium) and used a dual-head gamma camera (DST-XL SOPHA with LEHR collimator). We used filtered back projection (FBP) for image reconstruction. No correction for attenuation was made.

We prepared 3D SPECT brain scans in six consecutive operations: (i) image smoothing, (ii) normalization, (iii) background elimination, (iv) fuzzy edge detection, (v) watershed segmentation, and (vi) region counting.

Image smoothing (i), used a traditional method of noise suppression and was performed with a Gaussian 3D filter with radius as the first parameter.

The second step was oriented toward image intensity normalization (ii) in an interval (0, 1), where unit intensity corresponded to maximum brain activity.

Background elimination (iii) was the next image-processing step. The normalized intensity was compared with a threshold value as the second parameter of data processing. Positive differences were passed while negative ones were set to zero.

The fourth step was fuzzy edge detection (iv) based on Lukasiewicz BL-algebra [12]. Every voxel of the previous 3D image (after step iii) has 6 neighboring voxels; the fuzzy edge intensity (for a given voxel) was defined as the aggregate fuzzy non-equivalence between the voxel and its neighbors. The fuzzy equivalence of two voxel intensities was realized as a bi-residuum in Lukasiewicz BL-algebra. Bi-residuum reaches its unit maximum when the intensities are equal and the value falls to zero when they are opposite. The fuzzy non-equivalence is only a fuzzy negation of equivalence as a complement to the unit value. The fuzzy aggregation of six pairwise non-equivalences was performed via a fuzzy "OR" operator as the maximum function. Applying this procedure to every voxel and its neighbors, we obtain a 3D image of fuzzy edges (iv), which depicted structures with maximum morphological gradients of brain activity.

Edge contours with high intensity can help in image decomposition based on brain activity. The process of segmentation was automated using a standard 3D watershed transform (v) and constituted step five. The watershed method [13] is a tool for the digital image segmentation, which is based on the study of local minima and their basins of attraction. Watershed shapes in 3D consists of points where two basins of attraction are at least in their neighborhood. Sub-results of this procedure are demonstrated in Figure 1 for a central slice of the whole SPECT image of typical AD and control brains. The resulting 3D image of a parietal ROI was labeled to demarcate the regions and watershed borderlines (Figures 2, 3).

The last image processing step (vi) counts the total number of separated 3D regions into regions-of-interest (ROIs) centered in the left and right parietal lobes.

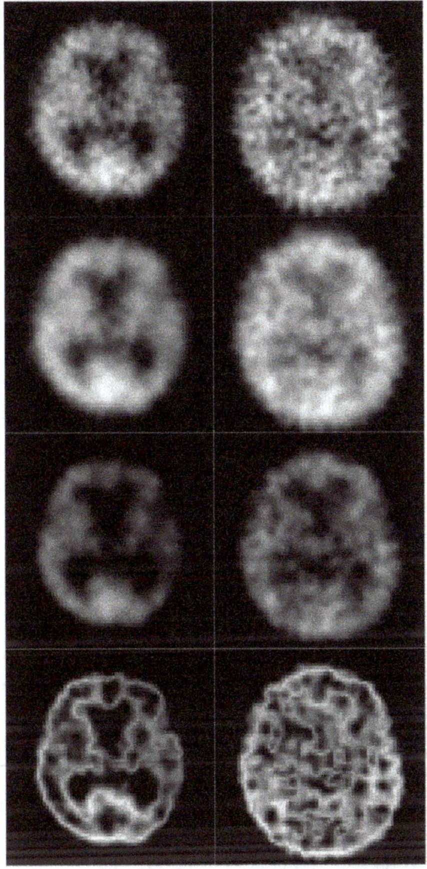

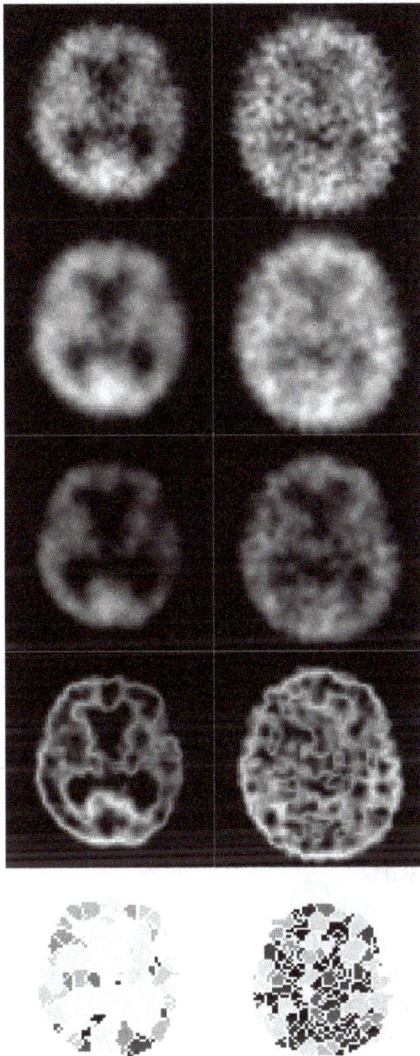

Figure 1 Processing steps for typical AD patients (left) and controls (right): original SPECT (1st - above), smoothing and normalization (2nd), thresholding (3rd), fuzzy edge detection (4th), watershed (5th - bottom).

All statistical calculations were performed using Matlab Statistical Toolbox from MathWorks Inc. Statistical characteristics were evaluated as point estimates together with 95% confidence intervals. The null hypothesis of the mean value equity was tested using the two-sample Student's t-test. Due to the relatively small groups of AD patients and controls, the 'leave-one-out' method [14] of cross-validation was used to obtain mean values of processing parameters and their standard deviations. Finally, the null hypothesis of the mean value equity was tested using the two-sample Student's t-test and the sensitivity and specificity of proposed method were estimated.

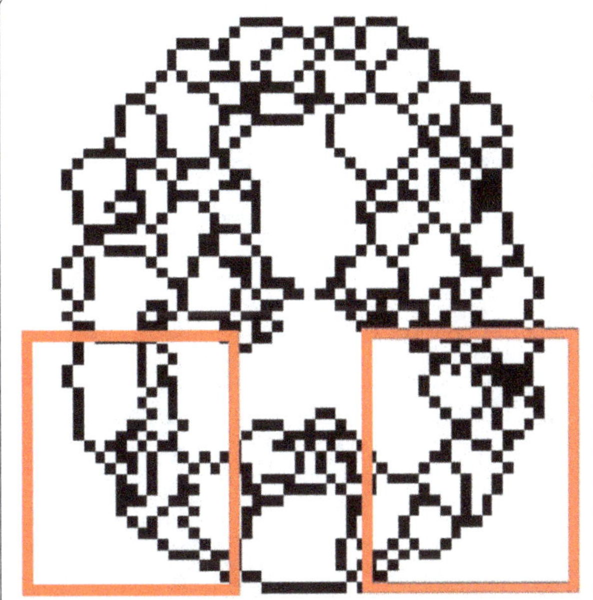

Figure 2 Final 3D watershed in a typical AD patient with 40 spatial regions (central slice).

Results

The study included 17 adult patients, where definite Alzheimer's disease was confirmed by autopsy using the NIA-Reagan Institute criteria (neocortical tangles score Braak V-VI), as well as the Consortium to Establish a Registry for Alzheimer's Disease criteria (CERAD plaque score frequent), and confirmed using specific monoclonal

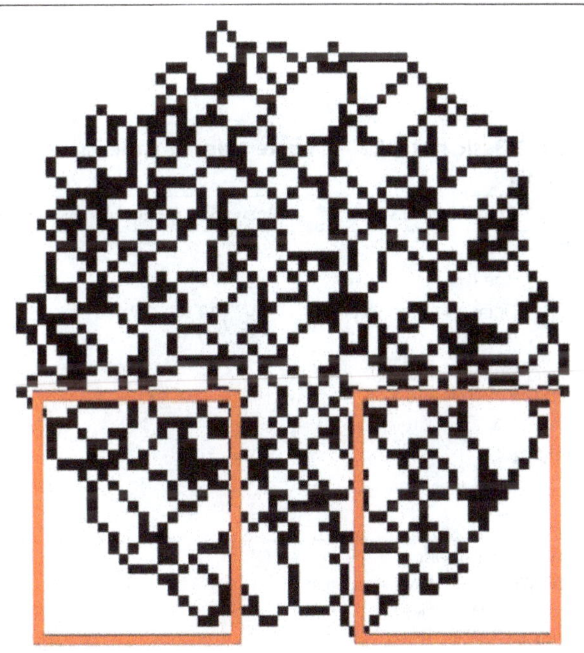

Figure 3 Final 3D watershed in a typical control with 70 spatial regions (central slice).

Table 1 Demographic data of patients and controls

Patient	Gender	Age (years)	MMSE	Braak stage	Comorbidity
1	M	78	23	VI	arterial hypertension
2	F	78	17	VI	alcohol abuse 10 years earlier
3	F	57	25	V	asthma, glaucoma
4	F	79	20	VI	arterial hypertension, coronary by-pass
5	M	74	19	VI	NA
6	M	76	20	VI	hypertension, minor stroke, diabetes, atrial fibrillation
7	F	83	10	VI	NA
8	F	83	20	VI	arterial hypertension
9	M	68	20	VI	NA
10	M	84	18	VI	NA
11	M	83	16	V	arterial hypertension, diabetes, myocardial infarction, hyperlipidemia
12	M	80	18	VI	arterial hypertension, subarachnoidal hemorrhage 30 years earlier
13	M	81	20	VI	NA
14	M	80	21	V	prostatic hypertrophy
15	F	86	16	VI	ischemic heart disease, diabetes
16	F	80	15	V	hypertension, atrial fibrillation
17	F	87	20	V	hypertension

antibodies against hyperphosphorylated tau protein and amyloid beta peptide. Basic patient characteristics are summarized in Tables 1, 2.

The 3D SPECT scans of 17 AD patients and 10 controls were analyzed as 3D matrices of 128×128×128 voxels using the described method with left and right parietal lobe ROIs having individual sizes of 22×29×3 voxels. Basic characteristics such as gender (F/M), age, Onset-Diagnosis, Diagnosis-Death, MMSE and the Braak stage are summarized in Tables 1, 2. The cross-validation using the 'leave-one-out' method had two main results.

Table 2 Basic statistical characteristics of patients and controls

Group	Characteristics	Mean	SD	Minimum	Maximum
AD	F/M	8/9			
	Age (years)	78.5	7.2	56	87
	Duration onset-diagnosis (months)	43	19	12	85
	Duration diagnosis-death (months)	19	13	1	50
	MMSE	18.7	3.4	10	25
Control	F/M	3/7			
	Age (years)	55.9	7.6	39	70
	MMSE	30	0	30	30

AD: Alzheimer's disease

MMSE: Mini Mental State Examination

F: female M: male subjects

NA: not applicable

Duration onset-diagnosis: time span from manifestation of first AD signs to clinical diagnosis confirmation

Duration diagnosis-death: time span from clinical diagnosis of AD to death

The mean values of processing parameters and their standard deviations were estimated. The optimum radius of Gaussian filtering was 0.8997 ± 0.0637, the threshold value was 0.2761 ± 0.0511 and the critical number of regions was 57.11 ± 0.32. There were 15 true positive cases and 8 true negative cases after cross-validation. Adequate sensitivity was 88.2% and the specificity reached 80.0%.

The mean values of parameters from cross-validation were used for the final statistical testing using the two-sided two-sample t-test. Results of posterior statistical analysis are presented in Table 3 and Figure 4 as the number of watershed regions in the ROIs.

SPECT data were recorded by one investigator (M.B.) while statistical analysis was performed separately two others (T.B., J.K.) anonymously without any information about the patients.

The testing criterion value was $t = 6.187$ and the probability value was $p = 3.8\times10^{-7}$ (i.e. $p < 0.01$), which means significantly fewer numbers of watershed regions in the AD group compared to controls. The optimum

Table 3 Number of watershed regions for AD and controls

Characteristics	AD patients Value [95% CI]	Controls Value [95% CI]
Mean	41.4 [33.7, 47.9]	68.1 [59.4, 76.8]
Std. deviation	9.9 [6.7, 17.9]	12.1 [8.3, 22.1]
Sensitivity (%)	94.1 [59.6, 98.3]	NA
Specificity (%)	NA	80.0 [44.4, 97.5]

NA: not applicable

CI: confidence interval

AD: Alzheimer's disease

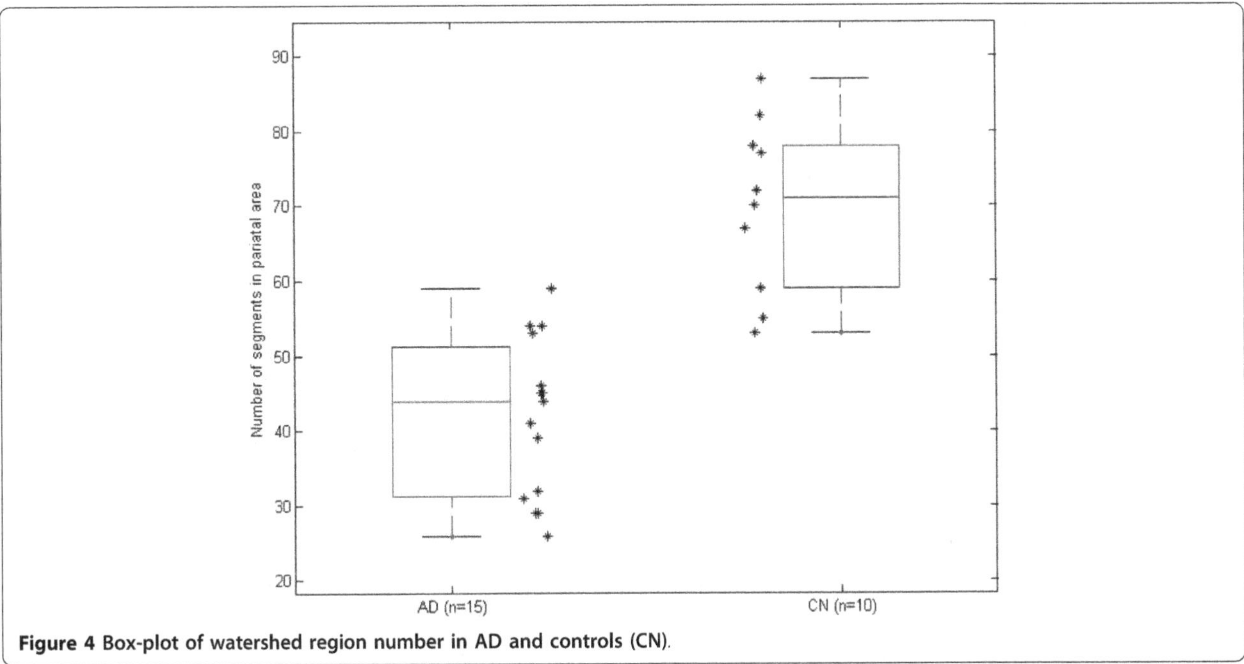

Figure 4 Box-plot of watershed region number in AD and controls (CN).

threshold for watershed regions was set to 57; the number of true positive cases was $TP = 16$ and the number of true negative cases was $TN = 8$. Thus, the method based on fuzzy edge detection and watershed transform reached a sensitivity of 94.1% and a specificity of 80.0% for AD patients and controls.

Discussion

AD diagnosis is based mainly on cognitive evaluation and a definite diagnosis requires neuropathological findings of beta amyloid deposits and neurofibrillary tangles.

AD is essentially a disease of the elderly and most patients have co-morbidities that may affect cognition. It is therefore important to emphasize that all our patients had neuropathologically proven "pure" Alzheimer's disease. In our retrospective study, we excluded all patients with vascular encephalopathy and other neurodegenerative brain disease. We also considered several co-morbidities in the patients selected to our study (listed in Table 1) but these were assessed as non-relevant in terms of their influence on the patient's cognitive performance.

Selection of controls involved two principal conditions: first, control cases had to have normal cognitive status and second, SPECT data needed to be available. Given the fact that SPECT utilizes a radioactive marker, it would be difficult to propose such an examination for healthy volunteers. We used post hoc data from an established register, which required taking into account that our controls might be younger than the AD patients (Table 1, 2) and could constitute a limitation of the study.

Finally, we decided to use data from 10 patients with amyotrophic lateral sclerosis (ALS) as controls. The patients were without noticeable co-morbidities, and had been assessed as part of a previously published study [11]. At the time of SPECT scanning, the cognitive status of the controls was normal and patients had no subjective memory and/or cognitive complaints. We considered them as cognitively normal subjects. Five control patients died before the end of the study and selected autopsies showed no significant AD related pathology.

In order to avoid possible bias, SPECT data acquisition and diagnostic evaluation were strictly separated from SPECT data analysis. The investigators (TB, JK) involved in SPECT data treatment were blinded and did not have access to any clinical and/or imaging details about the patients.

We propose a new method of SPECT image processing that could enhance the accuracy of an AD diagnosis. We developed a new approach for treating 'raw' SPECT data. The combination of digital filtering, fuzzy edge detection and watershed method facilitates detection of hypo-perfusion in a smaller number of localized segments.

Respecting the typical temporo-parietal SPECT pattern of AD, we hypothesized that critical differences between AD patients and controls could be found in the parietal regions. Focusing SPECT analysis on the parietal regions substantially increases both sensitivity and specificity, and approaches the 80% levels recommended by the Reagan Biomarker Working Group [15].

In SPECT of AD patients, perfusion in the posterior cingulate is also significantly decreased. However, it is difficult to distinguish a slight decrease in rCBF during early AD by visual inspection [16]. Moreover, according to a longitudinal SPECT study [17], decreases in rCBF adjusted for relative flow distribution, by normalization of global cerebral blood flow in the posterior cingulate gyrus and precuneus, became ambiguous as the disease progressed.

As demonstrated in Figure 1, the spatial resolution of our procedure is limited, therefore, and respecting the cited arguments, we decided to analyze 'traditionally used' parietal regions. This decision was supported by a recent study [18] that described a significant correlation between tau or phospho-tau concentrations in cerebrospinal fluid and perfusion in the left parietal cortex in AD patients.

In our study, the total number of regions was the only criterion for patient classification. The novelty and efficiency of our method is based on a combination of a fuzzy edge detector, watershed transform, and orientation toward activity separation of parietal lobe domains; other operations were necessary to reduce sensitivity to noise and artifacts.

Conclusions

SPECT data can be easily manipulated using available software; underscoring that extra software and/or manual corrections of raw SPECT data is not required; therefore, our method can be easily used by clinicians. Additionally, it offers earlier and more precise AD diagnoses with the associated patient benefits, and it can be done without significantly increased costs.

Abbreviations

The list of abbreviations used is as follows: SPECT: single photon emission computerized tomography; AD: Alzheimer's disease; ROI: regions-of-interest; rCBF: regional cerebral blood flow; CERAD: Consortium to Establish a Registry for Alzheimer's disease; ALS: amyotrophic lateral sclerosis

Acknowledgements

This study was partially supported by the Czech Ministry of Education (research program MŠM 0021620849, LA 08015 and SGS10/092/OHK4/1T/14) and the Czech Science Foundation (grant GAČR 309/09/P204). The authors thank Thomas Secrest for revision of the English version of this article.

Author details

[1]Department of Neurology, Thomayer Teaching Hospital and Institute for Postgraduate Education in Medicine, Prague, Czech Republic. [2]Department of Software Engineering in Economy, Faculty of Nuclear Science and Physical Engineering, Czech Technical University, Prague, Czech Republic. [3]Department of Nuclear Medicine, Institute for Clinical and Experimental Medicine, Prague, Czech Republic. [4]Department of Pathology and Molecular Medicine, Thomayer Teaching Hospital, Prague, Czech Republic.

Authors' contributions

RR and JK made substantial conceptual contributions to the design of the study, analysis and interpretation of data, and contributed to drafting of the manuscript. TB was involved in data analysis and interpretation, and developed mathematical tools for SPECT data analysis. MB was involved in acquisition of SPECT data, and RM performed neuropathological verifications and gave critical revision of the manuscript regarding important intellectual content. All authors have read and approved the final version of the manuscript.

Competing interests

The authors declare that they have no competing interests.

References

1. Blennow K, Hampel H: **CSF markers for incipient Alzheimer's disease.** *Lancet Neurol* 2003, **2**:605-13.
2. Engelborghs S, Sleegers K, Cras P, Brouwers N, Serneels S, De Leenheir E, Martin JJ, Vanmechelen E, Van Broeckhoven C, De Deyn PP: **No association of CSF biomarkers with APOEepsilon4, plaque and tangle burden in definite Alzheimer's disease.** *Brain* 2007, **130**:2320-6.
3. Dougall NJ, Bruggink S, Ebmeier KP: **Systematic review of the diagnostic accuracy of 99mTc-HMPAO-SPECT in dementia.** *Am J Geriatr Psychiatry* 2004, **12**:554-570.
4. Bonte FJ, Weiner MF, Bigio EH, White CL: **Brain blood flow in the dementias: SPECT with histopathologic correlation in 54 patients.** *Radiology* 1997, **202**:793-797.
5. Nagy Z, Hindley NJ, Braak H, Braak E, Yilmazer-Hanke DM, Schultz C, Barnetson L, Jobst KA, Smith AD: **Relationship between clinical and radiological diagnostic criteria for Alzheimer's disease and the extent of neuropathology as reflected by "stages": a prospective study.** *Dement Geriatr Cogn Disord* 1999, **10**:109-114.
6. Knopman DS, DeKosky ST, Cummings JL, Chui H, Corey-Bloom J, Relkin N, Small GW, Miller B, Stevens JC: **Practice parameter: diagnosis of dementia (an evidence-based review). Report of the Quality Standards Subcommittee of the American Academy of Neurology.** *Neurology* 2001, **56**:1143-1153.
7. Friston KJ, Ashburner J, Kiebel SJ, Nichols TE, Penny WD: **Statistical Parametric Mapping: The Analysis of Functional Brain Images.** Academic Press 2007.
8. Salas-Gonzalez D, Górriz JM, Ramírez J, López M, Álvarez I, Segovia F, *et al*: **Computer aided diagnosis of Alzheimer's disease using support vector machines and classification trees.** *Phys Med Biol* 2010, **55**:2807-17.
9. Imabayashi E, Matsuda H, Asada T, Ohnishi T, Sakamoto S, Nakano S, *et al*: **Superiority of 3-dimensional stereotactic surface projection analysis over visual inspection in discrimination of patients with very early Alzheimer's disease from controls using brain perfusion SPECT.** *J Nucl Med* 2004, **45**:1450-1457.
10. Ishii S, Shishido F, Miyajima M, Sakuma K, Shigihara T, Tameta T, *et al*: **Comparison of Alzheimer's disease with vascular dementia and non-dementia using specific voxel-based Z score maps.** *Ann Nucl Med* 2009, **23**:25-31.
11. Rusina R, Ridzoň P, Kulišťák P, Keller O, Bartoš A, Buncová M, *et al*: **Relationship between ALS and the degree of cognitive impairment, markers of neurodegeneration and predictors for poor outcome. A prospective study.** *Eur J Neurol* 2010, **17**:23-30.
12. Novák V, Perfilieva I, Močkoř J: **Mathematical Principles of Fuzzy Logic.** Kluwer Academic Publishers, Norwell, MA 1999.
13. Beucher S, Meyer F: **The morphological approach to segmentation: the watershed transformation.** In *Mathematical Morphology in Image Processing* Edited by: Dougherty ER 1993, 433-481.
14. Martens HA, Dardenne P: **Validation and verification of regression in small data sets.** *Chemometr Intell Lab* 1998, 4499-121.

15. Consensus report of the Working Group: **Molecular and Biochemical Markers of Alzheimer's Disease".** *Neurobiol Aging* The Ronald and Nancy Reagan Research Institute of the Alzheimer's Association and the National Institute on Aging Working Group 1998, **19**:109-116.
16. Minoshima S, Giordani B, Berent S, Frey KA, Foster NL, Kuhl DE: **Metabolic reduction in the posterior cingulate cortex in very early Alzheimer's disease.** *Ann Neurol* 1997, **42**:85-94.
17. Kogure D, Matsuda H, Ohnishi T, Asada T, Uno M, Kunihiro T, *et al*: **Longitudinal evaluation of early Alzheimer's disease using brain perfusion SPECT.** *J Nucl Med* 2000, **41**:1155-1162.
18. Habert MO, de Souza LC, Lamari F, Daragon N, Desarnaud S, Jardel C, *et al*: **Brain perfusion SPECT correlates with CSF biomarkers in Alzheimer's disease.** *Eur J Nucl Med Mol Imaging* 2010, **37**:589-93.

2

Brain computer tomography in critically ill patients

Ilse M Purmer[1], Erik P van Iperen[1], Ludo F M Beenen[2], Michael J Kuiper[3], Jan M Binnekade[1], Peter W Vandertop[4], Marcus J Schultz[1] and Janneke Horn[1*]

Abstract

Background: Brain computer tomography (brain CT) is an important imaging tool in patients with intracranial disorders. In ICU patients, a brain CT implies an intrahospital transport which has inherent risks. The proceeds and consequences of a brain CT in a critically ill patient should outweigh these risks. The aim of this study was to critically evaluate the diagnostic and therapeutic yield of brain CT in ICU patients.

Methods: In a prospective observational study data were collected during one year on the reasons to request a brain CT, expected abnormalities, abnormalities found by the radiologist and consequences for treatment. An "expected abnormality" was any finding that had been predicted by the physician requesting the brain CT. A brain CT was "diagnostically positive", if the abnormality found was new or if an already known abnormality was increased. It was "diagnostically negative" if an already known abnormality was unchanged or if an expected abnormality was not found. The treatment consequences of the brain CT, were registered as "treatment as planned", "treatment changed, not as planned", "treatment unchanged".

Results: Data of 225 brain CT in 175 patients were analyzed. In 115 (51%) brain CT the abnormalities found were new or increased known abnormalities. 115 (51%) brain CT were found to be diagnostically positive. In the medical group 29 (39%) of brain CT were positive, in the surgical group 86 (57%), *p* 0.01. After a positive brain CT, in which the expected abnormalities were found, treatment was changed as planned in 33%, and in 19% treatment was changed otherwise than planned.

Conclusions: The results of this study show that the diagnostic and therapeutic yield of brain CT in critically ill patients is moderate. The development of guidelines regarding the decision rules for performing a brain CT in ICU patients is needed.

Keywords: Computer tomography, Critically ill, Brain imaging, Diagnostic value

Background

Brain computer tomography (brain CT) is an important imaging tool in patients with suspected or proven intracranial disorders. Reasons to perform a brain CT in patients admitted to the intensive care unit (ICU) are failure to wake up after wearing off of sedative medication, neurological deterioration, follow up of known intracranial pathology or evaluation of a neurosurgical intervention. In the fast majority of ICUs, a brain CT implies an intrahospital transport of which the inherent risks are well known [1-4]. The proceeds and consequences of a brain CT in a critically ill patient should outweigh these risks. Therefore, the request for a brain CT in an ICU-patient with minor changes in the neurological condition or in a patient who is doing well clinically after surgery, frequently leads to a debate about the importance of that brain CT in terms of expectations and treatment consequences.

We prospectively collected all brain CT requests, the brain CT results and resulting changes in treatment during one year in two hospitals in order to determine the diagnostic and therapeutic impact of a brain CT in ICU patients. The aim of this study was to critically evaluate

* Correspondence: j.horn@amc.nl
[1]Department of Intensive Care Medicine, Academic Medical Center, PObox 226601100DD, Amsterdam, The Netherlands
Full list of author information is available at the end of the article

the diagnostic and therapeutic yield of brain CT in ICU patients.

Methods

Study design

This prospective observational study was performed in two ICUs in the Netherlands – one tertiary 16–bed mixed medical–surgical ICU, and one 30–bed university mixed medical–surgical ICU including neurosurgery. From May 2007 until June 2008 all consecutive brain CTs were included. The study was approved by the local medical ethics committees of the Academic Medical Center (Amsterdam, the Netherlands) and Medical Center Leeuwarden (Leeuwarden, the Netherlands) and was conducted in concordance with the principles of the declaration of Helsinki and good clinical practice. Informed consent from patients or relatives was not deemed necessary by the medical ethical committees given the observational nature of the study.

The decision to perform a brain CT was at the discretion of the attending neurologist, neurosurgeon or intensivist. The physician requesting the brain CT completed a standardized radiological request form, specifying the indication for the brain CT, the expectations regarding results and possible treatment consequences. Options that could be chosen from as expected abnormalities were "hydrocephalus", "ischaemia", "vascular occlusion or dissection", "intracranial hematoma", "edema (diffuse or local)", "midline shift", "herniation" or "other". More than one expected abnormality could be ticked. Possible treatment options were "insertion of intracranial pressure (ICP) monitor", "placement of ventricular catheter", "lumbar puncture", "craniectomy/craniotomy", "hematoma removal", "mannitol infusion ", "observation", or "other".

All brain CTs were evaluated by an independent radiologist. All abnormalities reported by the radiologist, irrespective whether they were old or new, were noted. In case of old abnormalities it was reported if they were increased, unchanged or decreased. The actually applied treatment on the ICU was evaluated by the members of the research team. Possible consequences were "treatment as planned", "treatment changed, not as planned", "treatment unchanged".

Patients were divided in two groups: surgical and medical. Surgical patients were admitted with a subarachnoid or intracerebral hemorrhage, traumatic brain injury, or after neurosurgical intervention. Medical patients were admitted to the ICU for a non- neurosurgical reason.

Other data collected: age, gender, ICU admission type (acute or elective), specialism (medical (including neurology), surgical (including neurosurgery)), APACHE II–score, neurological/neurosurgical diagnosis, and, if available, ICP data. Ventilation and administration of vasopressive medication during transport was recorded.

Definitions

An "expected abnormality" was any finding (or worsening of a previously noted finding) that had been predicted by the physician requesting the brain CT. A brain CT was "diagnostically positive", if the abnormality found was new or if an already known abnormality was increased. It was "diagnostically negative" if an already known abnormality was unchanged or if an expected abnormality was not found. A brain CT with more than one expected abnormality could only be "diagnostically negative" if all expectations were unconfirmed. The treatment consequences of the brain CT, which were collected from the medical files, were registered as "treatment as planned", "treatment changed, not as planned", "treatment unchanged". To determine the positive predictive value of a diagnostically positive brain CT on patient's treatment, "treatment as planned" and "treatment changed, not as planned", were considered as "treatment changed" versus "treatment unchanged".

Statistical analysis

Descriptive statistics were used to characterize the study cohort. The chance that a brain CT was followed by a change of treatment policy was expressed as relative risk (RR). Statistical uncertainty was expressed using 95% confidence intervals (CI). A statistical software package (Statistical Package for the Social Sciences, version 16; SPSS Inc., Chicago, IL) was used for the statistical analyses.

Results

Data of 225 brain CT obtained in 175 patients were collected and analyzed (see Figure 1). The majority of brain CT (207) were made in the university ICU, 18 in the tertiary mixed medical – surgical ICU. Patient characteristics are shown in Table 1. Seventy-four brain CT were performed in 72 medical patients, 151 in 103 surgical patients. In some patients more than one brain CT was performed (23 patients had two, 7 patients three brain CT and 3 patients had four, five and eight respectively). During brain CT transport mechanical ventilation was needed in 188 (83%) transports, vasopressive medication was administered during 80 (35%) transports.

Overall, 115 (51%) brain CT were found to be diagnostically positive, i.e. the abnormalities reported by the radiologist were new or increased known abnormalities. In the medical brain CT, 29 (39%) were positive, in the surgical group 86 (57%), p 0.01. Tables 2 and 3 displays the abnormalities as expected by the requesting physicians and the abnormalities as reported by the radiologist. All abnormalities, irrespective whether they are old or new, are shown. In most brain CT more than one abnormality was expected. In the medical group a brain CT was often made to exclude an intracranial hemorrhage, this

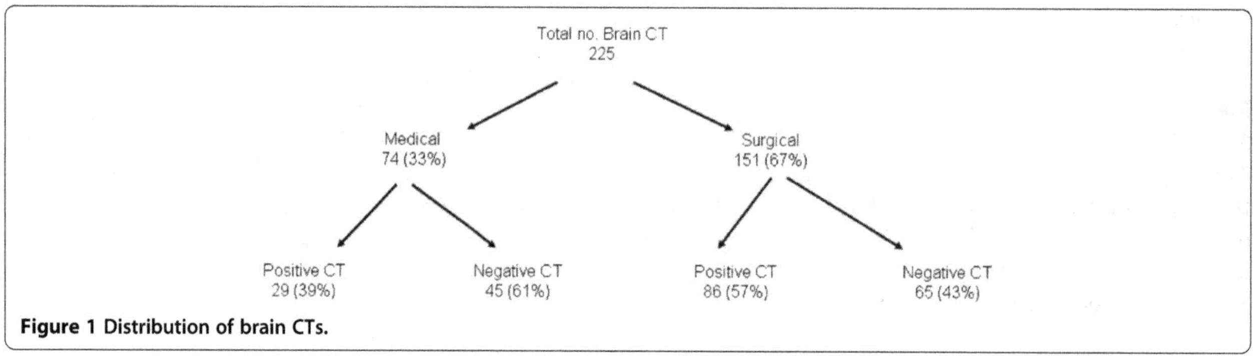

Figure 1 Distribution of brain CTs.

was expected in 36 brain CT, but found in 2 (5%). In surgical patients more brain CT (38%) than expected (23%) showed midline shift. Medical brain CT showed no abnormalities in 45%, in surgical brain CT no abnormalities were reported in 4%.

Table 4 shows the treatment strategies considered when requesting the brain CT. In medical patients, limitation or withdrawal of treatment as possible treatment strategy was mentioned in 16%, in surgical patients in 1%. A large number of surgical patients were treated with an external ventricular drainage system, and brain CT were requested to be informed about the position and effect of the drainage system.

After a positive brain CT, in which the expected abnormalities were found, treatment was changed as planned in 33%, and in 19% treatment was changed otherwise than planned (Table 5). In 73% of the negative brain CT (in which the expected abnormalities were not found) treatment remained unchanged. Despite such a negative brain CT the treatment was changed as was planned in 16%. The positive predictive value, i.e. the chance that a positive CT scan led to a change in treatment was 0.52 (95% CI 0.42 – 0.61), the negative predictive value, i.e. that chance that treatment was not changed after a negative CT scan was 0.73 (95% CI 0.64 – 0.80).

Table 1 Patient characteristics, n = 175

Treatment group	n (%)
Surgical	103 (58)
Medical	72 (42)
Age	Mean (Sd)
All patients	57.3 (15.5)
Surgical patients	53.1 (15.9)
Medical patients	63.2 (12.9)
Gender	n (%)
Male	111 (63)
Reason for admission ICU	n (%)
SAH	30 (17)
Intracerebral hematoma	20 (11)
TBI	44 (25)
Cerebral infarction	4 (2)
Post CPR	14 (8)
Sepsis / pneumonia	17 (10)
Cardiopulmonary surgery	13 (7)
Other	33 (19)
Apache II score	Mean (Sd)
All patients	23.6 (8.2)
Surgical patients	23.6 (7.7)
Medical patients	27.5 (8.9)

Abbreviations: *Sd*, standard deviation, *ICU*, intensive care unit, *SAH*, subarachnoid haemorrhage, *TBI*, traumatic brain injury, *CPR*, cardiopulmonary resuscitation.

Discussion

This is the largest cohort study sofar, investigating the results and consequences of brain CT in patients admitted to an ICU. The diagnostic value of brain CT is low, in only half of the brain CT the abnormalities as expected by the requesting physicians were found. In a brain CT performed in medical patients this is the case in less than fifty percent. The therapeutical consequences of the brain CT are also low, treatment was changed in little more than half of the brain CT.

From the fact that in this study only half of all brain CT showed the abnormalities that were expected, one

Table 2 Expected radiological abnormalities and results as reported by the radiologist in medical brain CT (n = 74)

Expected abnormalities	n (%)	Results radiologist	n (%)
Hematoma	36 (49)	Hematoma	2 (3)
Ischemia / infarction	49 (66)	Ischemia / infarction	34 (46)
Oedema	15 (20)	Oedema	5 (7)
Midline shift	1 (1)	Midline shift	2 (3)
Hydrocephalus	4 (5)	Hydrocephalus	7 (9)
Cerebral abscess	5 (7)	Cerebral abscess	0
No abnormalities	0	No abnormalities	33 (45)
Other	5 (7)	Other	5 (7)

Table 3 Expected radiological abnormalities and results as reported by the radiologist in surgical brain CT (n = 151)

Expected abnormalities	n (%)	Results radiologist	n (%)
Hematoma	97 (64)	Hematoma	105 (70)
Ischemia / infarction	33 (22)	Ischemia / infarction	33 (22)
Oedema	45 (30)	Oedema	55 (36)
Midline shift	35 (23)	Midline shift	57 (38)
Hydrocephalus	60 (40)	Hydrocephalus	58 (38)
(increase of) TBI	0	(increase of) TBI	0
Cerebral abscess	4 (3)	Cerebral abscess	0
No abnormalities	0	No abnormalities	4 (3)
Other	29 (19)	Other	53 (35)

could conclude that it is difficult for physicians who have performed clinical neurological assessment, to foretell what the brain CT will yield. It is known that neurological assessment of critically ill patients can be hampered due to a combination of the underlying disease, metabolic derangements and (sedative) medication administered. The reason to request a brain CT was different in medical patients, where it was often performed to exclude severe intracranial pathology, such as an intracerebral hemorrhage. Our results showed that an intracerebral hemorrhage is only found in 3% of medical critically ill patients.

Similar results in medical patients were reported by Rafanan et al. and Salerno et al [5,6]. Rafanan reviewed the results of 297 brain CT scans and describes a percentage of 37% of these scans to show acute intracranial abnormalities [5]. Ischemic stroke was found most frequently (49%), which is comparable to the percentage of infarction or ischemia in our study (46%). Salerno et al. reported data of a retrospective study in 123 medical ICU patients in whom a brain CT was performed [6]. In 26 patients (21%) a new finding was described by the radiologist, most often an ischemic cerebral infarct (13). Both studies reported that no patient characteristics or clinical variables could, with certainty, identify patients with either a positive or a negative brain CT. This interesting topic was not addressed in our study.

Balachandran et al. also studied the results of brain CT performed in ICU patients who did not wake up after discontinuation of sedative drugs [7]. In 42 patients, only one patient (2%) with abnormalities explaining the persistent coma was identified.

In surgical ICU patients results and consequences of brain CT have not been published and therefore we were unable to compare our data regarding the diagnostic or therapeutic yield of brain CT in this subgroup. There has been discussion about the yield of repeated brain CT in patients with blunt traumatic brain injury (TBI). Kaups et al. reported that repeated brain CT was unnecessary in patients who did not show deterioration in mental status, elevation of ICP, hypotension or coagulopathy, as the results of the CT did not alter patient management in this group [8]. His results were contradicted by Bee et al., who concluded that in patients with mild TBI, repeated brain CT can identify increase of intracranial lesions even if the patient remains clinically stable [9]. In a systematic review including 30 mostly retrospective studies about the utility of repeated brain CT after blunt TBI, Wang et al. found that progression of injury found on the repeat CT was reported in 8-67% of patients [10]. The number of patients reported to need neurosurgical interventions after the repeated brain CT was 0-54%. Especially patients with severe TBI, presenting with a Glasgow Coma Score of ≤ 8, were at risk of progression of injury necessitating neurosurgical interventions. Despite the large number of manuscripts and therefore patients included in the review, the authors could not determine which subgroup of TBI patients would benefit from repeated brain CT.

Although the number of identified abnormalities in this study is low, it is higher than figures reported from emergency room brain CT results in patients admitted with mild TBI. Several large prospective cohort studies in this population found intracranial traumatic lesions in 6–11% of patients [11-13]. Based on these experiences, prediction rules have been formulated to allow emergency room physicians to work as efficient as possible, without exposing patients to the risk of missing important abnormalities. Given the risks of transports in critically ill patients, similar studies and guidelines would be useful for brain CT in (neuro)surgical and medical

Table 4 Considered treatments as indicated on brain CT request form

Medical brain CTs (74)	N, (%)	Surgical brain CTs (151)	N, (%)
Craniotomy	9 (12)	Craniotomy	65 (43)
CSF drainage	9 (12)	CSF drainage / reposition EVD	55 (36)
Change medication	16 (22)	Change medication	16 (11)
Continue current therapy	20 (27)	Continue current therapy	36 (24)
Withdraw / limit treatment	12 (16)	Withdraw / limit treatment	1 (0)
Other	4 (0.1)	Other	15 (10)

Table 5 Treatment after positive or negative brain CT

All brain CTs	Positive CT, n = 115 (%)	Negative CT, n = 110 (%)
Treatment as planned	38 (33)	18 (16)
Treatment changed, not as planned	22 (19)	12 (11)
Treatment unchanged	55 (48)	80 (73)
CTs in surgical patients	Positive CT, n = 86 (%)	Negative CT, n = 65 (%)
Treatment as planned	29 (34)	11 (17)
Treatment changed, not as planned	19 (22)	8 (12)
Treatment unchanged	28 (44)	46 (71)
CTs in medical patients	Positive CT, n = 29 (%)	Negative CT, n = 45 (%)
Treatment as planned	9 (31)	7 (16)
Treatment changed, not as planned	3 (10)	4 (9)
Treatment unchanged	17 (57)	34 (76)

critically ill patients. The development of a portable CT scan diminishes the needs for intrahospital transport which can be of great value [14]. Nevertheless, every brain CT leads to radiation exposure, and therefore clinicians should still consider the diagnostic yield of a brain CT and the consequences it will have for the treatment strategy [15].

Some limitations of this study should be discussed. First, in this study we did not collect data on the clinical condition of the patients at the moment the brain CT was requested. Collection of clinical data would have allowed us to correlate the clinical findings to the expectations of the requesting physician and the final results of the brain CT. By doing this, we might have been able to identify clinical warning signs indicative of serious intracranial problems. A future study should address this issue.

Also, the severity of the identified abnormalities on the brain CT and the possible consequences for patients if they had been missed were not recorded. Especially the clinical condition of the patient in the ICU can lead to situations necessitating brain CT, because neurological tests can not be performed, for example when sedative drugs are administered and can not be interrupted. In these patients a brain CT with no new abnormalities can be expected more often than in patients who deteriorate neurologically. The consequences of missed abnormalities on a brain CT would certainly be interesting to study, but this was not included in this project.

Conclusion

The results of this study show that the diagnostic and therapeutic yield of brain CT in critically ill patients is moderate. However, consequences of missing serious intracranial abnormalities were not addressed in this study. Given the fact that intrahospital transport has risks in critically ill patients, further research is needed to enable the development of guidelines regarding the decision rules for performing a brain CT in ICU patients.

Abbreviations

APACHE: Acute physiology and chronic health evaluation; CI: Confidence intervals; CPR: Cardiopulmonary resuscitation; CT: Computer tomography; ICP: Intracranial pressure; ICU: Intensive care unit; RR: Relative risk; SAH: Subarachnoid haemorrhage; Sd: Standard deviation; TBI: Traumatic brain injury.

Competing interests

The authors declare that they have no competing interests regarding this study

Authors' contributions

IP contributed to data collection, analyses and interpretation of the data and drafting and finalizing of the manuscript. EvI contributed to data collection (e.g. building of database), interpretation of the data, drafting and finalizing of the manuscript. LB contributed to data collection (e.g. reporting of CTs), drafting and finalizing of the manuscript. MK contributed to data collection, drafting and finalizing of the manuscript. JB contributed to analyses and interpretation of the data, drafting and finalizing of the manuscript. PV contributed to study design, data collection and drafting and finalizing of the manuscript. MS has made considerable contributions to conception and design of the study and helped finalization of the manuscript. JH contributed to conception and design of the study, collected data, interpreted data and drafted and finalized the manuscript. All authors have given final approval of the version to be published.

Acknowledgements

Mrs Matty Koopmans helped with the collection of data in the Medical Center in Leeuwarden.

Author details

[1]Department of Intensive Care Medicine, Academic Medical Center, PObox 226601100DD, Amsterdam, The Netherlands. [2]Department of Radiology, Academic Medical Center, PObox 226601100DD, Amsterdam, The Netherlands. [3]Department of Intensive Care, Medicine, Medical Center Leeuwarden, PObox 8888901BR, Leeuwarden, The Netherlands. [4]Neurosurgical Center Amsterdam, Academic Medical Center, PObox 226601100DD, Amsterdam, The Netherlands.

References

1. Waydhas C: **Intrahospital transport of critically ill patients.** *Crit Care* 1999, 3:R83–R89.

2. Lahner D, Nikolic A, Marhofer P, Koinig H, Germann P, Weinstabl C, Krenn CG: **Incidence of complications in intrahospital transport of critically ill patients-experience in an Austrian university hospital.** *Wien Klin Wochenschr* 2007, **119:**412–416.
3. Peerdeman SM, Girbes AR, Vandertop WP: **Changes in cerebral glycolytic activity during transport of critically ill neurotrauma patients measured with microdialysis.** *J Neurol* 2002, **249:**676–679.
4. Fanara B, Manzon C, Barbot O, Desmettre T, Capellier G: **Recommendations for the intra-hospital transport of critically ill patients.** *Crit Care* 2010, **14:**R87.
5. Rafanan AL, Kakulavar P, Perl J, Andrefsky JC, Nelson DR, Arroliga AC: **Head computed tomography in medical intensive care unit patients: clinical indications.** *Crit Care Med* 2000, **28:**1306–1309.
6. Salerno D, Marik PE, Daskalakis C, Kolm P, Leone F: **The role of head computer tomographic scans on the management of MICU patients with neurological dysfunction.** *J Intensive Care Med* 2009, **24:**372–375.
7. Balachandran JS, Jaleel M, Jain M, Mahajan N, Kalhan R, Balagani R, Donnelly HK, Greenstein E, Mutlu GM: **Head CT is of limited diagnostic value in critically ill patients who remain unresponsive after discontinuation of sedation.** *BMC Anesthesiol* 2009, **9:**3.
8. Kaups KL, Davis JW, Parks SN: **Routinely repeated computed tomography after blunt head trauma: does it benefit patients?** *J Trauma* 2004, **56:**475–480.
9. Bee TK, Magnotti LJ, Croce MA, Maish GO, Minard G, Schroeppel TJ, Zarzaur BL, Fabian TC: **Necessity of repeat head CT and ICU monitoring in patients with minimal brain injury.** *J Trauma* 2009, **66:**1015–1018.
10. Wang MC, Linnau KF, Tirschwell DL, Hollingworth W: **Utility of repeat head computed tomography after blunt head trauma: a systematic review.** *J Trauma* 2006, **61:**226–233.
11. Haydel MJ, Preston CA, Mills TJ, Luber S, Blaudeau E, DeBlieux PM: **Indications for computed tomography in patients with minor head injury.** *N Engl J Med* 2000, **343:**100–105.
12. Smits M, Dippel DW, Steyerberg EW, de Haan GG, Dekker HM, Vos PE, Kool DR, Nederkoorn PJ, Hofman PA, Twijnstra A, Tanghe HL, Hunink MG: **Predicting intracranial traumatic findings on computed tomography in patients with minor head injury: the CHIP prediction rule.** *Ann Intern Med* 2007, **146:**397–405.
13. Stiell IG, Wells GA, Vandemheen K, Clement C, Lesiuk H, Laupacis A, McKnight RD, Verbeek R, Brison R, Cass D, Eisenhauer ME, Greenberg G, Worthington J: **The Canadian CT Head Rule for patients with minor head injury.** *Lancet* 2001, **357:**1391–1396.
14. Carlson AP, Yonas H: **Portable head computed tomography scanner-technology and applications: experience with 3421 scans.** *J Neuroimaging* 2012, **22**(4):408–415.
15. Gelfand AA, Josephson SA: **Substantial radiation exposure for patients with subarachnoid hemorrhage.** *J Stroke Cerebrovasc Dis* 2011, **20:**131–133.

3

Multidetector-row computed tomography for evaluating the branching angle of the celiac artery

Hiroyuki Tokue[1,2*], Azusa Tokue[1] and Yoshito Tsushima[1]

Abstract

Background: We performed this study in order to investigate the shape of the origin of the celiac artery in maximum intensity projection (MIP) using routine 64 multidetector-row computed tomography (MDCT) data in order to plan for the implantation of an intra-arterial hepatic port system.

Methods: A total of 1,104 patients with hepatocellular carcinoma were assessed with MDCT. In the definition of the branching angle, the anterior side of the abdominal aorta was considered the baseline, and the cranial and caudal sides were designated as 0 and 180 degrees, respectively. The angles between 0 and 90 degrees and between 90 and 180 degrees from the cranial side were considered upward and downward, respectively, and the branching angle of the celiac artery was classified every 30 degrees. The subclavian arterial route was used for the implantation of an intra-arterial hepatic port system in patients with branching angles of 150 degrees or more (sharp downward).

Results: The median branching angle was (median ± standard deviation) 135 ± 23 (range, 51–174) degrees. The branching was upward in 77 patients (7%) and downward in 1,027 patients (93%). The branching was downward with an angle of 120 to150 degrees in most patients (n = 613). The branching was sharply downward with an angle of 150 degrees or more in 177 patients (16%). A total of 10 patients were referred for interventional placement of an intra-arterial hepatic port system. The subclavian arterial route was used for implantation of an intra-arterial hepatic port system in 2 patients with sharp downward branching.

Conclusions: The branching angle of the celiac artery can be easily determined by the preparation of MIP images from routine MDCT data. MIP may provide useful information for the selection of the catheter insertion route in order to avoid a sharp branching angle of the celiac artery.

Keywords: Multidetector-row computed tomography, Maximum intensity projection, Celiac artery, Branching angle, Intra-arterial hepatic port system

Background

Besides a hepatectomy, systemic chemotherapy and arterial chemoinfusion therapy are used to treat primary and liver metastatic cancers. Catheter insertion is necessary for arterial infusion chemotherapy, and there are surgical and percutaneous catheter insertion methods. The low invasiveness of catheter insertions is important. There have been many reports of percutaneous implantations of port-catheter systems, which are a superior choice as it is a less invasive method. Methods for the percutaneous implantation of a port-catheter system are roughly divided into the subclavian arterial route method and the femoral arterial/inferior epigastric arterial route method [1-4]. The catheter insertion route is selected depending on the branching angle (upward or downward) of the origin of the celiac artery in some cases, and assessments of the branching angle before catheter insertion may increase the reliability of the technique. There have been no reports in the English literature about the branching angle of the celiac artery.

* Correspondence: tokue@s2.dion.ne.jp
[1]Department of Diagnostic and Interventional Radiology, Gunma University Hospital, 3-39-22 Showa-machi, Maebashi, Gunma 371-8511, Japan
[2]Department of Radiology, Maebashi Red Cross Hospital, Maebashi, Gunma, Japan

In this study, we analyzed the branching angle of the celiac artery using multidetector-row computed tomography (MDCT) in the planning of radiological catheter placement for the implantation of an intra-arterial hepatic port system. We prepared a maximum intensity projection (MIP) of a multiple projection volume reconstruction (MPVR) from the volume data of 64 MDCT with regard to the shape (upward or downward) of the origin of the celiac artery in patients who underwent routine MDCT [5,6] and investigated prior evaluations of the shape of the celiac artery.

Patients and methods

Patients

Computed tomography (CT) was performed in 1,800 patients with hepatocellular carcinoma from Jan 1st, 2008 to Dec 31, 2010. The study was performed in 1,200 patients who were aged 19–91 years (median age: 62 years), and there were 687 males and 513 females. The patients were satisfied the following inclusion criteria: (a) contrast CT was done; (b) the origin of the celiac artery was in the imaged region; (c) no implantation of a port-catheter system had been performed; (d) the vascular anatomy was not of the celiacomesenteric type; (e) no history of abdominal operations; and (f) written informed consent was obtained. This study was approved by the institutional review board at Gunma University. This study was conducted in accordance with the amended Helsinki Declaration.

CT Technique

Routine CT was performed in all patients on MDCT (Aquilion 64, Toshiba Medical Systems Corporation, Tokyo, Japan) after mechanical injection (AutoenhanceA-250, Nemoto Kyorindo Co., Ltd., Tokyo, Japan) of l00–150 mL of nonionic iodinated contrast medium with a concentration of 300 mg/mL [Iopamiron300 (iopamidol), Nihon Shering K.K., Osaka, Japan, and Omunipaque 300 (iohexol), Daiichi Sankyo Co., Ltd., Tokyo, Japan]. The medium was administered at a dose of 2 mL/kg bodyweight to a maximum of 150 mL. The contrast material was injected at a rate of 1.5–4 mL/s through a 20- or 21-gauge intravenous cannula. The examinations were performed in a cephalocaudal direction starting at the top of the liver, and each examination included non-enhanced scanning and contrast-enhanced scanning in 3 phases: a hepatic-arterial phase, a portal venous phase and an equilibrium phase. The hepatic arterial phase was started 35 s after the start of injection, the portal phase at 70 s, and the equilibrium phase at 140 s.

Scanning was acquired during inhalation in all patients. The volume data that were obtained were reconstructed by setting the slice thickness to the collimation thickness (1 or 2 mm), the reconstruction field of view (FOV) to 150 mm, and the reconstruction interval to 1/2 of the collimation thickness (0.5 or 1 mm).

Image processing

The axial raw data images were processed on a commercially available image processing workstation (ZIO M900 QUADRA, Amin Co., Ltd., Tokyo, Japan). Vascular maps were generated from the processed axial date using MIP. The axial view at the level of the origin of the celiac artery was prepared, and a MPVR with the width of the abdominal aorta was prepared. The direction of the axial image was set to the relative direction of the region from the origin of the celiac artery to the branching of the hepatic and splenic artery. The branching angle of the origin of the celiac artery was measured in the MPVR image of the sagittal MIP.

Image analysis

In the definition of the branching angle, the anterior side of the abdominal aorta was regarded as the baseline, and the cranial and caudal sides were designated as 0 and 180 degrees, respectively. The angles between 0 and 90 degrees and between 90 and 180 degrees from the cranial side were regarded as upward and downward, respectively, and the branching angle of the celiac artery was classified every 30 degrees. Cases that were difficult to evaluate were presented as not evaluable (NE). The branching angle of the celiac artery was investigated based on this classification method (Figure 1).

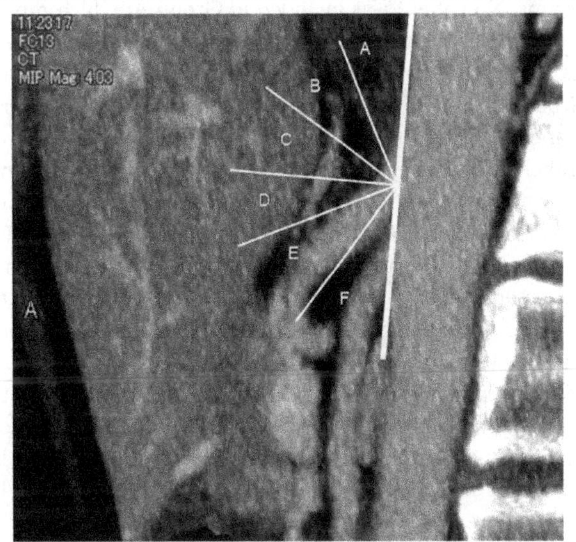

Figure 1 Classification of the branching angle. The anterior side of the abdominal aorta was regarded as the baseline, and the cranial and caudal sides were designated as 0 and 180 degrees, respectively. The branching angles between 0 and 90 and 180 degrees from the cranial side were regarded as upward and downward, respectively, and the celiac arterial branching angle was classified every 30 degrees.

Port implantation

The subclavian arterial route was used for implantation of an intra-arterial hepatic port system in patients with branching angles of 150 degrees or more (sharp downward). The femoral arterial route was used in patients with branching angles of 149 degrees or less. Technical success was defined as implantation of the catheter and port system.

Informed consent was obtained from each patient before of an intra-arterial hepatic port system was performed.

Results

The subjects were 1,200 patients. The branching angle of the origin of the celiac artery was measured in the MPVR of the sagittal MIP. All patients had hepatocellular carcinoma. Analysis and evaluation of the branching angle was difficult in 96 patients (8%) who were then excluded and presented as NE. The details of these NE cases are as follows: (a) allergic symptoms developed immediately after the administration of contrast medium, the images were acquired after treatment, or evaluation was difficult because of poor contrast: 3 patients; (b) identification of the branching site was difficult because of severe narrowing of the origin of the celiac artery: 31 patients; and (c) evaluation of the branching angle was difficult because of severe calcification of the origin of the celiac artery: 62 patients.

Analysis of the branching angle of the origin of the celiac artery was possible in 1,104 patients. The median branching angle was (median ± SD) 135 ± 23 (range, 51–174) degrees in these cases. These patients were divided into 6 groups. No patient was included in Group A, which represented cases with sharp upward branching with an angle less than 30 degrees, and 77 patients (7%) were included in Groups B and C, which represented cases with upward branching with an angle less than 90 degrees. The artery branched downward in most patients, and the branching was sharp downward with an angle of 150 degrees or more in 177 patients (16%) in group F (Figure 2).

A total of 10 patients were referred for interventional placement of an intra-arterial hepatic port system. There were no patients who were referred for interventional management in the NE cases. Technical success was 100% without any major adverse events that were associated with the procedure. The subclavian arterial route was used for the implantation of an intra-arterial hepatic port system in 2 patients with sharp downward branching (Figures 3a, b, and c). The femoral arterial route was used in the other 8 patients with branching angles of 149 degrees or less.

Discussion

This study showed that MDCT provides useful information of the branching angle of the celiac artery for selection of the catheter insertion route.

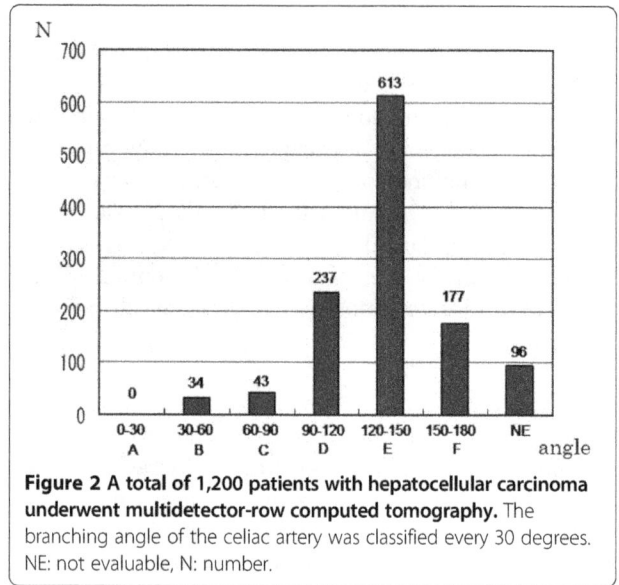

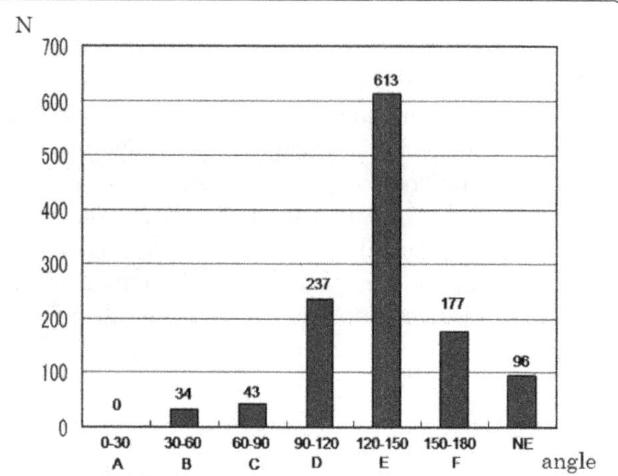

Figure 2 A total of 1,200 patients with hepatocellular carcinoma underwent multidetector-row computed tomography. The branching angle of the celiac artery was classified every 30 degrees. NE: not evaluable, N: number.

Less invasive implantation of a port-catheter system is important, and percutaneous insertion is recommended. The catheter insertion methods are roughly divided into the subclavian arterial route method and the femoral arterial/inferior epigastric arterial route method. The passing of large joints, such as the hip and shoulder joints, complications, such as cerebral infarction, and the skill of the operator are factors that are important in selecting the insertion method. However, in order to complete arterial chemoinfusion therapy, stable catheter insertion is necessary, and the branching angle of the celiac artery may contribute to the stability. Thus, MIP was prepared from routine MDCT data in order to investigate the branching angle of the origin of the celiac artery. Although breathing-induced changes were not investigated in this study, the celiac artery branched downward in 1,027 of the 1,104 patients analyzed (more than 90%). The median branching angle was 135 degrees, and the artery branched downward sharply with an angle of 150 degrees or more in 177 patients.

Evaluation was difficult in 96 patients, and the branching angle could not be measured in these patients. The number of patient excluded from analysis may be a high number in spite of using a 64 MDCT. The reason is unclear. There might be many patients who were affected by arteriosclerosis. However, the branching direction of the celiac artery was roughly confirmed. The branching was downward in most of these patients. If evaluation of the celiac angle was difficult, it may not affect the success of the implantation of the hepatic port system and the outcome.

The celiac artery branched downward in most cases, and compression of the celiac artery by the median arcuate ligament, which is located right above the celiac

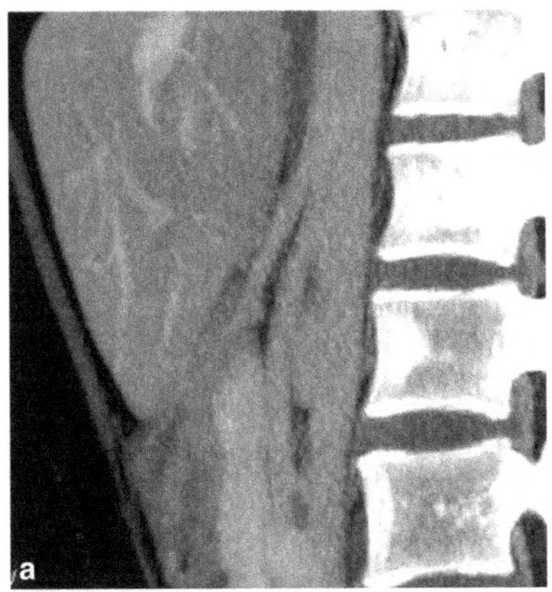

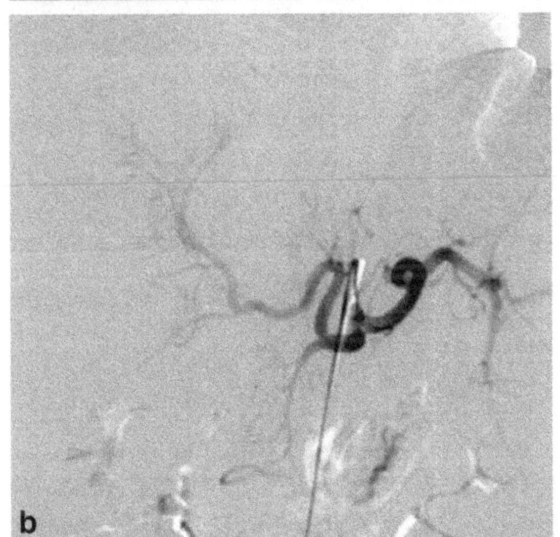

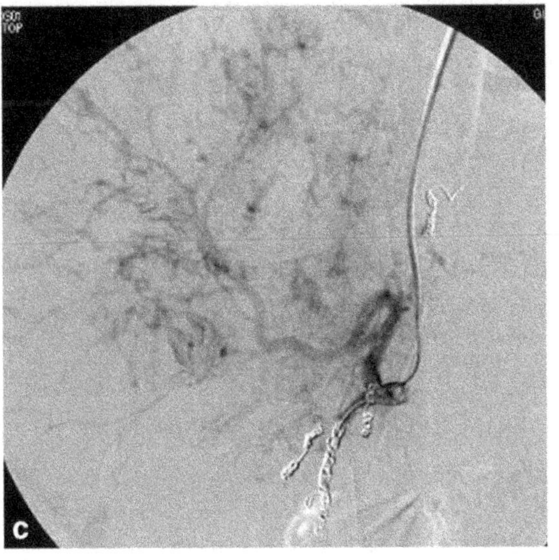

Figure 3 A case of a 58-year-old woman with hepatocellular carcinoma. The branching angle of the origin of the celiac artery was 168 degrees in the multiple projection volume reconstruction image of the sagittal maximum intensity projection (**a**). Digital subtraction angiography showed sharp downward branching of the celiac artery (**b**). The subclavian arterial route was selected for implantation of an intra-arterial hepatic port system (**c**).

artery, may be one reason. Lindner and Kemprud reported that the celiac artery branched right below the median arcuate ligament in 25 of 75 autopsy cases (33%). The rate of downward direction of the celiac artery may be high due to compression by this ligament [7,8]. In addition, breathing affects the angle of celiac artery. CT scans were obtained during deep inspiration, and, thus, the angle of the celiac artery may be exaggerated. However, there have been no reports in the English literature about the branching angle of the celiac artery.

As shown by this study, the celiac artery may branch downward sharply. For selection of the catheter insertion method of percutaneous implantation of a port-catheter system, the branching angle of the origin of the celiac artery should be considered. This branching angle can be readily investigated by preparation of sagittal MIP from routine MDCT data. The course of the celiac axis affects the technique of catheter placement. When a transfemoral or transepigastric approach is used, a caudal course of the celiac axis tends to be more difficult than a cranial course because multiple inflection points result in a reduction in the torque of the catheter and the guide wire [9].

The limitations of our study include the insufficient long-term follow up. In addition, we did not show if the imaging technique is actually useful for enhancing the outcome or success rates, and we did not compare or contrast our technique with existing solutions, such as ultrasound. At our institute, contrast-enhanced CT is routinely used for the pretreatment evaluation of malignant hepatic tumors, and additional MDCT in the same study was considered to be adequate. We suggest that MDCT is accurate in the detection of abdominal arterial anatomy, variations, and abnormalities. In addition, CT provides information about the number, size, and location of hepatic tumors and the presence of an extrahepatic disease. These are advantages over ultrasound and other imaging methods. A longer follow-up period in a larger sample of patients would improve the evidence for the efficacy. However, prior information of the branching angle before catheter insertion may increase the reliability of the insertion technique and the completion rate of the therapy.

Imaging of the celiac artery can make the process of implantation of hepatic port systems less invasive by enabling a percutaneous catheter insertion method and thereby avoiding surgery.

Conclusion

The branching angle of the celiac artery can be easily determined by the preparation of MIP images from routine MDCT data. MIP may provide useful information for the selection of the catheter insertion route in order to avoid sharp branching angles of the celiac artery.

Competing interests

The authors declare that they have no competing interests.

Authors' contributions

HT participated in the design of the study and carried out the clinical examination. All authors read and approved the final manuscript.

References

1. Herrmann KA, Waggershauser T, Sittek H, Reiser MF: **Liver intraarterial chemotherapy: use of the femoral artery for percutaneous implantation of catheter-port systems.** *Radiology* 2000, **215**:294–299.
2. Oi H, Kishimoto H, Matsushita M, Hori M, Nakamura H: **Percutaneous implantation of hepatic artery infusion reservoir by sonographically guided left subclavian artery puncture.** *Am J Roentgenol* 1996, **166**:821–822.
3. Ikebe M, Itasaka H, Adachi E, Shirabe K, Maekawa S, Mutoh Y, Yoshida K, Takenaka K: **New method of catheter-port system implantation in hepatic arterial infusion chemotherapy.** *Am J Surg* 2003, **186**:63–66.
4. Kuroiwa T, Honda H, Yoshimitsu K, Irie H, Aibe H, Tajima T, Shinozaki K, Masuda K: **Complications encountered with a transfemorally placed port-catheter system for hepatic artery chemotherapy infusion.** *Cardiovasc Intervent Radiol* 2001, **24**:90–93.
5. Sahani DV, Krishnamurthy SK, Kalva S, Cusack J, Hahn PF, Santilli J, Saini S, Mueller PR: **Multidetector-row computed tomography angiography for planning intra-arterial chemotherapy pump placement in patients with colorectal metastases to the liver.** *J Comput Assist Tomogr* 2004, **28**:478–484.
6. Kapoor V, Brancatelli G, Federle MP, Katyal S, Marsh JW, Geller DA: **Multidetector CT arteriography with volumetric three-dimensional rendering to evaluate patients with metastatic colorectal disease for placement of a floxuridine infusion pump.** *Am J Roentgenol* 2003, **181**:455–463.
7. Lindner HH, Kemprud E: **A clinicoanatomical study of the arcuate ligament of the diaphragm.** *Arch Surg* 1971, **103**:600–605.
8. Lee VS, Morgan JN, Tan AG, Pandharipande PV, Krinsky GA, Barker JA, Lo C, Weinreb JC: **Celiac artery compression by the median arcuate ligament: a pitfall of end-expiratory MR imaging.** *Radiology* 2003, **228**:437–442.
9. Sone M, Kato K, Hirose A, Nakasato T, Tomabechi M, Ehara S, Hanari T: **Impact of multislice CT angiography on planning of radiological catheter placement for hepatic arterial infusion chemotherapy.** *Cardiovasc Intervent Radiol* 2008, **31**:91–97.

4

Defining the mid-diastolic imaging period for cardiac CT – lessons from tissue Doppler echocardiography

James M Otton[1,2], Justin Phan[2], Michael Feneley[1,2], Chung-yao Yu[1], Neville Sammel[1] and Jane McCrohon[1,2*]

Abstract

Background: Aggressive dose reduction strategies for cardiac CT require the prospective selection of limited cardiac phases. At lower heart rates, the period of mid-diastole is typically selected for image acquisition. We aimed to identify the effect of heart rate on the optimal CT acquisition phase within the period of mid-diastole.

Methods: We utilized high temporal resolution tissue Doppler to precisely measure coronary motion within diastole. Tissue-Doppler waveforms of the myocardium corresponding to the location of the circumflex artery (100 patients) and mid-right coronary arteries (50 patients) and the duration and timing of coronary motion were measured. Using regression analysis an equation was derived for the timing of the period of minimal coronary motion within the RR interval. In a validation set of 50 clinical cardiac CT examinations, we assessed coronary motion artifact and the effect of using a mid-diastolic imaging target that was adjusted according to heart rate vs a fixed 75% phase target.

Results: Tissue Doppler analysis shows the period of minimal cardiac motion suitable for CT imaging decreases almost linearly as the RR interval decreases, becoming extinguished at an average heart rate of 91 bpm for the circumflex (LCX) and 78 bpm for the right coronary artery (RCA). The optimal imaging phase has a strong linear relationship with RR duration ($R^2 = 0.92$ LCX, 0.89 RCA). The optimal phase predicted by regression analysis of the tissue-Doppler waveforms increases from 74% at a heart rate of 55 bpm to 77% at 75 bpm. In the clinical CT validation set, the optimal CT acquisition phase similarly occurred later with increasing heart rate. When the selected cardiac phase was adjusted according to heart rate the result was closer to the optimal phase than using a fixed 75% phase. While this effect was statistically significant ($p < 0.01$ RCA/LCx), the mean effect of heart-rate adjustment was minor relative to typical beat-to-beat variability and available precision of clinical phase selection.

Conclusion: High temporal resolution imaging of coronary motion can be used to predict the optimal acquisition phase in cardiac CT. The optimal phase for cardiac CT imaging within mid-diastole increases with increasing heart rate although the magnitude of change is small.

Keywords: Cardiac CT, Image quality, Heart rate, Tissue Doppler, Echocardiography

Background

Improvements in cardiac computed tomography technology have enabled fast and reliable imaging of the coronary arteries. Nevertheless, temporal resolution remains a limiting factor and the timing of image acquisition is critical for optimal imaging quality. While various empiric principles have been adopted to guide coronary image acquisition, to date, studies of timing strategies have generally focused on preferable timing bands of CT acquisition [1-4] during systole or diastole according to heart rate. Mid-diastole is typically selected at lower heart rates. Precise guidance as to the optimal phase within this period has been limited due to the temporal resolution of coronary tracking techniques available.

Echocardiography, and in particular tissue Doppler, is particularly suited due to its high temporal resolution, accuracy and ability to interrogate the myocardial motion at the arterial segments most vulnerable to imaging

* Correspondence: jmccrohon@stvincents.com.au
[1]Cardiology Department, St Vincent's Hospital, Darlinghurst, Sydney 2010, AUSTRALIA
[2]University of New South Wales, Sydney, NSW, Australia

artifact [5]. Tissue Doppler provides motion assessment of the coronary arteries with a temporal resolution of less than 5 ms [6] as opposed to the much poorer 30-50 ms resolution of invasive angiography [7,8], 10-20 ms resolution for MRI [9] or the 70-160 ms temporal resolution of CT imaging itself [10]. Tissue Doppler may therefore be used to distinguish between coronary motion present at single-percentage phase intervals within the diastolic period.

Optimal timing of cardiac CT is important firstly to minimize or eliminate motion artifact, and secondly to guide imaging parameters with regards to aggressive dose minimization strategies, which frequently employ limited cardiac phases [11,12]. It is well recognized that the fraction of the cardiac cycle occupied by diastole decreases with increasing heart rate and comes proportionally later in the cardiac cycle. It would therefore be expected that the optimal window for cardiac imaging may vary with heart rate and that small adjustments to the acquired phase may result in improved image quality.

We sought to investigate the motion of the coronary arteries throughout the cardiac cycle in order to provide both a qualitative and mathematical description of the period of optimal diastolic cardiac image acquisition in order to guide coronary imaging by low-dose, limited-phase cardiac CT. We compared the resultant analysis and prediction equations to motion artifact outcomes within a clinical cardiac CT cohort.

Methods

Echocardiographic measurements were obtained from anonymised routine clinical data and participants within the CT cohort gave written consent for the use of clinical data for research purposes. The study was performed in accordance with the principles of the Helsinki declaration and was approved by the St Vincent's Hospital Human Ethics Committee (approval number 10/044).

In order to record physiological motion of the coronary arteries, consecutive clinical echocardiograms performed at our institution were retrospectively reviewed from June 2010. Echocardiograms were performed using either a Philips ie33 or Sonos 7500 echocardiography system by an experienced technician. One hundred echocardiograms with clear tissue Doppler traces of the left ventricular lateral wall and fifty with right ventricular lateral wall tissue Doppler were selected from a sequential cohort of 324 patients. Patients were referred from both inpatient and outpatient settings for standard indications including the assessment of ischemic heart disease, heart failure and valvular pathology. Exclusion criteria were poor image quality and the presence of a cardiac rhythm other than sinus rhythm.

The tracked volume was selected to encompass the lateral tricuspid annulus corresponding to the course of the mid right coronary artery and the lateral mitral valve annulus, corresponding to the mid-distal position of the circumflex artery.

Tissue Doppler provides the motion of the area of tissue selected, relative to the transducer, typically at approximately 4 ms time intervals with the velocity displayed as per the left hand scale in cm/s. The tissue Doppler signal (Figure 1) is formed initially by the S' wave, corresponding to ventricular systole, a short period of little to no movement reflecting the isovolumic relaxation time (IVRT) and shift from systolic to diastolic phases. The E' corresponds to rapid ventricular filling due to ventricular relaxation. A short period of almost no cardiac motion then follows at low heart rates- the period of minimal cardiac motion (PMCM)- and then the A' wave reflective of atrial contraction. This PMCM is indicative of the ideal period of mid-diastolic coronary CT acquisition.

Utilizing the recorded ECG trace simultaneous to echocardiographic image acquisition, the time interval from the mid-point of the QRS trace to the start and end of the isovolumic relaxation time (IVRT), center of the E' and A' waves and start and end of the period minimal cardiac motion (PMCM) was measured. The period of minimal cardiac motion was defined as the diastolic phase between the E' and A' during which time the spectrum of the tissue Doppler velocity trace indicated tissue velocity of less than 2 cm/s. The duration of the QRS interval, current and preceding RR interval and ejection fraction were also noted.

Clinical CT validation study

In a validation cohort of 50 consecutive cardiac CT studies we prospectively assessed motion artifact within mid-diastole. The prospective cohort of 50 consecutive clinical cardiac CT patients included all scans performed for standard clinical indications, and included a broad range of heart rates. Patients were excluded from the validation cohort if the underlying rhythm was not sinus rhythm. Patients within the derivation echocardiography set were not included within the CT validation cohort.

All CT scans were obtained utilizing a 320 detector-row CT (Toshiba Aquilion One) with z-axis coverage adjusted to ensure complete cardiac coverage within a single gantry rotation and image acquisition of the entire coronary tree at identical cardiac phase. The x-ray tube current (mA), voltage (kV) and contrast volume (Ultravist370) were adjusted according to body size and standard clinical protocols. A FC03 filter kernel was used for reconstruction, without the use of iterative noise reduction. The resultant CT images were displayed at 0.5 mm [3] isotropic resolution. Where multiple cardiac cycles were acquired (for example due to very high heart rates or multiple

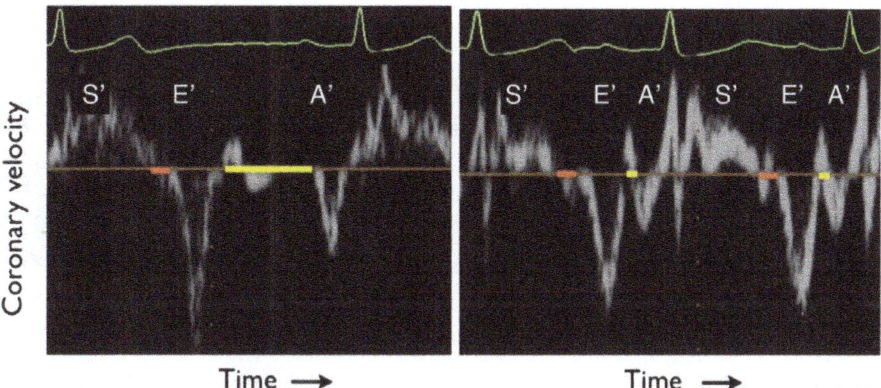

Figure 1 Tissue Doppler waveforms of the left atrio-ventricular groove (circumflex artery) at low (left) and high (right) heart rate. Coronary motion occurs throughout systole (S'). At the end of systole there is a short period of relative stasis between the closing of the aortic valve and the opening of the mitral valve (isovolumic relaxation time, IVRT), shown in red. This period varies little with heart rate. The period of minimal cardiac motion (yellow band) occurs between the E' and A' waves. The PMCM shortens with increasing heart rate. Images have been resized and edited for clarity.

volume acquisition), only the first RR interval was used for timing analysis.

The acquired cardiac phase was defined as the percentage of the RR interval corresponding to the midpoint of the half-scan reconstruction. All scans were acquired with a minimum of 170 ms of widened data acquisition, enabling reconstruction of a range of 70-80% of cardiac phase or greater, during which the mid-diastolic period is expected to occur at all physiological heart rates. In patients with a baseline heart rate of greater than 65 beats per minute or greater, a 30-80% range of cardiac phases were acquired. In all scans it was anticipated that the period of mid-diastole would be fully captured.

Motion artifact was defined as any blurring or loss of clear delineation of the coronary lumen and was assessed by a single reader (Figure 2). The cardiac phases at which motion artifact was absent was noted at both the mid right coronary artery and within the left coronary circulation at the bifurcation of the proximal left anterior descending artery and circumflex arteries. The ideal imaging target was selected separately for each artery as the mid-point between the first and last phases of artifact-free images. Where no motion free phase occurred, the phase containing the least motion artifact was selected as the ideal imaging target.

Statistical methods

Tissue Doppler analysis

Utilizing separate ordinary least squared linear regression models within STATA statistical software v10, StataCorp, USA we assessed the relationship between the RR interval and the dependent variables: time to the center of the IVRT, time to the E' wave, time to the A' wave and time to center of the period of minimal cardiac motion. The relationship and regression residuals were inspected visually. In addition, non-linearity was assessed using the Ramsay RESET test for omitted variables. Using simple algebraic substitution (noting Heart Rate = 60 seconds/RR interval) the regression equation relating the RR interval and the time to the center of the PMCM was used to form a prediction equation relating heart rate to the ideal target of cardiac imaging. This heart rate adjusted ideal phase equation was subsequently tested in the CT validation cohort.

As the duration of the PMCM, or imaging window, is limited by a lower bound of zero, truncated linear regression was used to generate an equation relating the RR interval and PMCM. This equation was used to forecast the PMCM based on the RR interval. The standard deviation of the forecast was calculated and used to create 90% confidence intervals of the forecast, which was then graphically displayed. The forecast equation of the PMCM was then displayed against heart rate within heart rates clinically relevant to diastolic imaging. This allowed the relationship between the CT acquisition time and the probability that the acquisition time falls within the PMCM to be graphically demonstrated.

CT validation cohort

The relationship between heart rate and ideal imaging target (the mid-point of the artifact free CT image time period) was assessed using ordinary least square regression. The null hypothesis, that there was no relationship between heart rate and ideal imaging target, was tested using a two-sided T test of the regression slope coefficient.

The timing error, or the absolute difference in time between the ideal imaging phase as judged by CT and

a) A fixed 75% phase
b) The heart-rate predicted ideal imaging phase

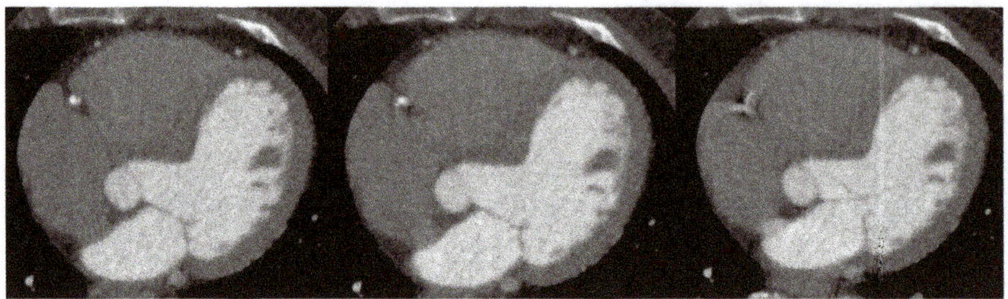

Figure 2 Examples of motion artifact definitions at the mid-right coronary artery. (Left) No artifact (Middle) Mild artifact (Right) Severe motion artifact. Phases containing no motion artifact were assigned to the period ideal cardiac imaging.

was measured. The error of each method of phase selection was compared using a paired t-test. The two-sided threshold for significance of the T-test was set at $p < 0.05$.

Results

Timing of tissue Doppler features and the cardiac imaging window

Visual examination of the relationship between the RR interval and the time to the E' wave, time to the A' wave, time to the IVRT and time to the center of the PMCM for the circumflex and right coronary arteries (Figures 3 and 4) indicated that the relationship between the variables did not demonstrate evident non-linearity, except at very low heart rates. This finding was mirrored by examination of the regression residuals. When heart rates < 50 where excluded, the Ramsay RESET test for omitted variables, indicative of non-linearity, were non-significant ($p > 0.3$) for all variables.

The center of the right coronary IVRT showed only a modest correlation with heart rate ($R^2 = 0.38$) irrespective of QRS duration or ejection fraction. The center of the IVRT occurred within the range (95% confidence interval) 32–63% of the RR duration, occurring later as a percentage of the RR interval as the heart rate increased

Correlation of the time to E' was strongly related to the RR duration (LCX $R^2 = 0.60$; RCA $R^2 = 0.52$ $p < 0.001$ for both). The A' was very strongly related to the RR duration (LCX $R^2 = 0.96$; RCA $R^2 = 0.92$. $P < 0.001$ for both). (Figure 4).

The coefficient of determination (R^2) of the relationship between the ideal imaging target and the RR interval was 0.92 for the circumflex and 0.86 for the right coronary artery. The regression equation for the optimal target of CT acquisition was found to be:

Optimal CT trigger time(ms) Circumflex = RR interval x 0.67 + 80 ms.

Optimal CT trigger time(ms) Right Coronary Artery = RR interval x 0.68 + 70 ms.

Heart rates outside the clinical range for diastolic imaging, 50–90 bpm, were excluded due to the excessive leverage of outlying values on regression analysis. The resultant heart rate targets, which are the same for both the circumflex and right coronary arteries are shown in Table 1.

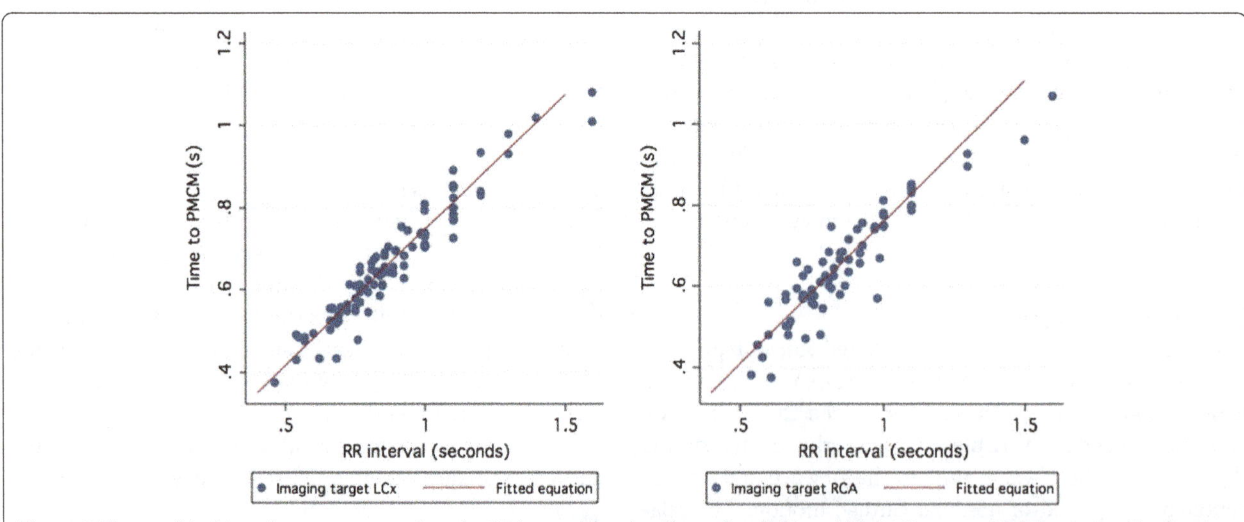

Figure 3 Time to ideal imaging target accord to the RR interval for the Circumflex (left) and Right Coronary (right) arteries. The fitted regression equation is also illustrated.

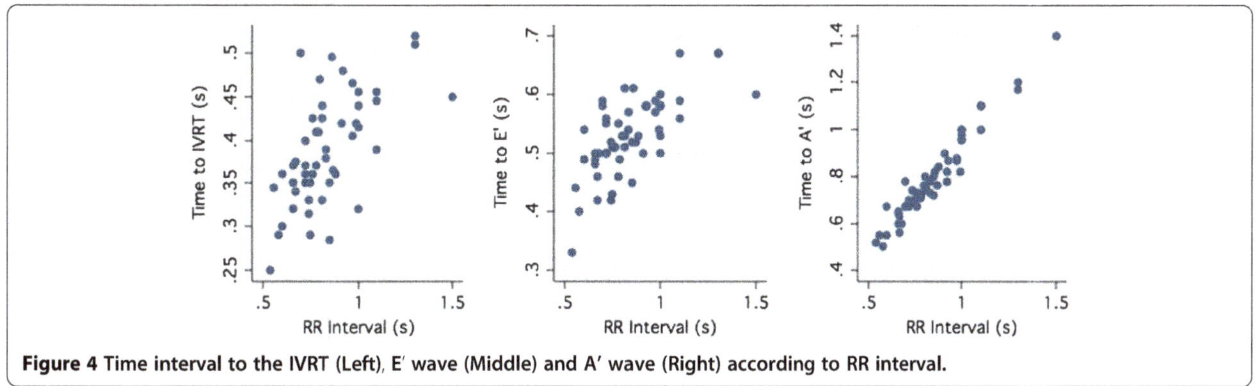

Figure 4 Time interval to the IVRT (Left), E′ wave (Middle) and A′ wave (Right) according to RR interval.

Doppler study of the duration of the cardiac imaging window in mid-diastole

As expected, tissue Doppler recording of both the right and left atrio-ventricular groove demonstrated greatest motion during systole. The mean duration of the IVRT, or end-systolic imaging window, was 55 ms and only a weak positive relation with the RR interval was noted ($R^2 = 0.28$, $p < 0.001$).

By contrast, the duration of diastolic PMCM is highly dependent on the heart rate extending almost linearly with increased RR interval (Figure 5A,B). At shorter RR intervals, the PMCM becomes progressively shorter, approaching zero above heart rates averaging 91 bpm for the circumflex and 78 bpm for the right coronary artery.

The duration of the circumflex PMCM averages 260 ms at a heart rate of 60, 150 ms at a heart rate of 70 and 77 ms at a heart rate of 80 bpm. The right sided PMCM is of shorter duration (Figure 6), reflecting the narrower imaging window and resultant greater chance of imaging motion artifact as illustrated in Figure 5C and D.

CT validation

Basic demographic details of patients studied are presented in Table 2. Ninety percent of patients received a rate controlling medication to achieve a target heart rate of 65 beats per minute or lower. 82% received oral beta-blockers, 4% IV beta-blockers and 2% received ivabradine or diltiazem respectively. Metoprolol was used in the large majority of cases and the median beta-blocker dose was 75 mg (range 25-200 mg). Due to extensive rate control, the median heart rate was 60 and only 3 patients recorded a heart rate of greater than 75 at the time of the CT scan.

In 38% of patients the stated reason for referral for CT was assessment due to cardiovascular risk factors or equivocal prior investigations. In 34% of patients the stated reason for referral for cardiac CT was of chest pain, and 14% were referred for prior arrhythmia. No referral reason was recorded for 14% of patients. The median radiation dose of all scans was 6.2 mSv.

The ideal cardiac phase for both the right and left coronary arteries increased with heart rate. The regression coefficient for the circumflex was 0.17 (95% CI 0.090-0.25, T-test $P < 0.01$) and 0.15 (95% CI 0.038-0.27, T-test $P < 0.05$) for right coronary artery indicating a 1.7% or 1.5% increase in the ideal imaging target in mid-diastole for every 10 beat increase in heart rate.

Analysis of time between the ideal cardiac imaging target, 75% phase target and the heart rate adjusted target (as per Table 1) demonstrated that the heart rate adjusted target was statistically closer to the ideal target than the fixed 75% target for both the right coronary artery and left anterior descending/circumflex arteries, ($p < 0.01$ for both). The absolute benefit of the heart rate adjusted strategy was 0.5% (SD 0.14%) for the circumflex and 0.4% (SD 0.13%)for the RCA. This partially reflects minor differences between the two prediction models at the most common heart rate 55–65 bpm. At heart rates greater than 65 the heart rate adjusted strategy was a mean of 1% for the RCA and 0.6% for the circumflex, closer to the ideal imaging phase.

While the heart rate guided phase target was statistically superior to the fixed target, both approaches demonstrated more motion artifact than could be predicted on the basis of coronary physiology alone (Figures 7 and 8). In 29 cases, no motion artifact was present in either artery at either the heart rate adjusted target or at the 75% phase. In 19 cases (38%), including 8 cases where no motion artifact free images occurred, image artifact was present with both timing strategies. The use of heart rate adjustment of CT timing would have led to the elimination of motion artifact in a net of 2 (4%) of patients within the validation cohort.

Table 1 Heart rate adjusted phase targets for both the right and circumflex coronary arteries

Heart Rate	50	55	60	65	70	75	80	85	90
Optimal diastolic target (% phase)	74%	74%	75%	76%	76%	77%	78%	78%	79%

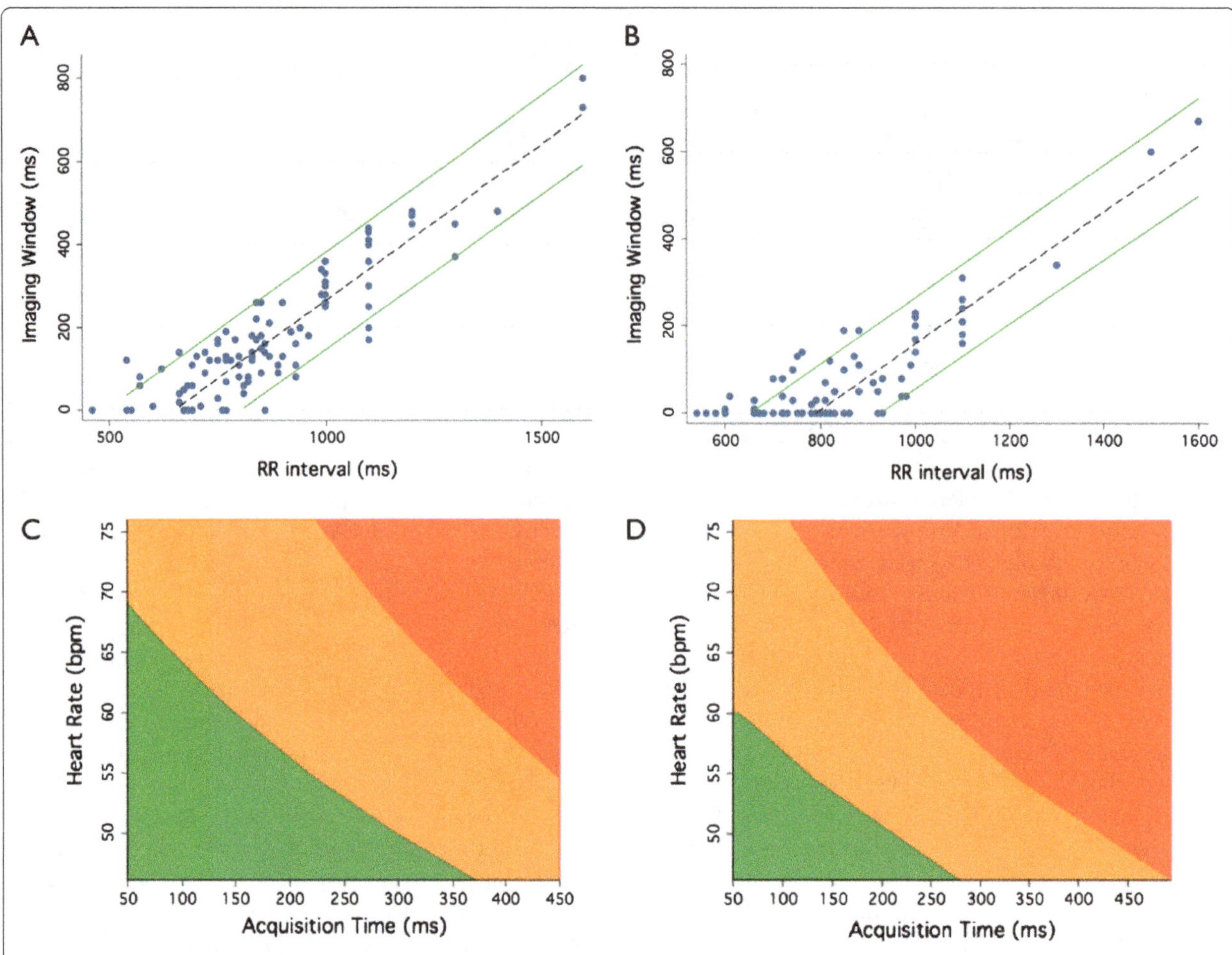

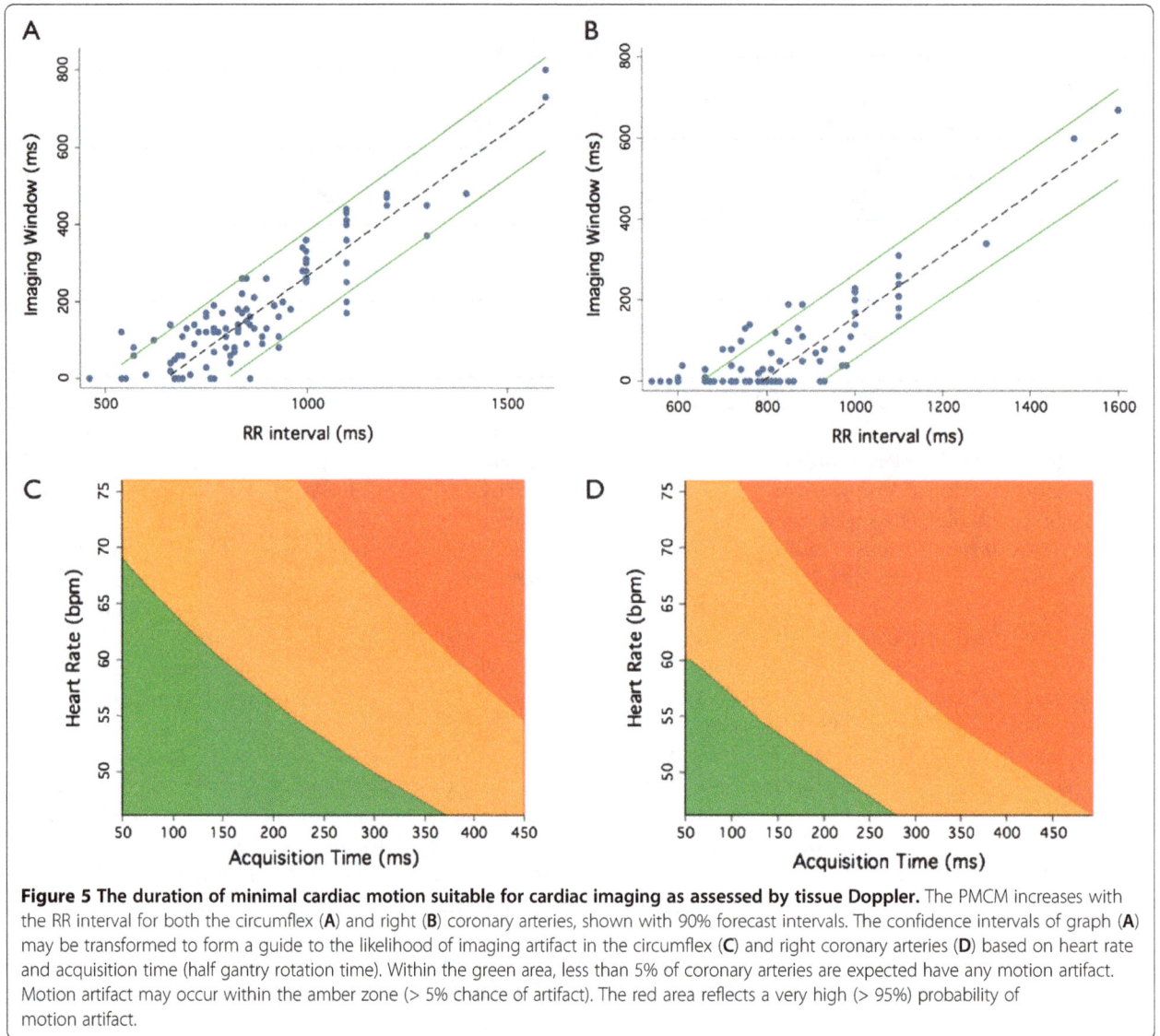

Figure 5 The duration of minimal cardiac motion suitable for cardiac imaging as assessed by tissue Doppler. The PMCM increases with the RR interval for both the circumflex (**A**) and right (**B**) coronary arteries, shown with 90% forecast intervals. The confidence intervals of graph (**A**) may be transformed to form a guide to the likelihood of imaging artifact in the circumflex (**C**) and right coronary arteries (**D**) based on heart rate and acquisition time (half gantry rotation time). Within the green area, less than 5% of coronary arteries are expected have any motion artifact. Motion artifact may occur within the amber zone (> 5% chance of artifact). The red area reflects a very high (> 95%) probability of motion artifact.

Discussion

This study demonstrates the role of careful examination of the physiology of coronary motion in understanding the optimal timing of cardiac CT within diastole and the impact of image acquisition speed on motion artifact. The study also demonstrates the difficulties of cardiac imaging timing given the inherent physiological variability in coronary motion. While we primarily assessed the effects of coronary motion on cardiac CT, the research may also have a role in other gated imaging modalities such as cardiovascular MRI.

The temporal resolution of half-scan reconstruction of current generation single source cardiac CT lies between 140 and 175 ms. While current dual-source imaging reduces the temporal resolution to 70 ms-83 ms [1,13], in its lowest dose, high-pitch exemplification, the time taken to image the entire axial cardiac volume remains in the order of 280 ms. Retrospective gating of cardiac CT, and increasing the window of acquisition can go some way towards reducing the effects of cardiac motion at higher heart rates, but at the cost of greatly increased radiation dose. Retrospective gated cardiac CT may deliver 4 or 5 times the ionizing radiation of prospective CT [14] and even when prospective cardiac CT protocols are used, for every extra 100 ms of the cardiac cycle acquired, radiation dose is increased by up to 45% [15]. On the other hand, very low dose prospectively gated cardiac CT acquired during minimal phase acquisition enables only one or a very narrow band of phases to be analyzed, compromising diagnosis in the case of motion artifact. Accurate timing of cardiac CT is therefore vital for both radiation dose reduction and prevention of imaging artifacts.

High temporal resolution imaging of coronary artery motion reveals interesting insights about coronary motion,

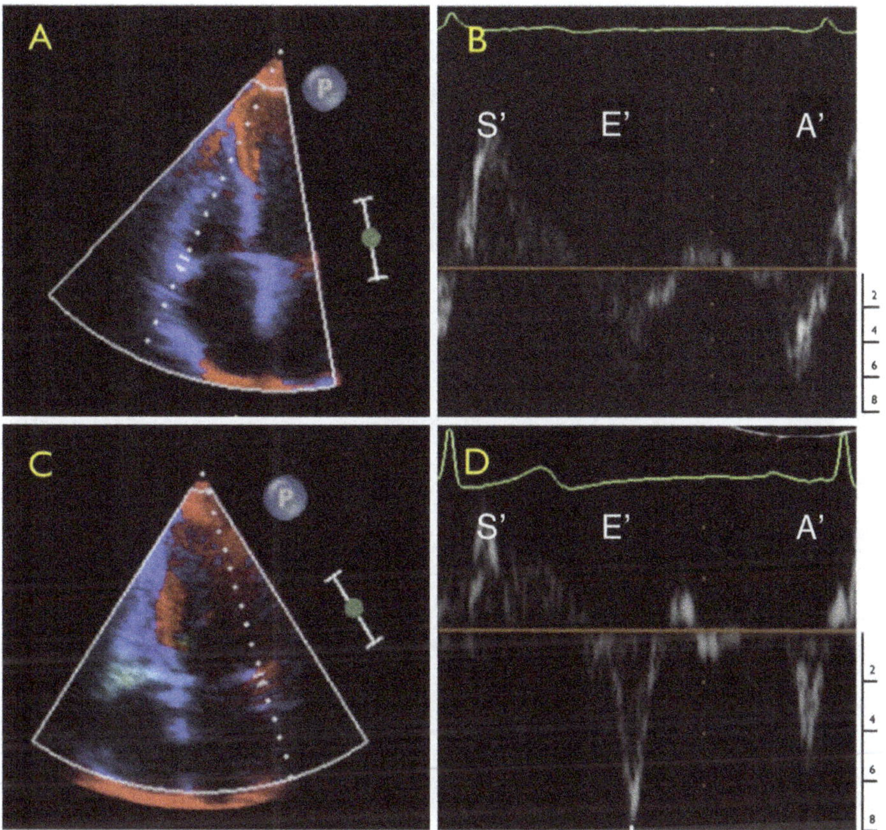

Figure 6 Tissue Doppler waveforms of the right (A) and left (C) atrio-ventricular grooves (Circumflex and Right coronary arteries). The right coronary artery E' and A' waves (**B**) tend to be broader leaving a shorter period of minimal cardiac motion. While the magnitude of each wave varies between individuals, the integral of the wave, or total motion is usually greater for the right than circumflex coronary arteries. This is the corollary of the rapid and more prolonged period of motion of the right coronary artery as may be seen during cine coronary angiography [7]. The duration of the PMCM of the right coronary between the E' and A' is also reduced relative to the Circumflex artery (**D**). Shown with indicative scale (cm/s). S' indicates systolic myocardial velocity.

which may be useful for effective cardiac imaging. Previous measurements of coronary artery motion using electron beam CT [16,17] or coronary angiography [7] are inadequate for the precise definition of the cardiac rest period within mid-diastole. This is because the low temporal resolution of these techniques can only provide information as to which broad band of phase acquisition is most appropriate according to heart rate. The issue as to whether end-systole or diastole is superior at a given heart rate is clinically important and has been previously studied [3,4,18-20]. Likewise the interaction of gantry rotation time, heart rate and image artifact requires careful attention in order to optimize image quality [21,22]. The current research adds to these prior works by further elucidating the nature, effects and variability of coronary motion during the imaging phase of mid-diastole.

Table 2 Validation patient demographic data

Variable	Median (Range)
Age, years	61 (24–75)
Weight (kg)	80 (44–135)
Body Mass Index	27 (18–37)
Heart rate	60 (43–102)

The equations and tables provided are intended as a guide for gated cardiac imaging across all CT types. They indicate the heart rates at which diastolic imaging becomes viable, the window available for imaging and the chance of motion artifact for given heart rates. In the validation cohort, a strategy of varying the targeted phase according to heart rate was statistically superior to a fixed percentage acquisition in terms of proximity to the ideal imaging phase, although the extent of benefit was small. These tools should prove useful for the achievement of high quality cardiac CT imaging. Nevertheless, there are several limitations to the formulas and conclusions provided and they should not be applied without consideration.

Firstly, it should be noted that even small differences in absolute timing make a large difference in the optimal phase selection. Variation can occur due to triggering

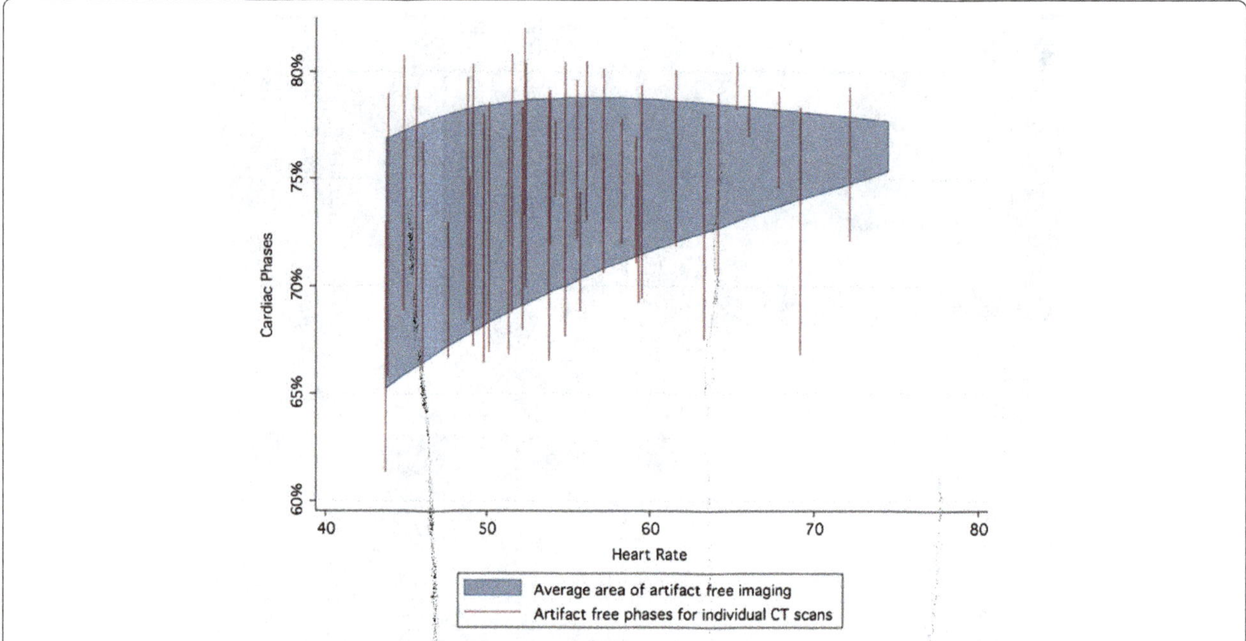

Figure 7 Motion-free acquisition windows for the circumflex artery from the CT validation set. Substantial variation in the motion-free period exists between individual studies. The fitted average of the motion-free period is shaded. While the upper bound of the area remains relatively constant with heart rate, the lower bound increases dramatically with heart rate.

parameters, QRS measurement and biological variability. Beat to beat variation of more than 50 ms can be expected at most heart rates and no system of CT triggering can ever account for the unpredictability associated with ectopic beats or atrial fibrillation. The wide variation in the ideal imaging target within the CT validation cohort may have reflected ectopy during the period of heart-rate assessment, although as we were only able to capture the two heartbeats immediately prior to imaging we were unable to assess the impact of ectopy in this study. While

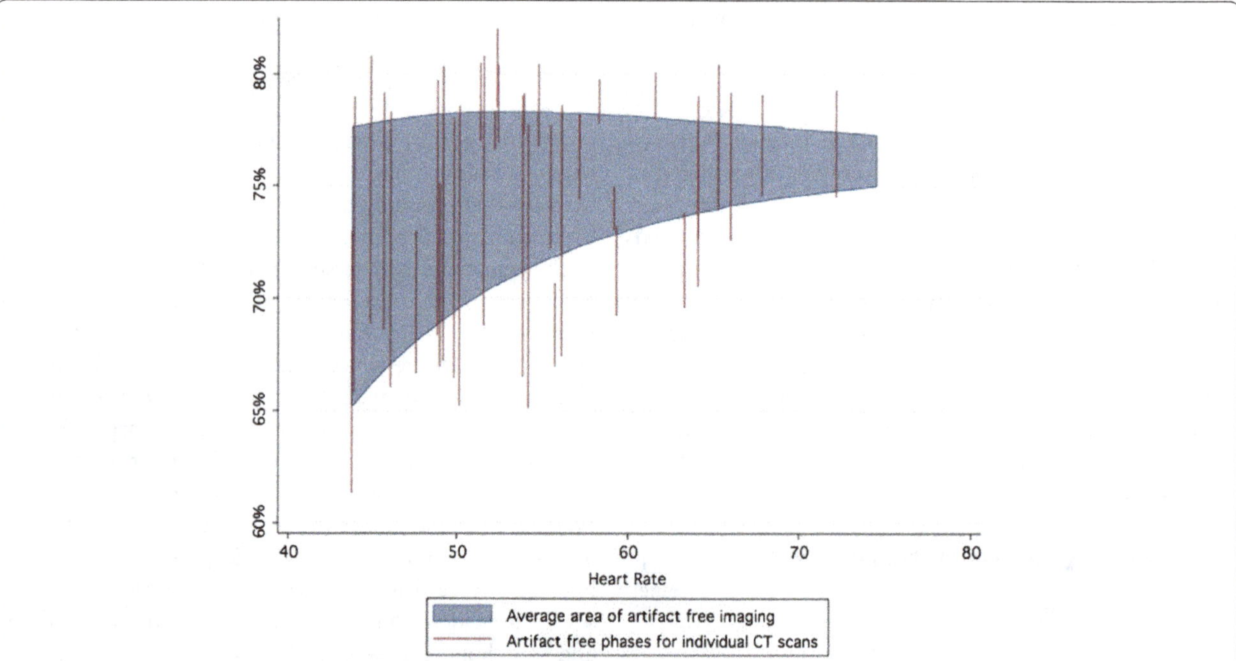

Figure 8 Motion free-acquisition window for the right coronary artery from the CT validation set. Very substantial variation in the motion-free period exists between individual studies. The acquisition window for the Right Coronary artery is relatively reduced and narrows more rapidly than the Circumflex artery.

measurement of time intervals on tissue Doppler has generally good reliability [23], the use of a single measurement in our study should also be considered a limitation and may have added to variability of tissue Doppler measurements.

Secondly, the definition of motion artifact used in this study was conservative and it is likely that a degree of motion artifact may be tolerated without affecting clinical interpretability. The effect of motion artifact on diagnosis is inherently subjective and the precise heart-rate boundaries of CT interpretability may vary from the predictions of this study.

Lastly, the difference between a fixed 75% phase trigger and a heart rate adjusted strategy was small, and both strategies benefit from a degree of extra phase acquisition at most heart rates and gantry speeds. CT coronary angiography performed as a part of this study was designed to ensure coverage of mid-diastole and analysis of systolic or end-systolic phases could not be performed. Adjustment of the precise imaging target within mid-diastole should be a consideration secondary to the more fundamental issue of whether end-systolic or diastolic imaging is required.

Conclusions

While the benefit of heart rate adjustment for coronary CT phase target selection within any individual patient is small, over a large cohort where dose minimization through single-phase acquisition is mandated, even minor adjustments in diastolic timing may result in a reduced chance of image motion artifact. Knowledge of physiological coronary motion reinforces the importance of heart rate control, acquisition time and phase selection in cardiac imaging.

Abbreviations

LCX: Left circumflex artery; RCA: Right coronary artery; PMCM: Period of minimal cardiac motion; IVRT: Isovolumic relaxation time.

Competing interests

The authors declare that they have no competing interests.

Authors' contributions

JO assisted with CT measurements, study design, data analysis and drafted the manuscript. JP performed CT and tissue Doppler measurements and critically edited the manuscript. MF participated in study conception and design. CYY critically edited the manuscript. NS critically edited the manuscript. JM participated in study design, conception, interpretation and helped draft the manuscript. All authors read and approved the final manuscript.

Acknowledgements

Grants and funding: Database infrastructure for the study was provided via a grant from the St Vincent's Clinic Foundation, Sydney Australia, a charitable medical research foundation. http://www.clinic.stvincents.com.au/clinic-foundation.

James Otton would like to acknowledge scholarship support from the National Health and Medical Research of Council of Australia, and grant support from the St Vincent's Clinic Foundation of Australia

Chung-Yao Yu is the current Swire Fellow in Advanced Cardiac Imaging and would like to acknowledge the Swire company for their generous financial support.

References

1. Achenbach S, Manolopoulos M, Schuhback A, Ropers D, Rixe J, Schneider C, Krombach GA, Uder M, Hamm C, Daniel WG, Lell M: **Influence of heart rate and phase of the cardiac cycle on the occurrence of motion artifact in dual-source CT angiography of the coronary arteries.** *J Cardiovasc Comput Tomogr* 2012, **6**:91–98.
2. Leschka S, Husmann L, Desbiolles LM, Gaemperli O, Schepis T, Koepfli P, Boehm T, Marincek B, Kaufmann PA, Alkadhi H: **Optimal image reconstruction intervals for non-invasive coronary angiography with 64-slice CT.** *Eur Radiol* 2006, **16**:1964–1972.
3. Seifarth H, Wienbeck S, Pusken M, Juergens KU, Maintz D, Vahlhaus C, Heindel W, Fischbach R: **Optimal systolic and diastolic reconstruction windows for coronary CT angiography using dual-source CT.** *AJR Am J Roentgenol* 2007, **189**:1317–1323.
4. Herzog C, Abolmaali N, Balzer JO, Baunach S, Ackermann H, Dogan S, Britten MB, Vogl TJ: **Heart-rate-adapted image reconstruction in multidetector-row cardiac CT: influence of physiological and technical prerequisite on image quality.** *Eur Radiol* 2002, **12**:2670–2678.
5. Zamorano J, Wallbridge DR, Ge J, Drozd J, Nesser J, Erbel R: **Non-invasive assessment of cardiac physiology by tissue Doppler echocardiography. A comparison with invasive haemodynamics.** *Eur Heart J* 1997, **18**:330–339.
6. Van de Veire NR, De Sutter J, Bax JJ, Roelandt JR: **Technological advances in tissue Doppler imaging echocardiography.** *Heart* 2008, **94**:1065–1074.
7. Wang Y, Vidan E, Bergman GW: **Cardiac motion of coronary arteries: variability in the rest period and implications for coronary MR angiography.** *Radiology* 1999, **213**:751–758.
8. Johnson KR, Patel SJ, Whigham A, Hakim A, Pettigrew RI, Oshinski JN: **Three-dimensional, time-resolved motion of the coronary arteries.** *J Cardiovasc Magn Reson: official journal of the Society for Cardiovascular Magnetic Resonance* 2004, **6**:663–673.
9. Tangcharoen T, Bell A, Hegde S, Hussain T, Beerbaum P, Schaeffter T, Razavi R, Botnar RM, Greil GF: **Detection of coronary artery anomalies in infants and young children with congenital heart disease by using MR imaging.** *Radiology* 2011, **259**:240–247.
10. Flohr TG, Raupach R, Bruder H: **Cardiac CT: how much can temporal resolution, spatial resolution, and volume coverage be improved?** *J Cardiovasc Comput Tomogr* 2009, **3**:143–152.
11. Husmann L, Valenta I, Gaemperli O, Adda O, Treyer V, Wyss CA, Veit-Haibach P, Tatsugami F, von Schulthess GK, Kaufmann PA: **Feasibility of low-dose coronary CT angiography: first experience with prospective ECG-gating.** *Eur Heart J* 2008, **29**:191–197.
12. Achenbach S, Marwan M, Ropers D, Schepis T, Pflederer T, Anders K, Kuettner A, Daniel WG, Uder M, Lell MM: **Coronary computed tomography angiography with a consistent dose below 1 mSv using prospectively electrocardiogram-triggered high-pitch spiral acquisition.** *Eur Heart J* 2010, **31**:340–346.
13. McCollough CH, Schmidt B, Yu L, Primak A, Ulzheimer S, Bruder H, Flohr TG: **Measurement of temporal resolution in dual source CT.** *Medical physics* 2008, **35**:764–768.
14. Maruyama T, Takada M, Hasuike T, Yoshikawa A, Namimatsu E, Yoshizumi T: **Radiation dose reduction and coronary assessability of prospective electrocardiogram-gated computed tomography coronary angiography: comparison with retrospective electrocardiogram-gated helical scan.** *J Am Coll Cardiol* 2008, **52**:1450–1455.
15. Labounty TM, Leipsic J, Min JK, Heilbron B, Mancini GB, Lin FY, Earls JP: **Effect of padding duration on radiation dose and image interpretation in prospectively ECG-triggered coronary CT angiography.** *AJR Am J Roentgenol* 2010, **194**:933–937.
16. Achenbach S, Ropers D, Holle J, Muschiol G, Daniel WG, Moshage W: **In-plane coronary arterial motion velocity: measurement with electron-beam CT.** *Radiology* 2000, **216**:457–463.
17. Mao S, Lu B, Oudiz RJ, Bakhsheshi H, Liu SC, Budoff MJ: **Coronary artery motion in electron beam tomography.** *J Comput Assist Tomogr* 2000, **24**:253–258.
18. Mok GS, Yang CC, Chen LK, Lu KM, Law WY, Wu TH: **Optimal systolic and diastolic image reconstruction windows for coronary 256-slice CT angiography.** *Acad Radiol* 2010, **17**:1386–1393.

19. Sun G, Li M, Li L, Li GY, Zhang H, Peng ZH: **Optimal systolic and diastolic reconstruction windows for coronary CT angiography using 320-detector rows dynamic volume CT.** *Clin Radiol* 2011, **66**:614–620.
20. Husmann L, Leschka S, Desbiolles L, Schepis T, Gaemperli O, Seifert B, Cattin P, Frauenfelder T, Flohr TG, Marincek B, Kaufmann PA, Alkadhi H: **Coronary artery motion and cardiac phases: dependency on heart rate – implications for CT image reconstruction.** *Radiology* 2007, **245**:567–576.
21. Greuter MJ, Dorgelo J, Tukker WG, Oudkerk M: **Study on motion artifacts in coronary arteries with an anthropomorphic moving heart phantom on an ECG-gated multidetector computed tomography unit.** *Eur Radiol* 2005, **15**:995–1007.
22. Greuter MJ, Flohr T, van Ooijen PM, Oudkerk M: **A model for temporal resolution of multidetector computed tomography of coronary arteries in relation to rotation time, heart rate and reconstruction algorithm.** *Eur Radiol* 2007, **17**:784–812.
23. Fraser AG, Payne N, Madler CF, Janerot-Sjoberg B, Lind B, Grocott-Mason RM, Ionescu AA, Florescu N, Wilkenshoff U, Lancellotti P, Wutte M, Brodin LA: **Feasibility and reproducibility of off-line tissue Doppler measurement of regional myocardial function during dobutamine stress echocardiography.** *Eur J Echocardiogr* 2003, **4**:43–53.

5

Automated measurement of heterogeneity in CT images of healthy and diseased rat lungs using variogram analysis of an octree decomposition

Richard E Jacob* and James P Carson

Abstract

Background: Assessing heterogeneity in lung images can be an important diagnosis tool. We present a novel and objective method for assessing lung damage in a rat model of emphysema. We combined a three-dimensional (3D) computer graphics method–octree decomposition–with a geostatistics-based approach for assessing spatial relationships–the variogram–to evaluate disease in 3D computed tomography (CT) image volumes.

Methods: Male, Sprague-Dawley rats were dosed intratracheally with saline (control), or with elastase dissolved in saline to either the whole lung (for mild, global disease) or a single lobe (for severe, local disease). Gated 3D micro-CT images were acquired on the lungs of all rats at end expiration. Images were masked, and octree decomposition was performed on the images to reduce the lungs to homogeneous blocks of $2 \times 2 \times 2$, $4 \times 4 \times 4$, and $8 \times 8 \times 8$ voxels. To focus on lung parenchyma, small blocks were ignored because they primarily defined boundaries and vascular features, and the spatial variance between all pairs of the $8 \times 8 \times 8$ blocks was calculated as the square of the difference of signal intensity. Variograms–graphs of distance vs. variance–were constructed, and results of a least-squares-fit were compared. The robustness of the approach was tested on images prepared with various filtering protocols. Statistical assessment of the similarity of the three control rats was made with a Kruskal-Wallis rank sum test. A Mann-Whitney-Wilcoxon rank sum test was used to measure statistical distinction between individuals. For comparison with the variogram results, the coefficient of variation and the emphysema index were also calculated for all rats.

Results: Variogram analysis showed that the control rats were statistically indistinct ($p = 0.12$), but there were significant differences between control, mild global disease, and severe local disease groups ($p < 0.0001$). A heterogeneity index was calculated to describe the difference of an individual variogram from the control average. This metric also showed clear separation between dose groups. The coefficient of variation and the emphysema index, on the other hand, did not separate groups.

Conclusion: These results suggest the octree decomposition and variogram analysis approach may be a rapid, non-subjective, and sensitive imaging-based biomarker for characterizing lung disease.

Keywords: Lung imaging, Disease detection, COPD, Emphysema, Pulmonary, Octree, Variogram

* Correspondence: richard.jacob@pnnl.gov
Biological Sciences Division, Pacific Northwest National Laboratory, 902 Battelle Blvd., Richland, WA 99352, USA

Background

Emphysema is an obstructive pulmonary disease that results in airway expansion and tissue destruction. Early and accurate detection of emphysema is important for disease management and improved patient outcomes [1]. Emphysema typically results in heterogeneous air trapping and increased ventilation-perfusion inequality. Thus, signatures of tissue heterogeneity or regional air trapping may facilitate earlier and/or more accurate diagnoses of emphysema [2,3].

It has been shown in many studies that CT is a reproducible and predictive modality for diagnosing and assessing emphysema [2,4-7]. The most common way to quantify moderate to severe emphysema from CT images is to measure the emphysema index: the percentage of voxels below a preset Hounsfield Unit (HU) threshold. However, this index may not detect subtle or early onset emphysema [7], or, conversely, it may identify "false positive" regions that appear emphysematous in asymptomatic healthy young subjects with no smoking history [8]. In addition, threshold values vary between studies, typically within a range of-900 to-980 HU, with factors other than disease influencing CT densitometry [2,4,9,10].

An approach to assessing heterogeneity that has been applied to myriad types of medical images is fractal analysis [11]. This approach exploits the scale-independent nature of fractals in systems, such as lung vasculature, whose variation in form or regularity is thought to be similar through different degrees of magnification [12]. Typically, a region (or regions) of interest (ROI) is selected, which is then evaluated for a mean value and/ or repeatedly subdivided to relate differences in signal intensity across space and across ROI size. If the relationship is characterized by a power law, then the exponent, or fractal dimension, is taken as an indication of complexity, texture, or heterogeneity [13-15]. However, this method is based on an a priori assumption that power law relationship exists and that a fractal dimension can be determined. Furthermore, because this approach requires ROI selection, it is often subjective and can result in omission of large sections of the lung [13,16].

A promising new approach, detailed in recent work by Subramaniam et al. [17], demonstrates the use of analysis of CT image slices using a quadtree decomposition. This approach iteratively divides a 2D image into increasingly small squares. Division occurs whenever the range of intensities within the quadrant are above a pre-defined threshold. In this way, regions with homogenous intensity are characterized by larger squares. Their work measures heterogeneity by counting the number of squares-per-area in the lung or in a local region of the lung.

We propose to extend the quadtree decomposition to 3D by using octrees. In this way, the entire lung CT image volume is used. An octree iteratively divides a cubic volume into eight evenly sized cubes, or octants. The octree method is well-developed and is used, for example, in 3D mesh generation and computer graphics [18,19], medical image registration [20], and finite element meshing in CT images [21]. The advantages of the octree here is that it facilitates a speed-up in 3D lung tissue analysis by non-subjectively subdividing the lungs into homogeneous regions, thereby allowing for focus on parenchyma by reducing partial volume averaging and eliminating edges [22].

To incorporate spatial information across the lung, we propose to couple the octree image decomposition approach with variogram analysis. Variograms are a spatio-statistical approach for measuring spatial variability by comparing sample value variances to the distance of separation [23,24]. Variograms are well-established in geostatistics, but have also recently attracted interest in biomedical applications, such as characterizing magnetic resonance images of white matter [25]. In this pilot study using our approach, we are able to significantly differentiate from each other the three groups of elastase-dosed rats: control, distributed mild emphysematous disease, and region-specific severe disease.

Methods

Disease model

An elastase-induced model of emphysema was used in this study. Nine male Sprague-Dawley rats with an average weight of 212 ± 11 g were orally intubated and dosed intratracheally with: 250 U/kg elastase dissolved in 200 μL saline to the whole lung (n = 3), or 50 U/kg elastase in 200 μL saline to a single lobe (n = 3), or 200 μL saline as a control (n = 3). Dosing levels were based on our previous work in which emphysematous changes were detected using ^{3}He diffusion MRI and histology [26]. All animal use was approved by the Institutional Animal Care and Use Committee at Pacific Northwest National Laboratory.

CT imaging

Three weeks following dosing, the rats were imaged using micro-CT. At this time, rats weighed 357 ± 10 g. The imaging procedure is described in detail in [27]. Briefly, rats were anesthetized, intubated, and mechanically ventilated at 1 Hz with 40% inhale and 60% exhale durations. Peak inhalation pressure was ~8 cmH_2O, and no peak end expiratory pressure was used so that images could be acquired at functional residual capacity. Anesthesia was maintained by providing 3-4% isoflurane in air (30% O_2, balance N_2). Sigh breaths were delivered periodically to maintain lung recruitment. A respiratory-gated GE eXplore 120 micro-CT scanner was employed with the following settings: 100 kV peak voltage, 50 mA tube current, 16 ms exposure time, and 360 projections with 1 degree angular steps. Images were reconstructed with supplied software to 150 μm isotropic resolution. Total imaging time was about 90 minutes due to the collection of multiple images throughout the breathing cycle; however, only the images acquired at full exhalation were used for the analyses herein. Post-mortem histology and tissue analysis were not possible due to *in situ* lung casting for other research purposes (i.e. supplying airway tree geometries for computational fluid dynamics models [28,29]).

Image preparation

A lung mask image was semi-automatically generated from the above-mentioned reconstructed images using ImageJ [30] and the ImageJ 3D Toolkit plug-in [31]. Starting from a seed-point inside the lung, a 3D connected threshold was applied with a threshold value empirically selected to exclude major vasculature and all external tissue, so that only lung tissue would be included in analysis. Mask boundaries were smoothed using the Region Dilate and Region Erode functions in succession. Applying the mask to the reconstructed images, all background was thus assigned an intensity value of 0, and all unmasked lung tissue retained original HU values. A five pixel diameter 3D median filter was then applied in order to reduce noise while contributing minimal blurring. Finally, the image canvas size was increased to $512 \times 512 \times 512$ by zero-filling in each direction. We note that zero-filling to a power of 2 served to conveniently restrict all octants in the octree decomposition to isotropic cubes.

Octree decomposition

An automated octree decomposition was performed by iteratively subdividing an image, with each division producing eight evenly sized octants (e.g., the initial $512 \times 512 \times 512$ image was decomposed into eight $256 \times 256 \times 256$ octant regions, and so on; see Figure 1) [32]. After each division, the maximum, minimum, mean, and standard deviation of the signal intensity were calculated for each octant region. Then, iterative octant subdivision of a region occurred if either the standard deviation of that region exceeded a user-defined threshold, or if the region contained at least one voxel–but not all voxels–with intensity equal to the background signal (i.e. 0). However, regions reaching a minimum size of $2 \times 2 \times 2$ were not subdivided. At the end of the decomposition, all boxes with a mean HU value $\neq 0$ and dimensions greater than $2 \times 2 \times 2$ represented portions of lung with relatively uniform HU values. Following decomposition, results were binned according to HU and box size for histogram display. Boxes containing at least one 0 were not included in the binning. Octree decomposition was implemented in Python and executed on a MacPro model 3.1. We note that we have modified our Python code to integrate ImageJ to minimize user interaction, although that was done subsequent to this work. The only interactive user-initiation required is the manual selection of a seed-point for the 3D connected threshold.

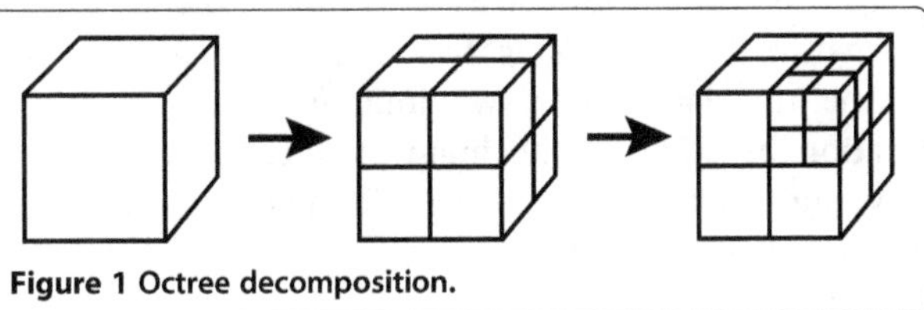

Figure 1 Octree decomposition.

There are multiple approaches to selecting the aforementioned user-defined threshold criteria. For example, in [17] boxes were subdivided if the HU range in the box exceeded 10% of the range of values in the entire image. Because our rats had different ranges of HU values depending on disease severity, we chose to use the standard deviation as the threshold criterion, as it does not require normalization. We describe how the threshold range was determined in Section Threshold range.

Variogram analysis

The purpose of using variograms in this context was to determine the spatial relationships between regions of the lung that are relatively homogeneous. The octree decomposition isolated regions of relatively high homogeneity; therefore, each resulting box was treated as a homogeneous "voxel" using the mean value of the box as the voxel intensity. Furthermore, it was important to use octree boxes that were all the same size. The largest box sizes that resulted from the octree decompositions were mostly $8 \times 8 \times 8$ with a few $16 \times 16 \times 16$ boxes. In order to ensure a sufficient number of boxes that were distributed throughout the lung and to enhance statistical power [25], each $16 \times 16 \times 16$ box was further broken down into $8 \times 8 \times 8$ boxes, and all $8 \times 8 \times 8$ boxes were used in the variogram analysis. This approach assumed that emphysematous disease was manifest on a scale greater than an $8 \times 8 \times 8$ box, which for these images is 1.2 mm on a side–this is consistent with what we observed in this disease model in previous work [26]. Importantly, excluding the smaller boxes largely eliminated vasculature, conducting airways, boundaries, and other features that had high spatial variability [22].

The calculation of the variance (or semi-variance) $\gamma(d)$ of the differences in signal intensity I is described in detail in many geostatistics texts, such as [23,24], and is given by:

$$y(d) = -\frac{1}{2N(d)}\sum_{i}^{N(d)}[I(x_i) - I(x_i - d)]^2 \quad (1)$$

where d is the distance between voxel centroids, x is the voxel location in 3D, and $N(d)$ is the number of voxel pairs for a given d. $\gamma(d)$ is calculated for all values of d. For an image with n voxels, the total number of voxel pairs (for all existing values of d) is given by

$$N = n(n-1)/2. \quad (2)$$

We then calculated the average semi-variance at each distance. Results were plotted on a distance vs. variance graph, or variogram, which graphically represents the spatial dissimilarity within the image.

The purpose of the variograms was to characterize spatial relationships between boxes of relatively high homogeneity that were dispersed throughout the lung. However, as described by [25] in work with brain images, increased distances between voxels, or octants, lead to decreased likelihood that the voxels are related in any way. This is especially true in the lung, which is composed of largely independent lobes (five in the rat). Moreover, the spatial relationship between parenchymal signal intensity in different lobes is, in many contexts, most accurately described by a unique path up and back down the airway tree, potentially covering 20 or more orders of branching [33]. The spatial distances are analogous to the "regionalized variable" in the geological context of mineral distribution. Indeed, the regionalized variable, or the maximum distance d_{max} over which the variogram is expected to be reliable, is estimated to be one half of the diameter of a region [25], while beyond d_{max} any relationships between distance and variance are expected to be random. Therefore, we limited our variogram analysis to a region that represented half of the average dimension of the left lobe, which is typically the largest lobe in the rat. This assumes that the disease varies slowly compared to the box size but rapidly compared to the lobe size. Using the 3D images and a lung cast, d_{max} was measured to be ≈ 8 mm (53 pixels) in the healthy rats, which was rounded up to the equivalent of seven face-bordering $8 \times 8 \times 8$ boxes, or 56 pixels.

Octree decomposition tests

We performed the following evaluations of the appropriateness and robustness of the octree and variogram approach.

Threshold range

The octree decomposition compared the standard deviation of the lung signal within a box to a threshold range to determine whether the box should be subdivided. The optimal threshold range was determined semi-empirically. As a starting point, we calculated the typical standard deviation of the lung tissue of the three control rats. This was accomplished by producing a histogram of each masked image and then fitting the main lung peak to a Gaussian curve. The mean of the control rats' standard deviations (σ) was set as the initial threshold range. We then tested the effects of thresholds that were $\sigma/3$, $2\sigma/3$, $4\sigma/3$, and 2σ by rerunning the decomposition on the same images. We evaluated the effectiveness of each threshold range at grouping the control rats and at distinguishing the full-lung-dose rats from the control group in the variograms.

Image filtering

We examined the effects of image filtering by generating variograms from unfiltered images, images filtered with a five pixel diameter 3D median filter, images filtered with a 3D Gaussian blur of radius = 2, and images filtered with a 3D Gaussian blur of radius = 4. Filters were applied in ImageJ prior to applying the mask. The number of octree boxes and differences in the variograms were compared. Adjustments to the threshold range were made for each filter test based on the standard deviation of the filtered image.

Image translation

Rat positioning during imaging can vary from animal to animal, and the octree decomposition should be independent of this. Therefore, we tested the effects of image translation on the variogram results. For the variogram analysis, the largest unit box retained after decomposition was $8 \times 8 \times 8$; therefore, a shift in the image by 8 pixels in any (or all) dimensions should result in no change to the resulting variogram, since the original image had isotropic dimensions of 2^n. Conversely, maximum change would occur from a four-pixel shift. To test the significance of the effects of translation, the image of one rat was shifted in x, y, and z by four pixels and by eight pixels using ImageJ, and variogram results were compared to those of the original image.

Image rotation

Animal positioning can also have an apparent effect on image rotation, and octree decomposition should be insensitive to this. Using the same rat image as used in the translation test, we imitated an arbitrary 3D rotation by rotating the image $\pi/4$ radians about the x, y, and z axes using ImageJ. Results were compared to the original image and to the results of the translation test.

Image downsampling

To demonstrate the increased value of the combined octree and threshold approach for establishing the 8 × 8 × 8 boxes versus simply downsampling the image, we generated variograms using standard image downsampling as a comparison. For this, we applied a bilinear downsampling to the 512 × 512 × 512 image, creating a 64 × 64 × 64 image–each voxel the equivalent size of an 8 × 8 × 8 octree box. Then we generated variograms utilizing the intensity value of every voxel in the 64 × 64 × 64 image (excluding the background voxels, again defined as those voxels with intensities equal to zero).

Emphysema index, coefficient of variation, and heterogeneity score

The percentage of lung below a HU threshold value, or emphysema index, was calculated for each rat to compare this conventional measurement of disease severity with the variogram results. Because there is no established HU threshold level in rat models of emphysema, we chose to count the percentage of voxels with HU values below two standard deviations from the control-group mean. This level was determined to be–717 HU. Calculations were made on the same masked images used for octree decomposition.

The CoV was calculated for each rat by fitting a histogram of the masked lung images to a Gaussian curve and taking the ratio of the standard deviation to the mean.

For comparison, we defined a new metric, the heterogeneity score (Δ), as the average difference between the mean variance of the control group and the spatial variance of each individual rat, in the range $d \leq d_{max}$.

Statistical analysis

Comparisons of variograms of the three control group rats were made using the Kruskal-Wallis (KW) rank sum test with a null hypothesis of $\alpha = 0.05$. This indicated whether there were significant differences within the group. For pairwise comparisons, a Mann-Whitney-Wilcoxon (MWW) rank sum test was employed, also with a null hypothesis of $\alpha = 0.05$.

Results

CT images

Figure 2 shows a representative unfiltered coronal slice from a rat in each dose group: panel A is a control rat, panel B is a full-lung-dose rat, and panel C is a partial-lung-dose rat (the dose was delivered to the distal portion of the left lobe). The mean HU value (± standard deviation) of the control group was-544 ± 58 HU and the mean of the full-lung dose group was–594 ± 38 HU. In spite of marginally lower HU values that would be expected from emphysematous disease, an analysis of variance showed that the two groups were indeed not statistically different ($p = 0.26$). On the other hand, the partial-lung-dose rats showed a bimodal distribution of HU values because the diseased regions of the lung were distinct from the healthy regions. An example of this can be seen in the lower portion of the left lobe of the partial-lung-dosed rat (panel C) where the signal intensity is substantially lower than the rest of the lung (by ≈ 200 HU)–indicative of severe tissue destruction and air trapping, which are characteristics of emphysematous lungs [34]. Based on the overall HU measurements, we presume that the full-lung-dose rats developed a mild–and difficult to distinguish–emphysematous disease while the single-lobe-dose rats developed a more severe, albeit localized, disease.

Octree decomposition tests

Threshold

The starting octree decomposition threshold level determined from the standard deviations of the control rats (Section Threshold range) was 60 ± 1 HU; therefore, 60 HU was used as the initial threshold level. Thus, the

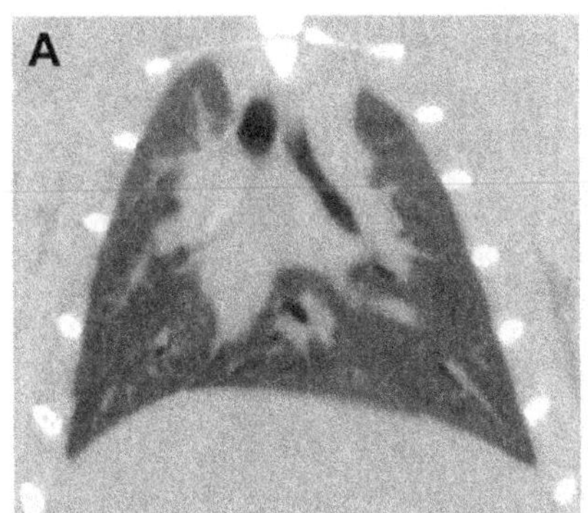

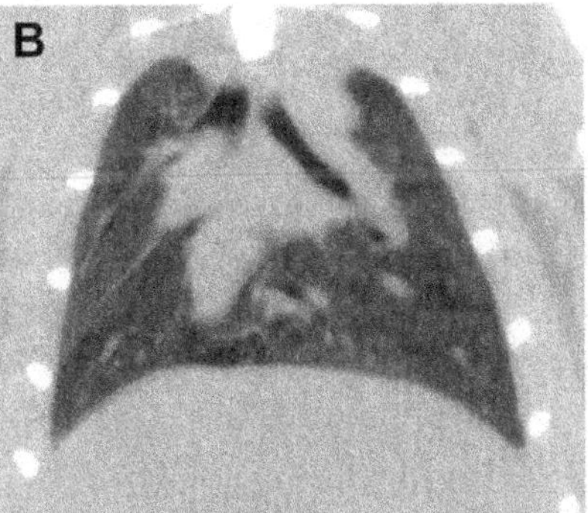

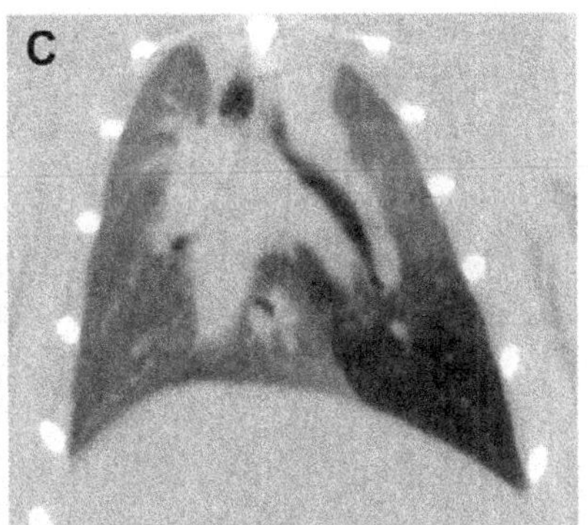

Figure 2 Unfiltered coronal slices from 3D images of A) a control rat, B) a full-lung-dose rat, and C) a single-lobe-dose rat. Only subtle differences between the full-lung-dose and control rats are evident; however, the distal region of the left lobe of the single-lobe-dose rat has considerably lower signal intensity, indicative of tissue destruction and/or air trapping characteristic of emphysematous disease.

other threshold levels tested were 20, 40, 80, and 120 HU. Octree decompositions were performed using the different threshold levels on the three control rats, and variograms were compared using a KW rank sum test. The threshold level that showed the least difference among the control rats was 40 HU ($p = 0.12$), with 60 HU also showing no significant differences ($p = 0.09$). The 20, 80, and 120 HU thresholds did have significant differences among the controls ($p = 0.02$, $p < 0.0001$, and $p < 0.0001$, respectively). Based on this result, we chose to use the threshold level of 40 HU for all subsequent octree decompositions (unless otherwise noted).

Image filtering

Results of applying the different filters showed that the variograms from the unfiltered image and the image with the median filter were indistinct in an MWW test ($p = 0.62$). However, the relatively noisy unfiltered image resulted in about 20% fewer 8 × 8 × 8 boxes than the filtered image. This was in spite of a higher threshold that was used, 48 HU, based on the unfiltered image's standard deviation. The radius = 2 and radius = 4 Gaussian filter results also did not differ significantly from the unfiltered image ($p = 0.41$ and $p = 0.48$, respectively) or from the median-filtered image ($p = 0.71$ and $p = 0.84$, respectively). A KW test showed that the radius = 2 filter resulted in control group variograms that were not distinct ($p = 0.16$), but the radius = 4 variograms were ($p = 0.0001$). However, because of the blurring caused by Gaussian filters, the number of 8 × 8 × 8 boxes that resulted from the Gaussian-filtered images was about 30% higher than the median filtered image, presumably because vascular structures and edges were not well preserved. Threshold levels used for the radius = 2 and radius = 4 images were 37 HU and 39 HU, respectively, based on the post-filtering standard deviations.

Effect of downsampling

Figure 3 shows an example of an original image (panel A), the image with the five voxel diameter 3D median filter (panel B), and the same image downsampled to 1/8 resolution, or 64 × 64 × 64 pixels (panel C). The variograms made from the downsampled images of the three control rats were statistically different in a KW rank sum test ($p < 0.0001$). On the other hand, the variograms made from only the 8 × 8 × 8 boxes that came out of the octree decomposition were not ($p = 0.12$; see Section Threshold).

Translation and rotation

Results of image translation and rotation were compared for one rat. For the eight-pixel translation, variogram results were exactly identical to that of the original image, as expected. The four-pixel shift was not statistically distinct from the original image as confirmed by a MWW test ($p = 0.96$). In addition, the result of the rotation showed no significant change from the original ($p = 0.56$) or from the four-pixel shift ($p = 0.59$). Thus, we confirm that shifts or rotations to the image (i.e. alternative positions of the lung during imaging) do not result in significant changes to the resulting variograms.

Octree decomposition

Figure 4 shows the results of the octree decomposition on a control rat and on one with severe disease in the lower left lobe (see Figure 2C). Column A shows the 2 × 2 × 2 boxes, and column B shows the 4 × 4 × 4 boxes. These box sizes largely define the fine structures and edge details, including the conducting airways and vasculature. For this reason, we ignored the 2 × 2 × 2 and 4 × 4 × 4 boxes for the variogram analysis. Column C shows the 8 × 8 × 8 boxes and their relatively uniform distribution throughout the lung. Conversely, the less uniform distribution of the considerably fewer 16 × 16 × 16 boxes–the largest that resulted from octree

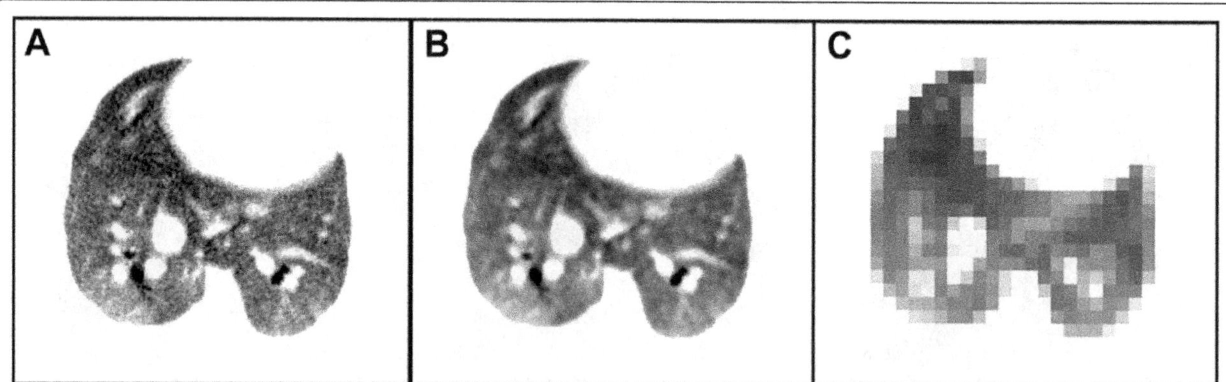

Figure 3 A masked axial slice from an original CT image with examples of different filtering. A: Unfiltered CT image. **B**: 3D median filter (5 pixel diameter). **C**: Downsampled by 8 ×.

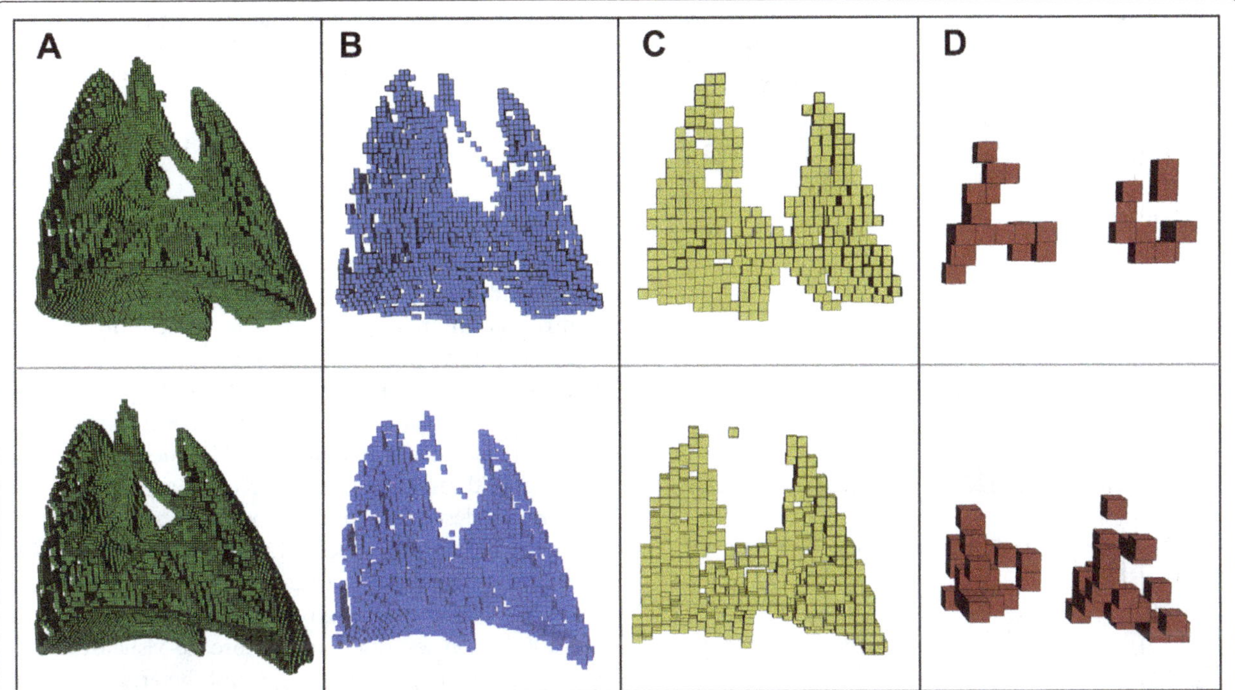

Figure 4 Octree decomposition results from two rats. The top row is a control rat and the bottom row is a single-lobe-dose rat (the same as those shown in Figure 2). Columns **A**, **B**, **C**, and **D** show the resulting 2 × 2 × 2, 4 × 4 × 4, 8 × 8 × 8, and 16 × 16 × 16 boxes, respectively.

decomposition–is shown in Column D. We point out, for example, that the lower left lobe of the treated rat (column D, bottom) has an approximately 2.5× higher density of 16 × 16 × 16 boxes than that of the control rat, indicating prevalence of localized homogeneous CT signal intensity.

Histograms of the octree decomposition for three rats are shown in Figure 5. The marker size corresponds to the box size. In the control and mild disease rats (panels A and B), the different sized boxes, other than the 2 × 2 × 2's, are approximately Gaussian distributed about the mean HU value of the lung, whereas the single-lobe-dose rat (panel C) shows a bimodal distribution, indicative of at least one large region of the lung with considerably lower HU values. These histograms show what percentage of the lung at each HU intensity is defined by the different box sizes, but they do not convey any information about the spatial relationships of the boxes.

Variograms

In order to visualize the spatial relationships between the 8 × 8 × 8 boxes (and decomposed 16 × 16 × 16 boxes), variograms were constructed. Figure 6 shows the average variograms from the three different dose groups. The dashed line in Figure 6 denotes the range of d_{max} (see Section Variogram analysis). For $d \leq d_{max}$ a KW test showed that the control rats were statistically similar ($p = 0.12$), and a MWW test showed that the dose groups were each statistically distinct from the control group ($p < 0.0001$) and from one another ($p < 0.0001$).

Emphysema index, coefficient of variation, and heterogeneity score

Results of the emphysema index are shown in the Figure 7A. Although the number of rats is too small to reliably calculate sensitivity and specificity, the graph shows that there is considerable overlap between subjects in each dose group, likely indicating poor sensitivity and specificity. The CoV for each rat is shown in Figure 7B. Similarly, there is no distinction between the control and full-lung dose groups. The part-lung dose group had considerably higher CoV values, because the standard deviation was enlarged due to a bimodal (and non-Gaussian) distribution of HU values.

For comparison, we calculated the heterogeneity score Δ of each rat's variance from that of the control group average; see Figure 7C. There is no overlap of Δ between dose groups (i.e. the highest Δ of the control group is lower than the lowest Δ of the full-lung group). This is not observed in Figure 7A or B, suggesting better sensitivity and specificity for Δ than the other metrics.

Discussion

This work combined two different data analysis tools, octree decomposition and variograms, to study tissue

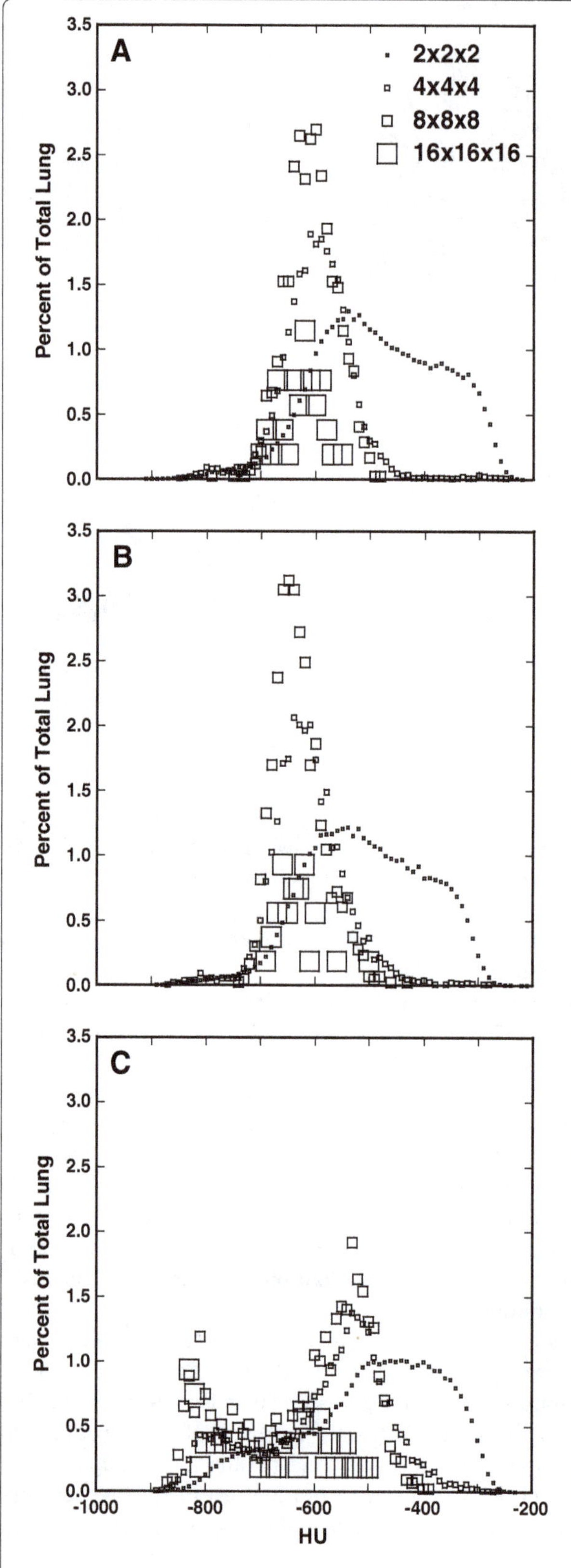

Figure 5 Octree decomposition histograms showing the relationship between box size, HU, and percentage of the lung by each box size at each HU level for three representative rats. **A**: Control (mean = -599 HU), **B**: Full-lung dose (mean = -634 HU), **C**: Single-lobe dose (mean of dosed region = -801 HU, mean of undosed region = -530 HU).

heterogeneity in lung disease. We showed that this merged approach was better able to differentiate rats with mild emphysematous disease from the healthy control group than methods that relied on absolute HU values. The main criterion for octree decomposition was based on the standard deviation of HU values within an octree box. An advantage to this approach is that it avoids thresholding according to HU values, although sophisticated thresholding algorithms may be useful [35-37]; rather, it focuses only on heterogeneity-based signatures that may characterize disease [2]. We propose that a heterogeneity score Δ, the average distance of a rat's variance from that of the control group average, may be useful to classify disease severity. Furthermore, to visualize the regions of the lung with the greatest heterogeneity, one could determine which boxes had the highest semivariance within d_{max} and map them back to the original image. This would provide 3D information about the spatial distribution of lung tissue heterogeneity and, potentially, disease distribution.

Another approach to a disease metric might be that of fitting the data to an established variogram model, most

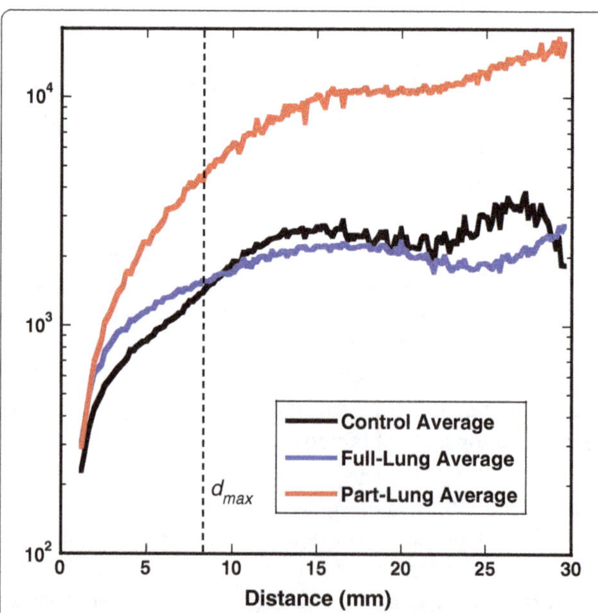

Figure 6 Variograms averaged for each dose group. The dashed line shows the extent of d_{max}, the characteristic lung distance to which variograms were analyzed for heterogeneous variations. The lines get "noisier" at higher distances, indicative of increased spatial variation even within the each group.

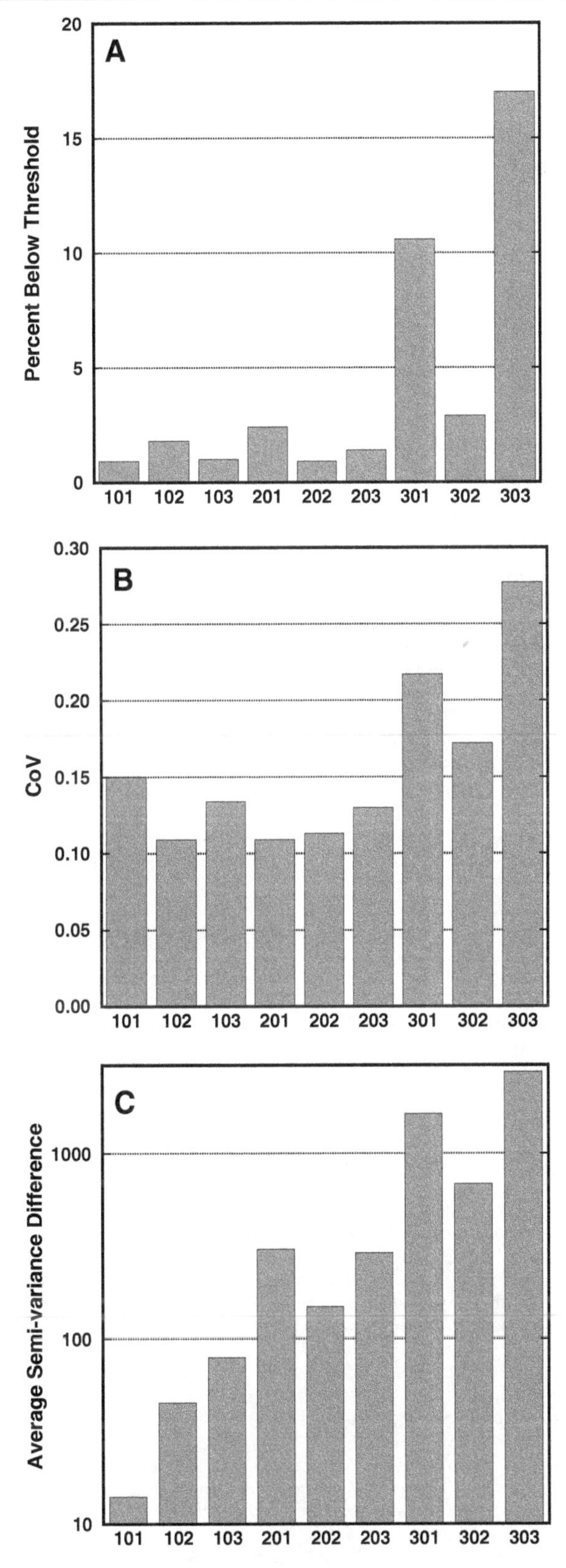

Figure 7 Graphs comparing the different metrics for detecting emphysema. A: Percentage of image pixels with HU values below two standard deviations from the mean of the control group. **B**: Coefficient of variation (CoV). **C**: The average distance of each individual rat's variogram from the mean of the control group. The x-axis labels are animal numbers: 100s are controls, 200s are full-lung-dose, and 300s are single-lobe-dose. 301 and 302 received the dose in the right caudal lobe, and 303 received the dose in the distal region of the left lobe (Figure 2C).

of which describe an asymptotic rise in variance (i.e. variance becomes independent of distance indicating that spatial relationships become random) [23]. This is seen to some degree in our data (see Figure 6). However, within the range of $d \leq d_{max}$, we found that a power law model generally fit our data better than other models. This model typically describes fractal behavior [38]. Our initial investigations into this model showed potential promise at using fit parameters to distinguish dose groups; however, results lacked statistical significance, and the full-lung dose group tended to not fit this model as well as the other two groups.

There was no single variogram model that satisfactorily fit the all the data over the entire range of distances, because the complex geometries found in the lung result in some problems for variograms. In particular, the direct linear path between two regions of the lung separated by large distances often crosses non-lung tissue, such as the heart, which are essentially treated as holes or voids in the geometry. Furthermore, neighboring lobes generally do not interact physiologically except through the vascular and airway trees, which may only connect regions through many orders of branching. As pointed out by Keil et al. [25], one could go to extraordinary measures to take into account structural distances (the physiological distance at which different regions interact) versus Euclidian (straight line) distances used herein. To limit the problem in this study, we constrained the distance of variogram analysis to approximately half the characteristic diameter of the largest lobe. However, to better understand the inter-and intra-lobe variance relationships, the lung could be segmented into lobes (if the image is of sufficient resolution to discern lobar boundaries), and the decomposition/variogram process repeated on the segmented images. Though, by ignoring inter-lobar variances, this approach would likely not capture information about disease that was confined to a single lobe, particularly if the entire lobe was affected homogeneously.

We employed octree decomposition prior to generating the variograms. In doing this, we assumed that the emphysematous disease is generally slowly varying over space, and that the disease causes changes to homogeneity on the order of or less than the lobar length scale but greater than the octree box length scale [4,34]. This is consistent with what we previously observed using ^{3}He MRI in the same disease model [26]. Without this assumption, variograms would have to be made directly from the raw images. This is possible but impractical, because the semi-variance computation time (and resulting file size) is proportional to the number of voxel pairs, which rises approximately as n^2 (see Eq. 2). We measured the variogram computation time for 1078 octree-decomposed boxes from one rat to be 6.6 seconds (on a MacPro model 3.1), and we verified experimentally that the computation time indeed rose in proportion to the square of the number of voxels. Therefore, to create a variogram on the entire masked 3D image, which consisted of 1.48×10^6 voxels (of lung tissue only), it would take us $\approx 1.25 \times 10^7$ seconds, or about 5 months–with a resulting file size on the order of 20 GB. Therefore, octree decomposition dramatically reduces the computation time while focusing non-subjectively on regions of the lung that are of greatest interest. We note that the octree decomposition itself was performed in ~2 minutes.

Image noise can confound octree decomposition and affect resulting variograms. Results of image filtering tests indicated that noise reduction using an edge-preserving filter resulted in more $8 \times 8 \times 8$ octree blocks without significantly affecting variogram results. An alternative to octree decomposition is downsampling, which is a quick and straightforward approach to reducing image noise and size. However, we verified that the octree decomposition approach performed much better at separating dose groups than simply downsampling the image and then calculating the semi-variance using every voxel. The octree decomposition assures that only the homogeneous regions of the lungs are singled out for comparison, whereas downsampling the image blurs together proximal voxels, including vasculature, airways, and lung boundaries irrespective of signal intensity or tissue type. Thus, the downsampling approach apparently causes a loss of information. The radius = 4 Gaussian filter had a result similar to downsampling.

One limitation of this pilot study was the small number of animals in each group, which did not allow the statistical evaluation of specificity and sensitivity. Therefore, follow-on work will be required to validate these results and establish specificity and sensitivity [2]. This might be accomplished in conjunction with pulmonary function tests, conventional morphometric measurements [39], and histological techniques particularly sensitive to early emphysematous changes [40]. Additional future work should evaluate the performance of this method on clinical CT images as well as test the effectiveness for distinguishing different diseases and disease models.

Conclusion

Results of this pre-clinical study of elastase-treated rats suggests that automated octree decomposition and variogram analysis based on image heterogeneity may provide a non-objective and sensitive metric for characterizing emphysematous lung disease, even in early disease stages. The method outperformed conventional approaches that utilize thresholding and absolute HU values. This approach may be applicable to human datasets and other diseases.

Competing interests

The authors have no conflicts of interest to disclose.

Authors' contributions

REJ designed the study, performed the experiments, analyzed the data, and drafted the manuscript. JPC developed Python code and participated in drafting the manuscript. Both authors read and approved the final manuscript.

Acknowledgements

The authors would like to thank T. Curry of PNNL for assistance with animal handling and B. Amidan of PNNL for helpful discussions. This project was supported by Award Number R01HL073598 from the National Heart, Lung, and Blood Institute and by PNNL through internal Laboratory Directed Research and Development LDRD DE-AC05-76RL01830. There was no involvement on the part of the sponsors in study design; in the collection, analysis, and interpretation of data; in the writing of the report; or in the decision to submit the paper for publication.

References

1. West JB: *Pulmonary Pathophysiology.* 5th edition. Philadelphia: Lippincott Williams & Wilkins; 1998.
2. Mets OM, De Jong PA, Van Ginneken B, Gietema HA, Lammers JW: **Quantitative computed tomography in COPD: possibilities and limitations.** *Lung* 2012, **190**(2):133–145.
3. Robertson HT, Buxton RB: **Imaging for lung physiology: what do we wish we could measure?** *J Appl Physiol* 2012, **113**(2):317–327.
4. Litmanovich D, Boiselle PM, Bankier AA: **CT of pulmonary emphysema–current status, challenges, and future directions.** *Eur Radiol* 2009, **19**(3):537–551.
5. Chong D, Brown MS, Kim HJ, Van Rikxoort EM, Guzman L, McNitt-Gray MF, Khatonabadi M, Galperin-Aizenberg M, Coy H, Yang K, *et al*: **Reproducibility of volume and densitometric measures of emphysema on repeat computed tomography with an interval of 1 week.** *Eur Radiol* 2012, **22**(2):287–294.
6. Uppaluri R, Mitsa T, Sonka M, Hoffman EA, McLennan G: **Quantification of pulmonary emphysema from lung computed tomography images.** *Am J Respir Crit Care Med* 1997, **156**(1):248–254.
7. Besir FH, Mahmutyazicioglu K, Aydin L, Altin R, Asil K, Gundogdu S: **The benefit of expiratory-phase quantitative CT densitometry in the early diagnosis of chronic obstructive pulmonary disease.** *Diagn Interv Radiol* 2012, **18**(3):248–254.
8. Irion KL, Marchiori E, Hochhegger B, Porto Nda S, Moreira Jda S, Anselmi CE, Holemans JA, Irion PO: **CT quantification of emphysema in young subjects with no recognizable chest disease.** *AJR Am J Roentgenol* 2009, **192**(3):W90–W96.
9. Reske AW, Busse H, Amato MB, Jaekel M, Kahn T, Schwarzkopf P, Schreiter D, Gottschaldt U, Seiwerts M: **Image reconstruction affects computer tomographic assessment of lung hyperinflation.** *Intensive Care Med* 2008, **34**(11):2044–2053.
10. Yuan R, Mayo JR, Hogg JC, Pare PD, McWilliams AM, Lam S, Coxson HO: **The effects of radiation dose and CT manufacturer on measurements of lung densitometry.** *Chest* 2007, **132**(2):617–623.
11. Chen CC, Daponte JS, Fox MD: **Fractal feature analysis and classification in medical imaging.** *IEEE Trans Med Imaging* 1989, **8**(2):133–142.

12. Glenny RW, Robertson HT: **Fractal properties of pulmonary blood flow: characterization of spatial heterogeneity.** *J Appl Physiol* 1990, **69**(2):532–545.
13. Copley SJ, Giannarou S, Schmid VJ, Hansell DM, Wells AU, Yang GZ: **Effect of aging on lung structure in vivo: assessment with densitometric and fractal analysis of high-resolution computed tomography data.** *J Thorac Imaging* 2012, **27**(6):366–371.
14. Kido S, Ikezoe J, Naito H, Tamura S, Machi S: **Fractal analysis of interstitial lung abnormalities in chest radiography.** *Radiographics* 1995, **15**(6):1457–1464.
15. Uppaluri R, Mitsa T, Galvin JR: **Fractal analysis of high-resolution CT images as a tool for quantification of lung disease.** In *Medical Imaging 1995: Physiology and Function from Multidimensional Images.* 2433rd edition. Edited by Hoffman EA. Bellingham, WA: SPIE; 1995:133–142.
16. Kido S, Sasaki S: **Fractal analysis for quantitative evaluation of diffuse lung abnormalities on chest radiographs: use of sub-ROIs.** *J Thorac Imaging* 2003, **18**(4):237–241.
17. Subramaniam K, Hoffman EA, Tawhai MH: **Quantifying tissue heterogeneity using quadtree decomposition.** *Conf Proc IEEE Eng Med Biol Soc* 2012, **2012:**4079–4082.
18. Shephard MS, Georges MK: **Automatic 3-dimensional mesh generation by the finite octree technique.** *Int J Numer Meth Eng* 1991, **32**(4):709–749.
19. Zhang JH, Owen CB: **Octree-based animated geometry compression.** *Comput Graph-Uk* 2007, **31**(3):463–479.
20. Szeliski R, Lavallee S: **Matching 3-D anatomical surfaces with non-rigid deformations using octree-splines.** *Int J Comput Vision* 1996, **18**(2):171–186.
21. Zhang YJ, Bajaj C, Sohn BS: **3D finite element meshing from imaging data.** *Comput Method Appl M* 2005, **194**(48–49):5083–5106.
22. Dua S, Kandiraju N, Chowriappa P: **Region quad-tree decomposition based edge detection for medical images.** *Open Med Inform J* 2010, **4:**50–57.
23. Clark I, Harper WV: *Practical Geostatistics 2000.* Columbus, Ohio: Ecosse North America, LLC; 2000.
24. Gringarten E, Deutsch CV: **Variogram interpretation and modeling.** *Math Geol* 2001, **33**(4):507–534.
25. Keil F, Oros-Peusquens AM, Shah NJ: **Investigation of the spatial correlation in human white matter and the influence of age using 3-dimensional variography applied to MP-RAGE data.** *Neuroimage* 2012, **63**(3):1374–1383.
26. Jacob RE, Minard KR, Laicher G, Timchalk C: **3D 3He diffusion MRI as a local in vivo morphometric tool to evaluate emphysematous rat lungs.** *J Appl Physiol* 2008, **105**(4):1291–1300.
27. Jacob RE, Lamm WJ: **Stable small animal ventilation for dynamic lung imaging to support computational fluid dynamics models.** *PLoS One* 2011, **6**(11):e27577.
28. Corley RA, Kabilan S, Kuprat AP, Carson JP, Minard KR, Jacob RE, Timchalk C, Glenny R, Pipavath S, Cox T, *et al*: **Comparative computational modeling of airflows and vapor dosimetry in the respiratory tracts of rat, monkey, and human.** *Toxicol Sci* 2012, **128**(2):500–516.
29. Minard KR, Kuprat AP, Kabilan S, Jacob RE, Einstein DR, Carson JP, Corley RA: **Phase-contrast MRI and CFD modeling of apparent (3)He gas flow in rat pulmonary airways.** *J Magn Reson* 2012, **221:**129–138.
30. **ImageJ.** http://imagej.nih.gov/ij/.
31. **ImageJ Plugins: 3D Toolkit.** http://ij-plugins.sourceforge.net/plugins/3d-toolkit/index.html.
32. Jackins CL, Tanimoto SL: **Oct-trees and their use in representing three dimensional objects.** *Computer Graphics and Image Processing* 1980, **14**(3):249–270.
33. Schulz H, Mühle H: **Respiration.** In *The Laboratory Rat.* Edited by Krinke GJ. San Diego. Academic Press; 2000:323 336.
34. Spencer H: **Pathology of the Lung.** In *Volume Volume 1.* 4th edition. New York: Pergamon Press; 1985:557–594.
35. El-Baz A, Gimel'farb G, Falk R, Holland T, Shaffer T: **A new stochastic framework for accurate lung segmentation.** In *Medical Image Computing and Computer-Assisted Intervention–MICCAI.* Edited by Metaxas D, Axel L, Szekely G. New York, NY: Springer; 2008:322–330.
36. Abdollahi B, Soliman A, Civelek AC, Li XF, Gimel'farb G, El-Baz A: **A novel 3D joint MGRF framework for precise lung segmentation.** In *Third International Workshop MLMI: 2012.* Nice, France: Springer; 2012:86–93.
37. El-Baz A, Beache GM, Gimel'farb G, Suzuki K, Okada K, Elnakib A, Soliman A, Abdollahi B: **Computer-aided diagnosis systems for lung cancer: challenges and methodologies.** *Int J Biomed Imaging* 2013, **2013:**942353.
38. Bohling GC: **Introduction to Geostatistics.** In *Kansas Geological Survey Open File Report no. 2007-26*; 2007:50.
39. Hsia CC, Hyde DM, Ochs M, Weibel ER: **An official research policy statement of the American Thoracic Society/European Respiratory Society: standards for quantitative assessment of lung structure.** *Am J Respir Crit Care Med* 2010, **181**(4):394–418.
40. Jacob RE, Carson JP, Gideon KM, Amidan BG, Smith CL, Lee KM: **Comparison of two quantitative methods of discerning airspace enlargement in smoke-exposed mice.** *PLoS One* 2009, **4**(8):e6670.

6

Specific CT 3D rendering of the treatment zone after Irreversible Electroporation (IRE) in a pig liver model: the "Chebyshev Center Concept" to define the maximum treatable tumor size

Dominik Vollherbst[1], Stefan Fritz[2], Sascha Zelzer[3], Miguel F Wachter[1], Maya B Wolf[4], Ulrike Stampfl[1], Daniel Gnutzmann[1], Nadine Bellemann[1], Anne Schmitz[1], Jürgen Knapp[5], Philippe L Pereira[6], Hans U Kauczor[1], Jens Werner[2], Boris A Radeleff[1] and Christof M Sommer[1*]

Abstract

Background: Size and shape of the treatment zone after Irreversible electroporation (IRE) can be difficult to depict due to the use of multiple applicators with complex spatial configuration. Exact geometrical definition of the treatment zone, however, is mandatory for acute treatment control since incomplete tumor coverage results in limited oncological outcome. In this study, the "Chebyshev Center Concept" was introduced for CT 3d rendering to assess size and position of the maximum treatable tumor at a specific safety margin.

Methods: In seven pig livers, three different IRE protocols were applied to create treatment zones of different size and shape: Protocol 1 (n = 5 IREs), Protocol 2 (n = 5 IREs), and Protocol 3 (n = 5 IREs). Contrast-enhanced CT was used to assess the treatment zones. Technique A consisted of a semi-automated software prototype for CT 3d rendering with the "Chebyshev Center Concept" implemented (the "Chebyshev Center" is the center of the largest inscribed sphere within the treatment zone) with automated definition of parameters for size, shape and position. Technique B consisted of standard CT 3d analysis with manual definition of the same parameters but position.

Results: For Protocol 1 and 2, short diameter of the treatment zone and diameter of the largest inscribed sphere within the treatment zone were not significantly different between Technique A and B. For Protocol 3, short diameter of the treatment zone and diameter of the largest inscribed sphere within the treatment zone were significantly smaller for Technique A compared with Technique B (41.1 ± 13.1 mm versus 53.8 ± 1.1 mm and 39.0 ± 8.4 mm versus 53.8 ± 1.1 mm; $p < 0.05$ and $p < 0.01$). For Protocol 1, 2 and 3, sphericity of the treatment zone was significantly larger for Technique A compared with B.

Conclusions: Regarding size and shape of the treatment zone after IRE, CT 3d rendering with the "Chebyshev Center Concept" implemented provides significantly different results compared with standard CT 3d analysis. Since the latter overestimates the size of the treatment zone, the "Chebyshev Center Concept" could be used for a more objective acute treatment control.

Keywords: Irreversible electroporation, Liver, CT 3d rendering, Segmentation, Chebyshev center

* Correspondence: christof.sommer@med.uni-heidelberg.de
[1]Department of Diagnostic and Interventional Radiology, University Hospital Heidelberg, Heidelberg, Germany
Full list of author information is available at the end of the article

Background

Focal tumor ablation is an accepted option for the treatment of primary and secondary malignant liver tumors. Irreversible electroporation (IRE) was introduced as a non-thermal technique for tissue destruction. After local application of high-voltage electrical pulses of microsecond duration, homogeneous areas of non-viable cells are induced [1]. In first clinical studies, IRE demonstrates promising results for the treatment of malignant liver lesions [2-4]. The routine use of IRE, however, is still not established [5,6]. Whereas radiofrequency ablation and microwave ablation induce cell death via thermal damage, the exact mechanisms for IRE are not entirely understood [7]. Nonetheless, IRE is attributed with potential advantages compared with thermal ablation (e.g. reduced collateral damage and insignificance of the heat-sink effect) [5]. Those advantages can be explained with the relative resistance of low lipid containing structures (e.g. extracellular matrix and endothelial cells) to the electrical pulses while high lipid containing structures (e.g. tumor cells) can be destroyed completely [8,9]. Accordingly, IRE should be a promising alternative especially if tumors are located near vulnerable structures.

As with thermal ablation, the treatment zone after IRE must cover the entire tumor in addition to a safety margin. As demonstrated by Wang et al., the size of the safety margin plays a key role for the oncological success of focal tumor ablation [10]. After radiofrequency ablation of colorectal liver metastases, they found that a safety margin uniformly larger than 5 mm, defined with post-interventional contrast-enhanced CT, is associated with better local tumor control. For the combination of optimal oncological outcome with liver-sparing tumor ablation, which is relevant for the minimization of procedure-related complications, another prerequisite is mandatory: congruency of tumor center and coagulation center [11]. Currently, there exists no clinically relevant software that can be used to determine whether the treated tumor and the intended safety margin are covered completely by the treatment zone. Standard CT 3d analysis of the treatment zone after focal tumor ablation consists of measurements based on standard CT image planes (e.g. axial), without meeting the clinical requirements of interventional radiologists in terms of objective treatment control. A major drawback of currently available 3d software is suboptimal assessment of the exact geometry of the treatment zone in relation to the tumor extent. For example indentations limiting the expansion of the treatment zone need to be assessed since those are likely to represent the site of incomplete tumor destruction and local recurrence. Since IRE can be performed with lots of different protocols (e.g. up to six applicators with a tip exposure of up to 40 mm) all affecting significantly size and shape of the treatment zone, the exact geometrical assessment is mandatory to further improve the procedural success. This issue was published by Adeyanju et al., who demonstrated that IRE protocols impact not only the extent of the treatment zone but also the maximum treatable tumor size [12].

With this background, the objective of our study was defined: to introduce the "Chebyshev Center Concept" for CT 3d rendering to assess size and position of the maximum treatable tumor size at a specific safety margin after IRE in a pig liver model, and to demonstrate better performance compared with standard CT 3d analysis. For our study, the "Chebyshev Center" of the treatment zone is the center of the largest inscribed sphere within the treatment zone. In geometry, the largest inscribed sphere is the sphere that bounds the edges of a three-dimensional body in such a manner that there is no other sphere that lies completely within that three-dimensional body and at the same time has a larger diameter than the largest inscribed sphere. The three-dimensional body corresponds to the treatment zone, and the largest inscribed sphere is the largest sphere that is covered completely by the treatment zone. The "Chebyshev Center Concept" can be used to quantify and visualize diameter and position of the largest inscribed sphere within the treatment zone after focal tumor ablation. This sphere is relevant since it allows the definition of the maximum treatable tumor size at a specific safety margin. Furthermore, the "Chebyshev Center Concept" is applicable to determine whether tumor and intended safety margin is located within the treatment zone (or in other words whether the concrete treatment zone is adequate for a specific tumor extent).

Methods

The experiments were performed in accordance with the "Guide for the Care and Use of Laboratory Animals". "State Animal Care and Ethics Committee" approval was obtained.

Animal preparation

Seven healthy landrace pigs with a body weight between 35 and 41 kg were sedated with an intramuscular cocktail consisting of 10 mg ketamine, 6 mg azaperone and 0.4mg midazolam per kg body weight. Peripheral and central venous catheters were installed. After intubation, anesthesia was maintained with isoflurane. Intravenous bolus injections with pancuronium were used to induce and maintain muscle relaxation. A continuous 4-lead electrocardiogram was performed throughout the procedure. Before and immediately after IRE, contrast-enhanced CT was performed with a 128-slice multi-detector row CT scanner (Somatom Definition Flash; Siemens Medical Solutions, Forchheim, Germany). The CT protocol consisted of a non-enhanced phase, and after intravenous injection of 70 ml of iodinated contrast material, arterial (delay of 5 s after reaching the trigger threshold of 100 HU), venous (delay of 50 s) and late (delay of 180 s) phases followed. Image reconstructions included axial image planes with a slice thickness of 1 mm and an overlap of 0.5 mm. The CT scan immediately after IRE was intended as acute treatment control according to best clinical practice. Animals were sacrificed subsequently.

IRE procedure

IRE was performed with a commercial generator (NanoKnife™ Electroporator; AngioDynamics® Inc., Queensbury, USA). Electrocardiogram synchronization was used to prevent cardiac arrhythmias. Commercial monopolar 19G applicators (NanoKnife™ Applicator; AngioDynamics® Inc., Queensbury, USA) served for local pulse application. A total of 15 IREs were carried out. Three different IRE protocols were used to obtain different extents of the treatment zone: Protocol 1 (three applicators, tip exposure of 20 mm, distance between pairs of applicators of 15 mm, pulse number of 90, pulse length of 90 μs, and electric field of 1500 V/cm; n = 5 IREs), Protocol 2 (three applicators, tip exposure of 25 mm, distance between pairs of applicators of 20 mm, pulse number of 90, pulse length of 90 μs, and electric field of 1500 V/cm; n = 5 IREs), and Protocol 3 (six applicators, tip exposure of 30 mm, distance between pairs of applicators of 15 mm, pulse number of 70, pulse length of 90 μs, and electric field of 1400 V/cm; n = 5 IREs). Based on the information of the manufacturer as well as on findings of published and own IRE experience, those protocols allow predicting the size of the treatment zone, with treatment zones between 1 and 5 cm. In this context, the different mechanisms of tissue destruction between IRE and thermal ablation are important to mention. In thermal ablation, heat expands from the tip of an applicator to the periphery, and power output and ablation time are major predictors for size and shape of the coagulation zone. On the contrary, size and shape of the treatment zone after IRE is determined by number and spatial configuration of applicators, tip exposure, pulse number, pulse length as well as electric field. The treatment zones expand between the different pairs of applicators, resulting finally in one overlapping treatment zone. According to our treatment plan, applicators were positioned standardized across all animals. In one pig, two IREs according to Protocol 1 were performed in the right liver and one IRE according to Protocol 2 was performed in the left liver. In another pig, one IRE according to Protocol 1 was performed in the left liver and one IRE according to Protocol 2 was performed in the right liver. In two other pigs, one IRE according to Protocol 1 was performed in the left liver and one IRE according to Protocol 3 was performed in the right liver. In the three remaining pigs, one IRE according to Protocol 2 was performed in the left liver and one IRE according to Protocol 3 was performed in the right liver. Consequently, in six pigs a maximum of 2 IREs per pig was realized, and in one pig a maximum of three IREs was realized. This proceeding avoided overlap and interaction between the IREs in the same liver (e.g. impact of microvascularization resulting in inaccurate CT enhancement patterns after application of intravenous contrast material). All applicators were positioned step-by-step in parallel fashion under CT guidance. The correct applicator configuration according to the treatment plan was confirmed with a non-enhanced CT scan using multi-planar image planes.

Analysis of size and shape of the treatment zone

The image data were extracted from our institutional prospective digital database (GE Centricity 4.1, GE Healthcare, Barrington, USA) and analyzed on a PC applying the software described in this study. Two techniques for the analysis of the treatment zone were compared: Technique A versus Technique B (not to be confused with the different IRE Protocols) (Figure 1). According to other publications, the treatment zone after IRE was defined as the hypodense area with sharp demarcation on contrast-enhanced CT images of the venous phase [13,14].

Technique A

Technique A consisted of a semi-automated software prototype for CT 3d rendering with the "Chebyshev Center Concept" implemented (MITK freeware "Geometric evaluation of ablations" http://www.mitk.org/AblationEvaluation; German Cancer Research Center (dkfz) Heidelberg, Heidelberg, Germany). Axial image planes with a slice thickness of 1 mm and an overlap of 0.5 mm were uploaded (Figure 2). Treatment zones were outlined manually by means of cursor in the sense of segmentation. After segmentation, parameters for size and shape (long, intermediate and short diameter, circularity and sphericity as well as the diameter of the largest inscribed sphere within the treatment zone and the diameter of the largest possible treatable tumor sphere for both applying the "Chebyshev Center") were obtained automatically. The geometrical center of the treatment zone (from now on the barycenter) was determined automatically by using a principal component analysis. The diameter of the treatment zone through the barycenter in direction of the eigenvector with the largest principal component was defined as the long diameter. The diameter of the treatment zone perpendicular to the long diameter and through the barycenter in direction of the second largest principal component eigenvector was defined as the intermediate diameter. The third diameter of the treatment zone perpendicular to the long and intermediate

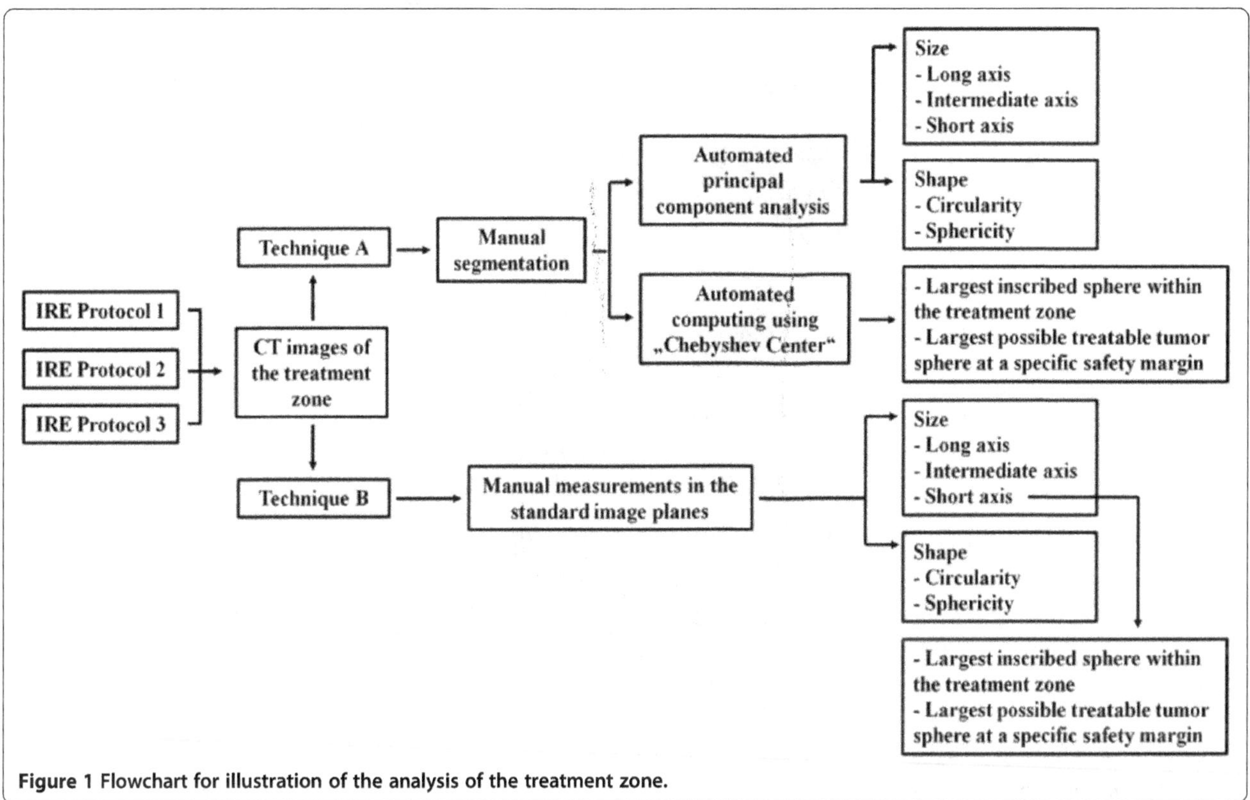

Figure 1 Flowchart for illustration of the analysis of the treatment zone.

diameter and through the barycenter was defined as the short diameter. Consequently, the barycenter is the intersection point of long, intermediate and short diameter of the treatment zone. Circularity and sphericity of the treatment zone are measures to describe the shape of the treatment zone applying long, intermediate and/or short diameter [15-17]:

(1) Circularity of the treatment zone = short diameter/long diameter (a number of "1" indicates a perfect roundness) and

(2) Sphericity of the treatment zone = long diameter/((intermediate diameter + short diameter)/2) (a number of "1" indicates a perfect roundness).

The largest inscribed sphere within the treatment zone was defined automatically. As mentioned above, the "Chebyshev Center" is the center of this sphere, and can be applied for the determination of diameter and position (barycenter offset) of the largest inscribed sphere within the treatment zone. Thereby, the barycenter offset is the distance between the barycenter and the "Chebyshev Center". The diameter of the largest possible treatable tumor sphere was defined automatically also. This sphere has the same center as the largest inscribed sphere within the treatment zone ("Chebyshev Center"). Moreover, the largest possible treatable tumor sphere has a diameter 10 mm smaller as the short diameter (corresponding to a uniform safety margin of 5 mm).

Technique B

Technique B consisted of standard CT 3d analysis without specific software assistance (such as principal component analysis). Axial image planes with a slice thickness of 1 mm and an overlap of 0.5 mm were uploaded in the "CTA Abdomen" workflow on a commercial work station (TeraRecon, INC., Aquarius, iNtuition™ Edition, Ver. 4.4.4.23.771, San Mateo, USA) (Figure 3). Applying the multi-planar mode, the absolute longest diameter of the treatment zone was measured manually on axial image planes. Perpendicular to this diameter, the longest diameter of the treatment zone was measured manually on axial image planes. On coronal image planes, the longest craniocaudal diameter of the treatment zone was measured manually. This proceeding is in line with current clinical practice for treatment control after radiofrequency ablation [15-17]. The three measured diameters were ordered by size, and defined as long, intermediate and short diameter of the treatment zone. Circularity and sphericity of the treatment zone were calculated according to equations (1) and (2). The diameter of the largest inscribed sphere within the treatment zone was defined equal to the short diameter. The diameter of the largest possible treatable tumor sphere was defined using a diameter 10 mm smaller as the diameter of the largest inscribed sphere within the treatment zone. For Technique B, the barycenter offset was not assessable.

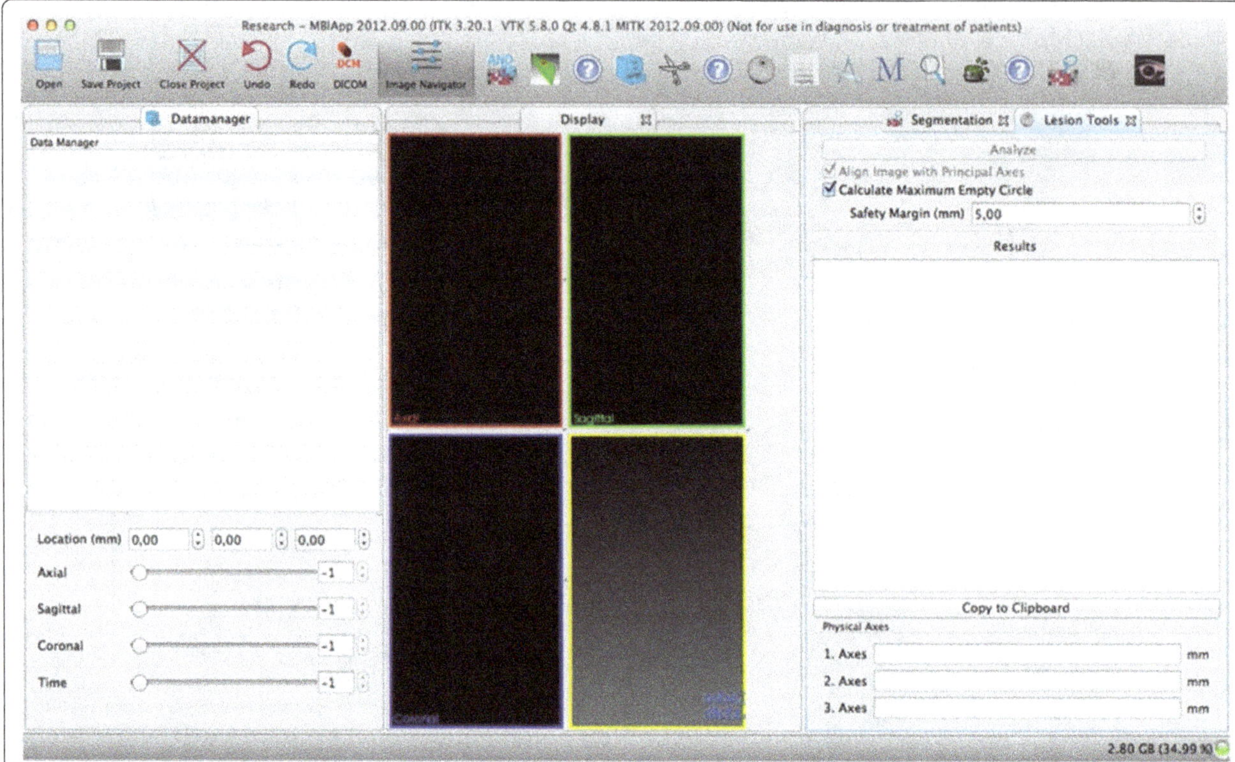

Figure 2 Technique A (Semi-automated Software Prototype for CT 3d Rendering with the "Chebyshev Center Concept" implemented) - User Interface. The MITK user interface consists of three work columns: "data manager" in the left column, "display" in the middle column, and post-processing tools ("Segmentation" and "Lesion Tools" in this case) in the right column. Images in different formats (e.g. DICOM or JPEG) can be uploaded and scrolled in the "data manager" column. Multi-planar image planes are visualized in the "display" column. In the post-processing tool column, the treatment zone can be outlined manually by means of cursor (in the sense of a segmentation) applying "Segmentation". Then, applying "Lesion Tools", long, intermediate and short diameter, circularity and sphericity as well as the diameter of the largest inscribed sphere within the treatment zone and the diameter of the largest possible treatable tumor sphere at a defined safety margin (in this case 5mm) inclusive of the barycenter offset can be calculated automatically.

Differences between technique A and technique B

To quantify the differences between Technique A and Technique B regarding the largest inscribed sphere within the treatment zone, the difference ratio was calculated:

(3) Difference ratio = Diameter of the largest inscribed sphere within the treatment zone$_{\text{Technique A}}$ - Diameter of the largest inscribed sphere within the treatment zone$_{\text{Technique B}}$.

The difference ratio indicates the absolute difference between Technique A and Technique B. A negative difference ratio means that the parameter for Technique A is smaller than for Technique B (or in other words that standard CT 3d analysis overestimates the extent of the treatment zone), whereas a positive difference ratio means that the parameter for Technique A is larger than for Technique B (or in other words that standard CT 3d analysis underestimates the extent of the treatment zone).

Statistics

Prism software (Version 6.00, GraphPad Software, LaJolla, USA) was used. Quantitative data were presented as mean ± standard deviation, and range. To evaluate statistical differences between Technique A and Technique B, the Wilcoxon signed-rank test was used. To describe statistical differences between IRE Protocol 1, Protocol 2 and Protocol 3, the Kruskal-Wallis test was applied. $P < 0.05$ was defined as the level of significance.

Results and discussion

The mean duration of the IRE procedures per pig was 37 ± 12 min (25-70 min).

Size of the treatment zone

Detailed data are presented in Table 1 (Figures 4, 5 and 6). For Protocol 1 and Protocol 2, long, intermediate and short diameters were not significantly different between Technique A and Technique B, respectively. There was a trend for a larger long diameter for Technique A for Protocol 1 as well as a trend for smaller short diameter for Technique A for Protocol 1 and Protocol 2, respectively. For Protocol 3, long and intermediate diameters were not significantly different

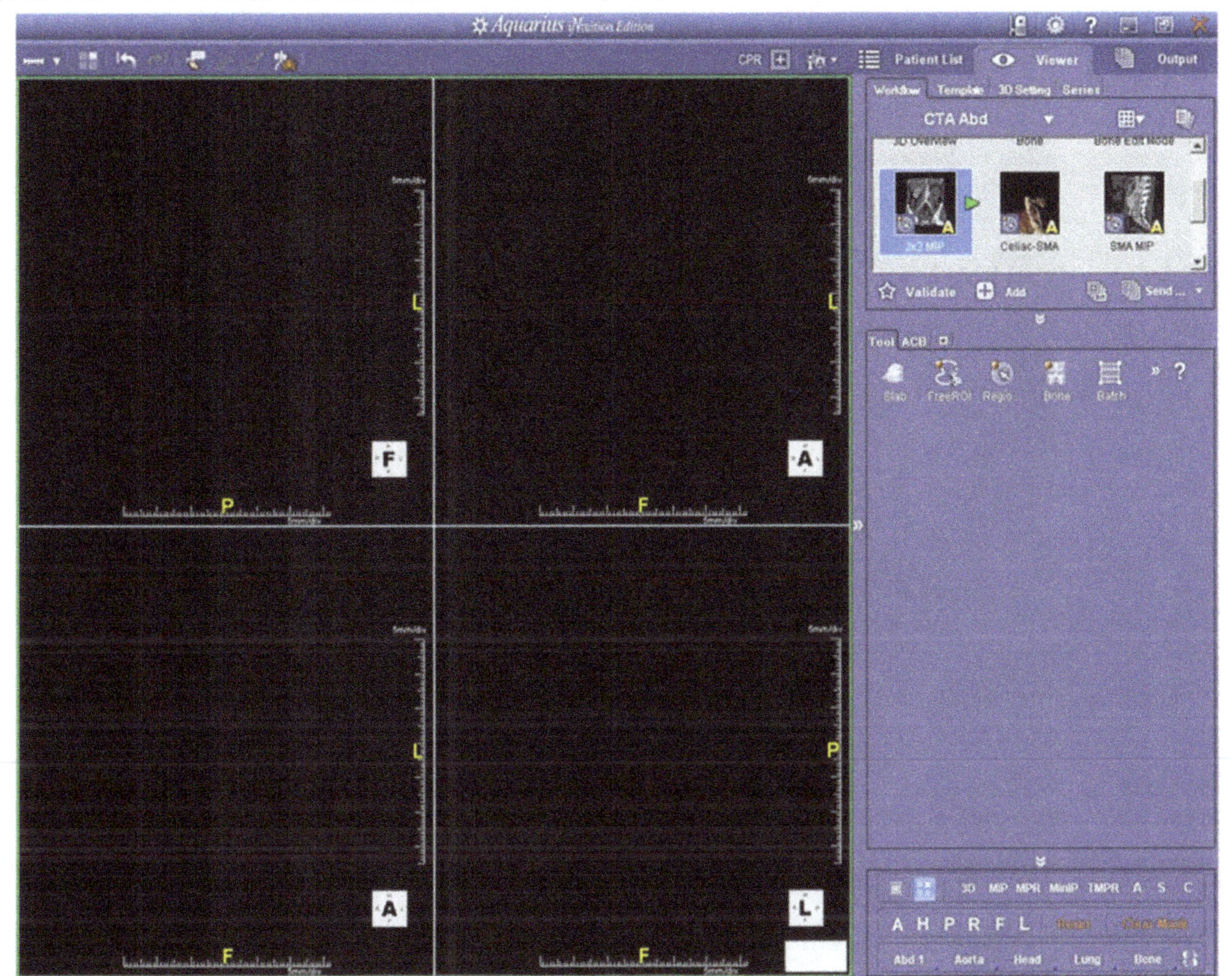

Figure 3 Technique B (Standard CT 3d Analysis) - User Interface. This user interface is clinically established, and provides the possibility to measure manually diameters on axial, coronal and sagittal image planes (CTA abdomen workflow, multi-planar mode).

Table 1 Size of the treatment zone

	Long diameter (mm)		Intermediate diameter (mm)		Short diameter (mm)	
	Technique A[1]	Technique B[2]	Technique A[1]	Technique B[2]	Technique A[1]	Technique B[2]
Protocol 1[3]	$42.1 \pm 3.2^{\#,*}$	$37.5 \pm 10.2^{\#,**}$	$30.1 \pm 3.2^{+,***}$	$27.9 \pm 5.5^{+,****}$	$17.2 \pm 6.0^{\circ,*****}$	$19.9 \pm 4.6^{\circ,******}$
	(39.3 - 47.2)	(29.4 - 48.6)	(26.6 - 33.7)	(22.0 - 32.7)	(10.9 - 24.4)	(15.4 - 26.4)
Protocol 2[4]	$43.7 \pm 8.6^{\#\#,*}$	$43.8 \pm 3.9^{\#\#,**}$	$35.7 \pm 8.2^{++,***}$	$37.1 \pm 6.2^{++,****}$	$27.9 \pm 4.2^{\circ\circ,*****}$	$31.1 \pm 10.5^{\circ\circ,******}$
	(30.4 – 52.8)	(40.1 - 50.2)	(26.1 – 44.8)	(30.6 - 46.0)	(25.3 - 35.3)	(17.5 - 42.1)
Protocol 3[5]	$74.5 \pm 6.1^{\#\#\#,*}$	$71.0 \pm 3.4^{\#\#\#,**}$	$56.3 \pm 5.3^{+++,***}$	$56.3 \pm 2.9^{+++,****}$	$41.1 \pm 13.1^{\circ\circ\circ,*****}$	$53.8 \pm 1.1^{\circ\circ\circ,******}$
	(63.7 - 78.1)	(67.3 - 75.1)	(47.2 - 60.1)	(52.7 - 59.2)	(20.7 - 52.6)	(52.4 - 54.9)

[1]semi-automated software prototype for CT 3d rendering with the "Chebyshev Center Concept" implemented;
[2]standard CT 3d analysis;
[3]Protocol 1 with n = 5 IREs (three applicators, tip exposure of 20 mm, distance between pairs of applicators of 15 mm, pulse number of 90, pulse length of 90 µs, and electric field of 1500 V/cm);
[4]Protocol 2 with n = 5 IREs (three applicators, tip exposure of 25 mm, distance between pairs of applicators of 20 mm, pulse number of 90, pulse length of 90 µs, and electric field of 1500 V/cm);
[5]Protocol 3 with n = 5 IREs (six applicators, tip exposure of 30 mm, distance between pairs of applicators of 15 mm, pulse number of 70, pulse length of 90 µs, and electric field of 1400 V/cm);
statistical differences between Technique A and Technique B were analyzed with the Wilcoxon signed-rank test: $^{\#}p > 0.05$; $^{\#\#}p > 0.05$; $^{\#\#\#}p > 0.05$; $^{+}p > 0.05$; $^{++}p > 0.05$; $^{+++}p > 0.05$; $^{\circ}p > 0.05$; $^{\circ\circ}p > 0.05$; $^{\circ\circ\circ}p < 0.05$;
statistical differences between Protocol 1, Protocol 2 and Protocol 3 were analyzed with the non-parametric Kruskal-Wallis test: $^{*}p < 0.01$; $^{**}p < 0.01$; $^{***}p < 0.01$; $^{****}p < 0.005$; $^{*****}p < 0.01$; $^{******}p < 0.005$.

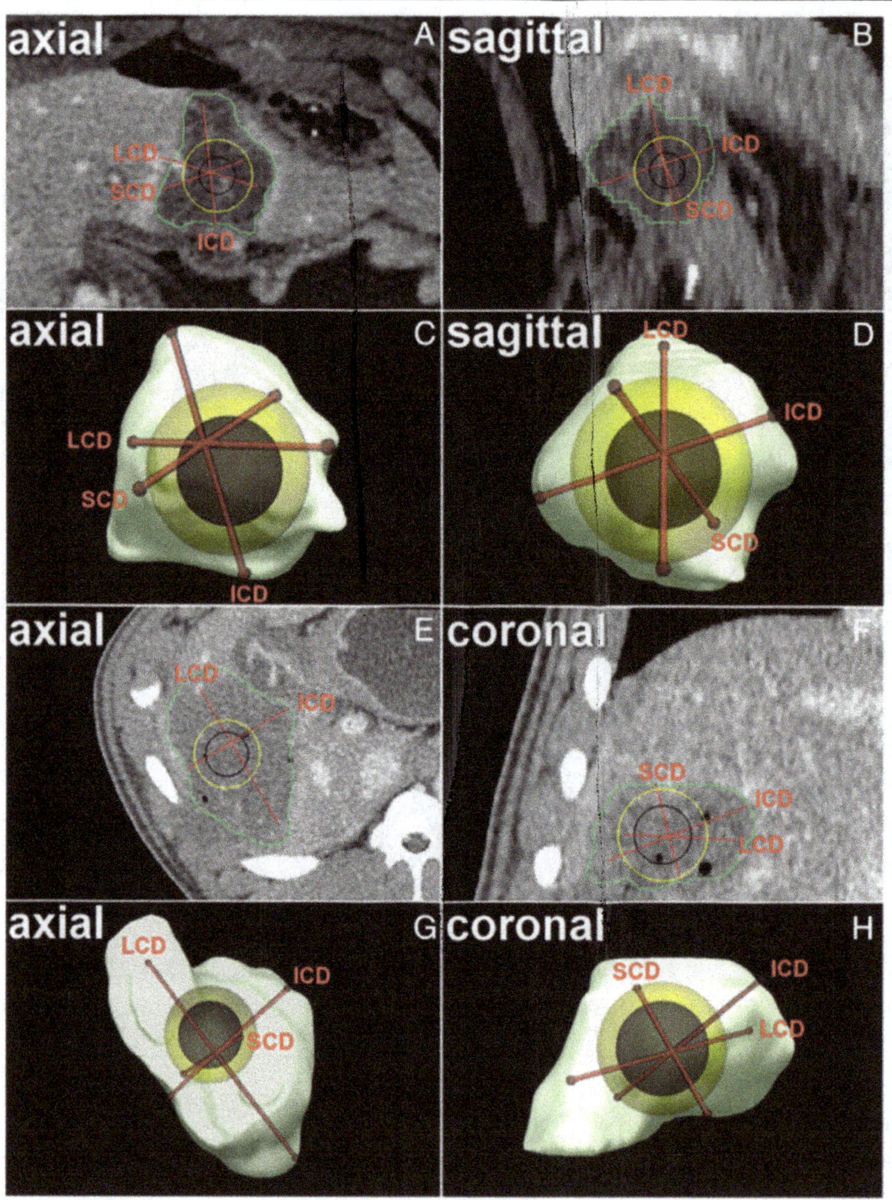

Figure 4 Technique A (Semi-automated Software Prototype for CT 3d Rendering with the "Chebyshev Center Concept" implemented) - Image Example. A-D Axial image plane **(A)** and sagittal image plane **(B)** as well as corresponding volume rendering **(C, D)** – IRE Protocol 2. **E-H** Axial image plane **(E)** and coronal image plane **(F)** as well as corresponding volume rendering **(G, H)** – IRE Protocol 3. Note: after manual segmentation of the treatment zone (green), long, intermediate and short diameter (LCD, ICD and SCD) as well as the largest inscribed sphere within the treatment zone (yellow) and the largest possible treatable tumor sphere (black) were defined automatically (in Figure 4E, SCD is not indicated since its craniocaudal course). The barycenter offset is the distance between the barycenter of the treatment zone (intersection point of long, intermediate and short diameter) and the "Chebyshev Center" (center of the largest inscribed sphere within the treatment zone = center of the largest possible treatable tumor sphere). Observe the conspicuous eccentricity of the "Chebyshev Center" within the treatment zone (which is quantified by the barycenter offset) on standard image planes (B and E) which is not assessable with standard CT 3d analysis (Figure 5). Visualization and quantification of size and position of the largest inscribed sphere within the treatment zone (as well as of the largest possible treatable tumor sphere) can be relevant for acute treatment control after IRE (e.g. confirmation of the intended safety margin size).

between Technique A and Technique B, respectively. There was a trend for a larger long diameter for Technique A for Protocol 3. For Protocol 3, the short diameter was significantly smaller for Technique A compared with Technique B (41.1 ± 13.1 mm versus 53.8 ± 1.1 mm; $p < 0.05$). All parameters for Technique A and Technique B were significantly different between Protocol 1, Protocol 2 and Protocol 3, respectively.

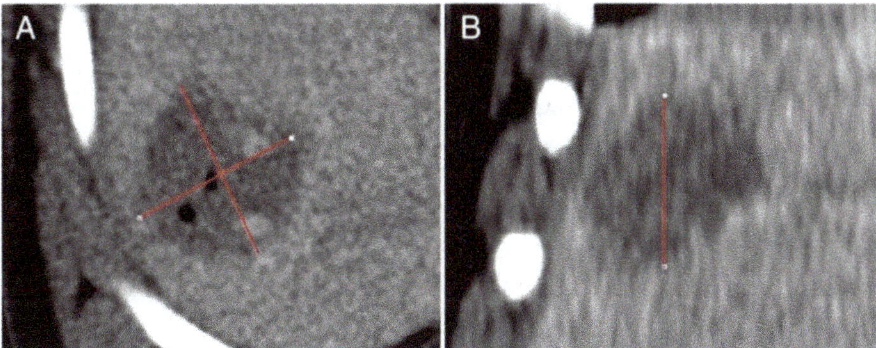

Figure 5 Technique B (Standard CT 3d Analysis) - Image Example. A, B axial image plane **(A)** as well as coronal image plane **(B)** – IRE Protocol 1. Note: in the axial image plane, the absolute longest diameter of the treatment zone was measured, and perpendicular to this parameter, the longest diameter of the treatment zone was determined. In the coronal image plane, the longest craniocaudal diameter of the treatment zone was determined. These three diameters were ordered by size and defined as long, intermediate and short diameter. The diameter of the largest inscribed sphere within the treatment zone was defined equal to the short diameter. The barycenter offset is not assessable applying this approach.

Shape of the treatment zone

Detailed data are presented in Table 2 (Figures 4, 5 and 6). For Protocol 1 and Protocol 2, circularity was not significantly different between Technique A and Technique B, respectively. Sphericity was significantly larger for Technique A compared with Technique B for Protocol 1 and Protocol 2, respectively (1.7 ± 0.3 versus 1.0 ± 0.2 and 1.4 ± 0.2 versus 0.9 ± 0.1; $p < 0.01$ and $p < 0.01$, respectively). For Protocol 3, circularity and sphericity were significantly different between Technique A and Technique B, respectively (0.5 ± 0.2 versus 0.8 ± 0.1 and 1.6 ± 0.2 versus 0.9 ± 0.1; $p < 0.01$ and $p < 0.01$, respectively). Circularity and sphericity for Technique A and Technique B were not significantly different between Protocol 1, Protocol 2 and Protocol 3, respectively.

Diameter and position of the largest inscribed sphere within the treatment zone

Detailed data are presented in Table 3 (Figures 4 and 6). For Protocol 1 and Protocol 2, the diameter of the largest inscribed sphere within the treatment zone as well as the diameter of the largest possible treatable tumor sphere were not significantly different between Technique A and Technique B, respectively. There was a trend for a smaller diameter of the largest inscribed sphere within the treatment zone as well as a trend for a smaller diameter of the largest possible treatable tumor sphere for Technique A for Protocol 2, respectively. For Protocol 3, the diameter of the largest inscribed sphere within the treatment zone as well as the diameter of the largest possible treatable tumor sphere were significantly different between Technique A and Technique B, respectively (39.0 ± 8.4 mm versus 53.8 ± 1.1 mm and 29.0 ± 8.4 mm versus 43.8 ± 1.1 mm; $p < 0.01$ and $p < 0.01$, respectively). The barycenter offset was not assessable for Technique B. All parameters but the barycenter offset for Technique A and Technique B were significantly different between Protocol 1, Protocol 2 and Protocol 3, respectively.

Differences between technique A and technique B

For Protocol 1, Protocol 2 and Protocol 3, the difference ratio was negative (-0.4 ± 1.5 mm (-1.8-1.2 mm), -6.4 ± 8.7 mm (-16.3-5.1 mm) and -14.9 ± 7.4 mm (-25.6–7.9 mm), respectively). Thereby, significant differences existed between Protocol 1, Protocol 2 and Protocol 3 ($p < 0.05$).

Discussion

In this in-vivo pig liver study, significant differences regarding the geometry of the treatment zone after IRE exist when CT 3d rendering with the "Chebyshev Center Concept" implemented (Technique A) is compared with standard CT 3d analysis (Technique B). In summary, the diameter of the largest inscribed sphere within the treatment zone and the diameter of the largest possible treatable tumor sphere either were identical (for IRE Protocol 1), tended to be smaller (for IRE Protocol 2), or were significantly smaller (for IRE Protocol 3) for Technique A compared with Technique B. For all IRE protocols, sphericity was significantly larger for Technique A compared with Technique B indicating rounder treatment zones for the latter. On contrary to Technique B, the position of the largest inscribed sphere within the treatment zone as well as the position of the largest possible treatable tumor sphere within the treatment zone could be quantified and visualized for Technique A.

Standard techniques for the evaluation of the treatment zone after focal tumor ablation are manual measurements of perpendicular diameters on axial, coronal and/or sagittal image planes [18,19]. With such a proceeding, however,

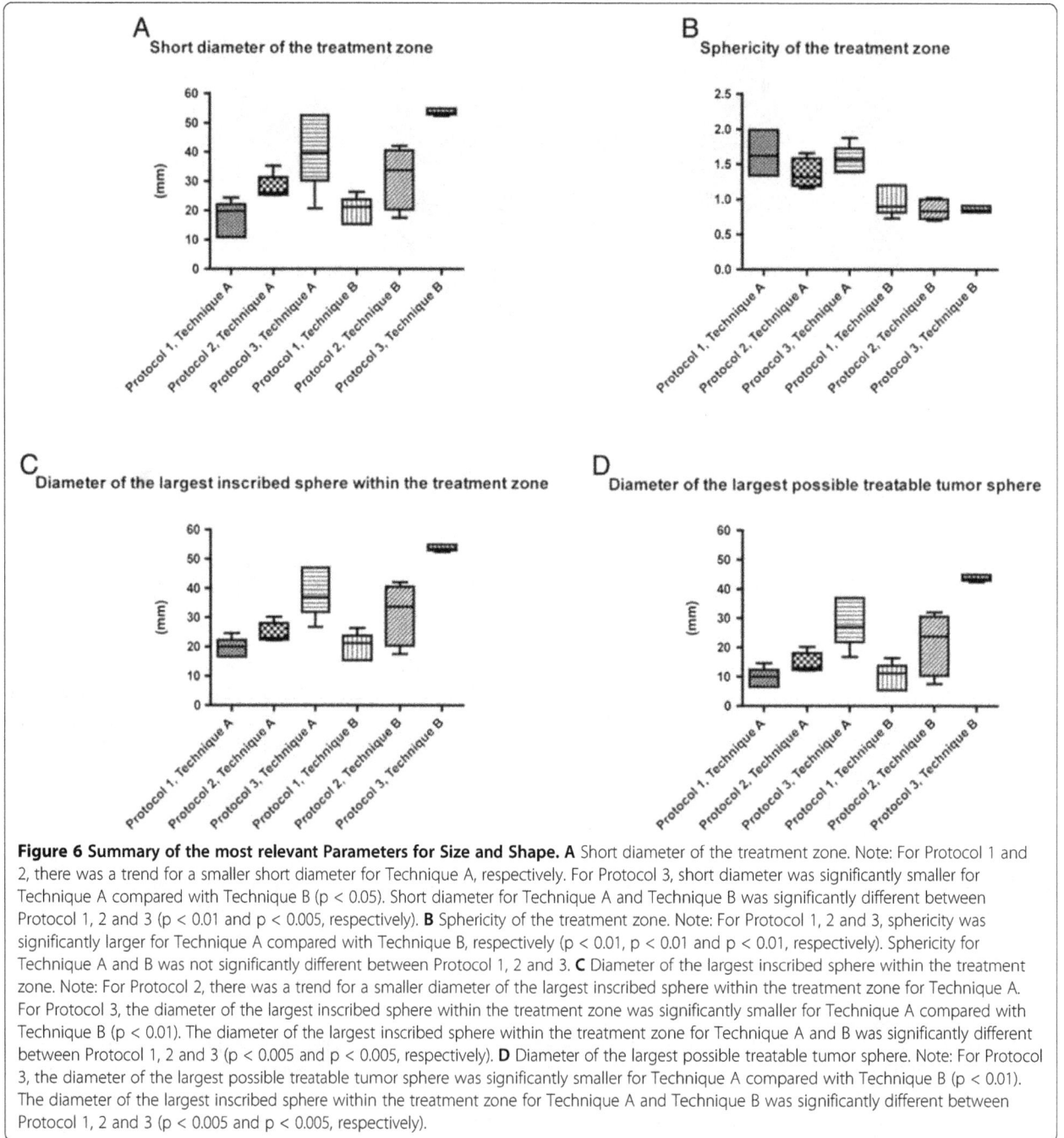

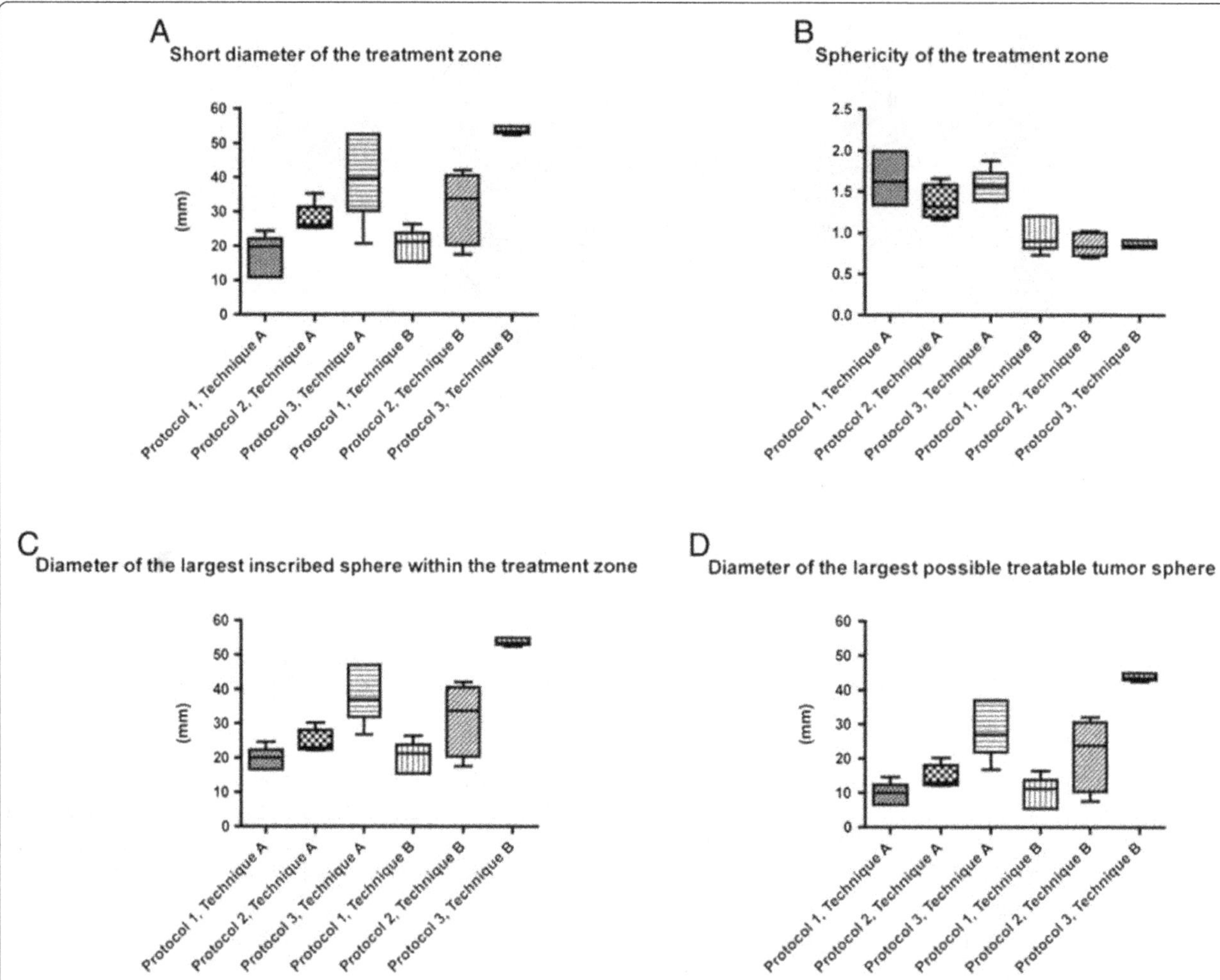

Figure 6 Summary of the most relevant Parameters for Size and Shape. A Short diameter of the treatment zone. Note: For Protocol 1 and 2, there was a trend for a smaller short diameter for Technique A, respectively. For Protocol 3, short diameter was significantly smaller for Technique A compared with Technique B ($p < 0.05$). Short diameter for Technique A and Technique B was significantly different between Protocol 1, 2 and 3 ($p < 0.01$ and $p < 0.005$, respectively). **B** Sphericity of the treatment zone. Note: For Protocol 1, 2 and 3, sphericity was significantly larger for Technique A compared with Technique B, respectively ($p < 0.01$, $p < 0.01$ and $p < 0.01$, respectively). Sphericity for Technique A and B was not significantly different between Protocol 1, 2 and 3. **C** Diameter of the largest inscribed sphere within the treatment zone. Note: For Protocol 2, there was a trend for a smaller diameter of the largest inscribed sphere within the treatment zone for Technique A. For Protocol 3, the diameter of the largest inscribed sphere within the treatment zone was significantly smaller for Technique A compared with Technique B ($p < 0.01$). The diameter of the largest inscribed sphere within the treatment zone for Technique A and B was significantly different between Protocol 1, 2 and 3 ($p < 0.005$ and $p < 0.005$, respectively). **D** Diameter of the largest possible treatable tumor sphere. Note: For Protocol 3, the diameter of the largest possible treatable tumor sphere was significantly smaller for Technique A compared with Technique B ($p < 0.01$). The diameter of the largest inscribed sphere within the treatment zone for Technique A and Technique B was significantly different between Protocol 1, 2 and 3 ($p < 0.005$ and $p < 0.005$, respectively).

the geometry of the treatment zone might be assessed not as precise as necessary. As it has been demonstrated for liver tumors, 3d segmentation showed a better depiction of tumor size and shape compared with conventional image analysis [20,21]. For hepatocellular carcinoma, Galizia et al. found that the maximum tumor diameter is significantly different between 3d analysis and control (32 ± 9 mm vs. 35 ± 12 mm; $p < 0.001$) [20]. Rothe et al. analyzed 102 liver metastases in 45 patients, and found significantly lower volumes for 3d analysis compared with 2d analysis, with relative differences up to 41.1% [21]. For focal tumor ablation, comparable data is very rare. In a work published by Elhawary et al., 3d volumetric non-rigid image registration during cryoablation could improve the ablation procedure relating to planning, targeting and evaluation of tumor coverage [22]. In another study, segmentation with image fusion results in a more accurate treatment control after radiofrequency ablation [23]. Accordingly, the depiction of the treatment zone after IRE should be more exact for Technique A compared with

Table 2 Shape of the treatment zone

	Circularity		Sphericity	
	Technique A[1]	Technique B[2]	Technique A[1]	Technique B[2]
Protocol 1[3]	$0.4 \pm 0.1^{\#,*}$	$0.6 \pm 0.3^{\#,**}$	$1.7 \pm 0.3^{+,***}$	$1.0 \pm 0.2^{+,****}$
	(0.3 - 0.5)	(0.3 - 0.8)	(1.3 - 2.0)	(0.7 - 1.2)
Protocol 2[4]	$0.7 \pm 0.1^{\#\#,*}$	$0.7 \pm 0.2^{\#\#,**}$	$1.4 \pm 0.2^{++,***}$	$0.9 \pm 0.1^{++,****}$
	(0.5 - 0.9)	(0.4 - 0.9)	(1.2 - 1.7)	(0.7 - 1.0)
Protocol 3[5]	$0.5 \pm 0.2^{\#\#\#,*}$	$0.8 \pm 0.1^{\#\#\#,**}$	$1.6 \pm 0.2^{+++,***}$	$0.9 \pm 0.1^{+++,****}$
	(0.3 - 0.7)	(0.7 - 0.8)	(1.4 - 1.9)	(0.8 - 0.9)

[1]semi-automated software prototype for CT 3d rendering with the "Chebyshev Center Concept" implemented;
[2]standard CT 3d analysis;
[3]Protocol 1 with n = 5 IREs (three applicators, tip exposure of 20 mm, distance between pairs of applicators of 15 mm, pulse number of 90, pulse length of 90 μs, and electric field of 1500 V/cm);
[4]Protocol 2 with n = 5 IREs (three applicators, tip exposure of 25 mm, distance between pairs of applicators of 20 mm, pulse number of 90, pulse length of 90 μs, and electric field of 1500 V/cm);
[5]Protocol 3 with n = 5 IREs (six applicators, tip exposure of 30 mm, distance between pairs of applicators of 15 mm, pulse number of 70, pulse length of 90 μs, and electric field of 1400 V/cm);
statistical differences between Technique A and Technique B were analyzed with the Wilcoxon signed-rank test: $^{\#}p > 0.05$; $^{\#\#}p > 0.05$; $^{\#\#\#}p < 0.01$; $^{+}p < 0.01$; $^{++}p < 0.01$; $^{+++}p < 0.01$;
statistical differences between Protocol 1, Protocol 2 and Protocol 3 were analyzed with non-parametric Kruskal-Wallis test: $^{*}p > 0.05$; $^{**}p > 0.05$; $^{***}p > 0.05$; $^{****}p > 0.05$.

Technique B since Technique A determines automatically the 3 perpendicular diameters after 3d segmentation without being limited to analyses in the standard image planes. Technique A allows not only assessment of the objective size of the treatment zone (especially definition of the short diameter, which is of paramount importance for the oncological success) but also of the objective shape of the treatment zone (which can be relevant to reduce procedure-related complications such as protection of viable structures) [19]. Technique A is independent of the tumor orientation with respect to the standard imaging planes. It is a reproducible automatic method based on a standard mathematical analysis (principal component analysis) of geometric shapes and also suitable for automatic comparisons of geometric features between imaging sessions. Our data suggest that the larger the treatment zone is, the larger the difference regarding size between Technique A and Technique B is. Regarding

Table 3 Diameter and position of the largest inscribed sphere within the treatment zone as well as of the largest possible treatable tumor sphere

	Diameter of the largest inscribed sphere within the treatment zone (mm)		Diameter of the largest possible treatable tumor sphere (mm)		Barycenter offset[1] (mm)	
	Technique A[2]	Technique B[3]	Technique A[2]	Technique B[3]	Technique A[2]	Technique B[3]
Protocol 1[4]	$19.6 \pm 3.3^{\#,*}$	$19.9 \pm 4.6^{\#,**}$	$9.6 \pm 3.3^{+,***}$	$9.9 \pm 4.6^{+,****}$	$9.1 \pm 2.1^{*****}$	n.a.
	(16.6 - 24.6)	(15.4 - 26.4)	(6.6 - 14.6)	(5.4 - 16.4)	(5.4 - 10.6)	
Protocol 2[5]	$24.8 \pm 3.4^{\#\#,*}$	$31.1 \pm 10.5^{\#\#,**}$	$14.8 \pm 3.4^{++,***}$	$21.1 \pm 10.5^{++,****}$	$5.4 \pm 3.6^{*****}$	n.a.
	(22.2 - 30.2)	(17.5 - 42.1)	(12.2 - 20.2)	(7.5 - 32.1)	(1.2 - 10.1)	
Protocol 3[6]	$39.0 \pm 8.4^{\#\#\#,*}$	$53.8 \pm 1.1^{\#\#\#,**}$	$29.0 \pm 8.4^{+++,***}$	$43.8 \pm 1.1^{+++,****}$	$5.9 \pm 3.8^{*****}$	n.a.
	(26.8 - 47.0)	(52.4 - 54.9)	(16.8 - 37.0)	(42.4 - 44.9)	(2.4 - 11.7)	

[1]distance between the barycenter of the treatment zone (intersection point of long, intermediate and short diameter) and the "Chebyshev Center"
[2]semi-automated software prototype for CT 3d rendering with the "Chebyshev Center Concept" implemented;
[3]standard CT 3d analysis;
[4]Protocol 1 with n = 5 IREs (three applicators, tip exposure of 20 mm, distance between pairs of applicators of 15 mm, pulse number of 90, pulse length of 90 μs, and electric field of 1500 V/cm);
[5]Protocol 2 with n = 5 IREs (three applicators, tip exposure of 25 mm, distance between pairs of applicators of 20 mm, pulse number of 90, pulse length of 90 μs, and electric field of 1500 V/cm);
[6]Protocol 3 with n = 5 IREs (six applicators, tip exposure of 30 mm, distance between pairs of applicators of 15 mm, pulse number of 70, pulse length of 90 μs, and electric field of 1400 V/cm);
statistical differences between Technique A and Technique B were analyzed with the Wilcoxon signed-rank test: $^{\#}p > 0.05$; $^{\#\#}p > 0.05$; $^{\#\#\#}p < 0.01$; $^{+}p > 0.05$; $^{++}p > 0.05$; $^{+++}p < 0.01$;
statistical differences between Protocol 1, Protocol 2 and Protocol 3 were analyzed with the Kruskal-Wallis test: $^{*}p < 0.005$; $^{**}p < 0.005$; $^{***}p < 0.005$; $^{****}p < 0.005$; $^{*****}p > 0.05$;
n.a. not assessable.

shape, Technique A and Technique B showed significantly different results for all IRE protocols. Both issues might emphasize the need for specific 3d rendering techniques for focal tumor ablation if one intends an optimal procedural outcome [24].

The spatial positioning of the multiple IRE applicators lead to complex treatment zones regarding shape, indentations and skip lesions compared with the rather predictable ellipsoid treatment zones after thermal ablation created with one straight needle design applicator [11,12,18]. Technique A can be used for a practicable and precise analysis of complex treatment zones after IRE. Per definition, the "Chebyshev Center" is the center of the largest inscribed sphere within a three dimensional body. In our study, this concept is used to define diameter and position of the largest inscribed sphere within the treatment zone. Technique A aligns automatically the largest inscribed sphere within the treatment zone, and calculates the barycenter offset. Due to the fact that the diameter of the largest possible treatable tumor sphere is smaller than the diameter of the largest inscribed sphere within the treatment zone by twice the safety margin, and since both spheres have the same center (the "Chebyschev Center"), the precise location of the largest possible treatable tumor sphere can be easily defined. For Technique B, the diameter of the largest possible treatable tumor sphere is determined with the short diameter, and the barycenter offset is not assessable. The presented differences between Technique A and Technique B result since only Technique A takes into account the exact geometry of the treatment zone including all shape irregularities (e.g. indentations). This means, if Technique B is applied for treatment control after focal tumor ablation, that (I) the operator can be fooled into believing that the achieved treatment zone is large enough to cover tumor and safety margin although in fact the treatment zone is too small (since Technique B overestimates the size of the treatment zone), and that (II) the correct positioning of the treatment zone in relation to the tumor can neither be confirmed nor denied objectively (since the barycenter offset is not quantified and visualized). Theoretically, the downloadable MITK freeware "Geometric evaluation of ablations" allows everyone to determine whether the intended safety margin was realized, or if another focal tumor ablation is necessary to destroy completely the tumor. At this point, the authors are obliged to point out that the use of this software is currently limited to research, and clinical decisions based on this software prototype are currently strictly forbidden. In this study, we detected differences between Technique A and Technique B in regards of the geometry of the treatment zone. Clinical superiority for one technique, however, was not proven since no clinical data were analyzed.

This study has limitations. First, IRE was performed in normal pig liver tissue, and the extent of the treatment zone might be different in human tumor tissue (e.g. since different cell density). CT datasets from patients before and after IRE could be analyzed applying our approach, and the results correlated to local tumor control during follow-up. Second, only three different IRE protocols were used. Although those were clinically relevant, alternative protocols (e.g. different number and different spatial order of electrodes) might result in treatment zones more difficult to determine geometrically especially applying standard CT 3d analysis. IRE protocols are just now being optimized for different tumor sizes and tissue characteristics (e.g. liver cirrhosis), and then should undergo 3d analysis of the treatment zone. For such protocols, the benefits of CT 3d rendering with the "Chebyshev Center Concept" implemented could be even more obvious. Third, the presented results were collected in an acute setting. Survival studies should further evaluate subacute and chronic effects after IRE (e.g. imaging findings correlated to homogeneity of cell death). Since cellular repopulation and tissue healing is likely to occur after IRE of healthy liver tissue with complete resolution of the treatment zone over weeks, the clinical feasibility of our approach for acute treatment control could be best evaluated for liver tumors. Only if the tumor and safety margin is completely covered by the largest inscribed sphere within the treatment zone on acute post-interventional CT images and the tumor disappears during follow-up, our concept can be regarded as clinically relevant. Fourth, the comparison between Technique A and B is not on the same level since an automatic technique is compared with a manual technique. For a better comparison, an automation of Technique B would have been required.

Conclusions

Regarding size and shape of the treatment zone after IRE, CT 3d rendering with the "Chebyshev Center Concept" implemented provides significantly different results compared with standard CT 3d analysis. Since standard CT 3d analysis cannot assess the extent of the treatment zone as precise as CT 3d rendering with the "Chebyshev Center Concept" implemented (especially since overestimation of the size of the treatment zone as well as the non-assessable position of the largest possible treatable tumor sphere within the treatment zone), the latter might be regarded as superior. The benefits could be used clinically to improve local tumor control due to a more objective acute treatment control.

Competing interests

The authors declare that this study was supported technically and financially by AngioDynamics® Inc., Queensbury, USA.

Authors' contributions

CMS, BAR, SF and JW were responsible for the study concept. CMS, MFW, DV, SF, US, SZ and PLP participated in the concrete design of the study. CMS, DV, MBW, NB, SU, AS, DG, JK and SF carried out the experiments and/or performed the data acquisition. Quality control of data and algorithms was performed by MFW, MBW, JK and SZ. CMS, DV, MFW, SF, DG and AS participated in data analysis and interpretation. Statistical analysis was performed by CMS, NB, DV and MFW. The manuscript was prepared by CMS, DV and MFW. BAR, SU and SF were responsible for manuscript editing. PLP, HUK, BAR and JW reviewed the manuscript. All authors approved submission of the final manuscript.

Acknowledgements

The authors of this manuscript express their gratitude to Roland Galmbacher and Markus Cattelaens for their excellent support during the experiments.

Author details

[1]Department of Diagnostic and Interventional Radiology, University Hospital Heidelberg, Heidelberg, Germany. [2]Department of General, Abdominal and Transplantation Surgery, University Hospital Heidelberg, Heidelberg, Germany. [3]Medical and Biological Informatics, German Cancer Research Center, Heidelberg, Germany. [4]Department of Radiology, German Cancer Research Center (dkfz) Heidelberg, INF 280, Heidelberg, Germany. [5]Department of Anesthesiology, University Hospital Heidelberg, Heidelberg, Germany. [6]Clinic for Radiology, Minimally-invasive Therapies and Nuclear Medicine, SLK Kliniken Heilbronn GmbH, Heilbronn, Germany.

References

1. Davalos RV, Mir IL, Rubinsky B: **Tissue ablation with irreversible electroporation.** *Ann Biomed Eng* 2005, **33**(2):223–231.
2. Edd JF, Horowitz L, Davalos RV, Mir LM, Rubinsky B: **In vivo results of a new focal tissue ablation technique: irreversible electroporation.** *IEEE Trans Biomed Eng* 2006, **53**(7):1409–1415.
3. Lee EW, Loh CT, Kee ST: **Imaging guided percutaneous irreversible electroporation: ultrasound and immunohistological correlation.** *Technol Cancer Res Treat* 2007, **6**(4):287–294.
4. Rubinsky B, Onik G, Mikus P: **Irreversible electroporation: a new ablation modality–clinical implications.** *Technol Cancer Res Treat* 2007, **6**(1):37–48.
5. Brace CL: **Radiofrequency and microwave ablation of the liver, lung, kidney, and bone: what are the differences?** *Curr Probl Diagn Radiol* 2009, **38**(3):135–143.
6. Charpentier KP: **Irreversible electroporation for the ablation of liver tumors: are we there yet?** *Arch Surg* 2012, **147**(11):1053–1061.
7. Thomson KR, Cheung W, Ellis SJ, Federman D, Kavnoudias H, Loader-Oliver D, Roberts S, Evans P, Ball C, Haydon A: **Investigation of the safety of irreversible electroporation in humans.** *J Vasc Interv Radiol* 2011, **22**(5):611–621.
8. Rubinsky B: **Irreversible electroporation in medicine.** *Technol Cancer Res Treat* 2007, **6**(4):255–260.
9. Wendler JJ, Pech M, Blaschke S, Porsch M, Janitzky A, Ulrich M, Dudeck O, Ricke J, Liehr UB: **Angiography in the isolated perfused kidney: radiological evaluation of vascular protection in tissue ablation by nonthermal irreversible electroporation.** *Cardiovasc Intervent Radiol* 2012, **35**(2):383–390.
10. Wang X, Sofocleous CT, Erinjeri JP, Petre EN, Gonen M, Do KG, Brown KT, Covey AM, Brody LA, Alago W, *et al*: **Margin Size is an Independent Predictor of Local Tumor Progression After Ablation of Colon Cancer Liver Metastases.** *Cardiovasc Intervent Radiol* 2013, **36**(1):166–175.
11. Sommer CM, Sommer SA, Sommer WO, Zelzer S, Wolf MB, Bellemann N, Meinzer HP, Radeleff BA, Stampfl U, Kauczor HU, *et al*: **Optimisation of the coagulation zone for thermal ablation procedures: a theoretical approach with considerations for practical use.** *Int J Hyperthermia* 2013, **29**(7):620–628.
12. Adeyanju OO, Al-Angari HM, Sahakian AV: **The optimization of needle electrode number and placement for irreversible electroporation of hepatocellular carcinoma.** *Radiology Oncol* 2012, **46**(2):126–135.
13. Lee YJ, Lu DS, Osuagwu F, Lassman C: **Irreversible electroporation in porcine liver: acute computed tomography appearance of ablation zone with histopathologic correlation.** *J Comput Assist Tomogr* 2013, **37**(2):154–158.
14. Lee YJ, Lu DS, Osuagwu F, Lassman C: **Irreversible electroporation in porcine liver: short- and long-term effect on the hepatic veins and adjacent tissue by CT with pathological correlation.** *Invest Radiol* 2012, **47**(11):671–675.
15. Sommer CM, Kortes N, Zelzer S, Arnegger FU, Stampfl U, Bellemann N, Gehrig T, Nickel F, Kenngott HG, Mogler C, *et al*: **Renal artery embolization combined with radiofrequency ablation in a porcine kidney model: effect of small and narrowly calibrated microparticles as embolization material on coagulation diameter, volume, and shape.** *Cardiovasc Intervent Radiol* 2011, **34**(1):156–165.
16. Laeseke PF, Lee FT Jr, Sampson LA, van der Weide DW, Brace CL: **Microwave ablation versus radiofrequency ablation in the kidney: high-power triaxial antennas create larger ablation zones than similarly sized internally cooled electrodes.** *J Vasc Interv Radiol* 2009, **20**(9):1224–1229.
17. Pereira PL, Trubenbach J, Schenk M, Subke J, Kroeber S, Schaefer I, Remy CT, Schmidt D, Brieger J, Claussen CD: **Radiofrequency ablation: in vivo comparison of four commercially available devices in pig livers.** *Radiology* 2004, **232**(2):482–490.
18. Mulier S, Ni Y, Frich L, Burdio F, Denys AL, De Wispelaere JF, Dupas B, Habib N, Hoey M, Jansen MC, *et al*: **Experimental and clinical radiofrequency ablation: proposal for standardized description of coagulation size and geometry.** *Ann Surg Oncol* 2007, **14**(4):1381–1396.
19. Goldberg SN, Grassi CJ, Cardella JF, Charboneau JW, Dodd GD 3rd, Dupuy DE, Gervais DA, Gillams AR, Kane RA, Lee FT Jr, *et al*: **Image-guided tumor ablation: standardization of terminology and reporting criteria.** *J Vasc Interv Radiol* 2009, **20**(7 Suppl):S377–S390.
20. Galizia MS, Tore HG, Chalian H, Yaghmai V: **Evaluation of hepatocellular carcinoma size using two-dimensional and volumetric analysis: effect on liver transplantation eligibility.** *Acad Radiol* 2011, **18**(12):1555–1560.
21. Rothe JH, Grieser C, Lehmkuhl L, Schnapauff D, Fernandez CP, Maurer MH, Mussler A, Hamm B, Denecke T, Steffen IG: **Size determination and response assessment of liver metastases with computed tomography-Comparison of RECIST and volumetric algorithms.** *Eur J Radiol* 2013, **82**(11):1831–1839.
22. Elhawary H, Oguro S, Tuncali K, Morrison PR, Tatli S, Shyn PB, Silverman SG, Hata N: **Multimodality non-rigid image registration for planning, targeting and monitoring during CT-guided percutaneous liver tumor cryoablation.** *Acad Radiol* 2010, **17**(11):1334–1344.
23. Passera K, Selvaggi S, Scaramuzza D, Garbagnati F, Vergnaghi D, Mainardi L: **Radiofrequency ablation of liver tumors: quantitative assessment of tumor coverage through CT image processing.** *BMC Med Imaging* 2013, **13**(1):3.
24. Tateishi R, Shiina S, Akahane M, Sato J, Kondo Y, Masuzaki R, Nakagawa H, Asaoka Y, Goto T, Otomo K, *et al*: **Frequency, risk factors and survival associated with an intrasubsegmental recurrence after radiofrequency ablation for hepatocellular carcinoma.** *PloS one* 2013, **8**(4):e59040.

7

Validation of a measuring technique with computed tomography for cement penetration into trabecular bone underneath the tibial tray in total knee arthroplasty on a cadaver model

Hennie Verburg[1*], Laurens C van de Ridder[1], Vincent WJ Verhoeven[2] and Peter Pilot[1]

Abstract

Background: In total knee arthroplasty (TKA), cement penetration between 3 and 5 mm beneath the tibial tray is required to prevent loosening of the tibia component. The objective of this study was to develop and validate a reliable *in vivo* measuring technique using CT imaging to assess cement distribution and penetration depth in the total area underneath a tibia prosthesis.

Methods: We defined the radiodensity ranges for trabecular tibia bone, polymethylmethacrylate (PMMA) cement and cement-penetrated trabecular bone and measured the percentages of cement penetration at various depths after cementing two tibia prostheses onto redundant femoral heads. One prosthesis was subsequently removed to examine the influence of the metal tibia prostheses on the quality of the CT images. The percentages of cement penetration in the CT slices were compared with percentages measured with photographs of the corresponding transversal slices.

Results: Trabecular bone and cement-penetrated trabecular bone had no overlap in quantitative scale of radio-density. There was no significant difference in mean HU values when measuring with or without the tibia prosthesis. The percentages of measured cement-penetrated trabecular bone in the CT slices of the specimen were within the range of percentages that could be expected based on the measurements with the photographs ($p = 0.04$).

Conclusions: CT scan images provide valid results in measuring the penetration and distribution of cement into trabecular bone underneath the tibia component of a TKA. Since the proposed method does not turn metal elements into artefacts, it enables clinicians to assess the width and density of the cement mantle *in vivo* and to compare the results of different cementing methods in TKA.

Keywords: Computed tomography, CT scan, Cement penetration, Total knee arthroplasty, TKA

Background

In total knee arthroplasty (TKA), up to ninety percent of the orthopaedic surgeons use cement to fixate the tibia component [1]. Despite this fixation, one of the main reasons for late failure of TKA is loosening of the tibia component [2]. This loosening is believed to be caused by micro motion at the cement-bone interface. The degree of fixation at the cement-bone interface, and hence the prevention of micro motion, is thought to depend on the penetration depth of cement into the trabecular bone underneath the tibial tray [3,4]. In a post-mortem retrieval analysis of fixation strength of cemented tibial trays, Gebert de Uhlenbrock et al. concluded that fixation is improved by greater cement penetration [5]. Other studies on tibia cement penetration in TKA have shown that cement penetration between 3 and 5 mm beneath the tibial tray appears to be the optimal depth [6,7]. Cement penetration to a depth of less than 3 mm results in a weak cement-bone interface, which predisposes for micro motion. However, penetration deeper

* Correspondence: hverburg@rdgg.nl
[1]Department of Orthopaedics, Reinier de Graaf Groep, Reinier de Graafweg 3, 2625 AD Delft, The Netherlands
Full list of author information is available at the end of the article

than 5 mm can lead to heat-induced necrosis of bone and does not increase the strength of the interface [8,9].

While these studies have demonstrated the importance of optimal cement penetration, measuring the cement mantle surrounding implants *in vivo* remains a challenge. In current clinical practice, cement penetration is measured *in vivo* by means of conventional radiographs [8]. However, the downside of conventional radiographs is that they merely provide a two dimensional view of the cement-bone interface. Moreover, it is difficult to shoot the X-ray beam exactly parallel to the prosthesis. Consequently, the measurement of the penetration depth will not always take place directly under the prosthesis, which is the place where an optimal interdigitation between bone and cement is required for fixation of the tibial tray when using the most common cementing technique, i.e. surface cementing.

Various authors used Computed Tomography (CT) imaging to examine the cement mantle around implants [5,10-14]. Goodheart et al. [11] and Mann et al. [13] used micro-CT image processing, a technique which cannot be used *in vivo*. CT images, on the other hand, can be used *in vivo*. The disadvantage of using CT images used to be that the metal prosthesis produced artefacts in the images, which made a good interpretation difficult. In 2009, Lui et al. [12] attempted to develop an algorithm for reducing metal artifacts in CT images of implanted metal orthopaedic devices. Since then, with the recent technical improvements of the CT equipment and software, this problem might have been solved, and CT images might have become a valid measuring technique for tibia cement penetration in TKA. We hypothesized that it might be possible to examine a cross section (i.e. a transversal CT slice) of the cancellous bone, and to assess the cement distribution on that cross section by calculating the percentage of the cement-penetrated cancellous bone versus the non-penetrated cancellous bone. By examining cross sections at consecutive depths, we might measure the width of the cement mantle as well as the density of the cement penetration at the required depth.

So far no measuring technique has been validated for measuring tibia cement penetration in TKA *in vivo* by means of CT imaging. Hence, the objective of this study was to develop and validate an *in vivo* measuring technique which provides a truthful indication of the percentage distributed and penetrated cement in the total scanned surface underneath a tibia prosthesis. We assessed the accuracy of using CT scan images to measure cement distribution, i.e. the amount of cement on a cross section of the bone, and cement penetration, i.e. the amount of cement in the depth of the bone just underneath the tibial tray, and we evaluated the influence of metal elements on the depiction of cement on the CT reconstruction.

Methods

To be able to discriminate between cement-penetrated cancellous bone and non-penetrated cancellous bone, we first defined the radiodensity (Hounsfield units, HU) ranges for trabecular tibia bone, polymethylmethacrylate (PMMA) cement and cement-penetrated trabecular bone. The calibration of the HU levels was checked by scanning a phantom with water, teflon and nylon compartments. The scan of this phantom was analyzed to determine uniformity between the measured HU levels of water, teflon and nylon. If a parameter exceeded its criteria, corrective measures were taken. Next, we measured cement penetration at various depths after cementing two tibia prostheses, one of which was subsequently removed again to examine the influence of the metal tibia prostheses on the quality of the CT images. This tibia prosthesis had been covered with a silicone layer to enable removal of the prosthesis after the first measurements without damage to the bone-cement interface. The other prostheses remained *in situ* and no silicone was required, therefore we did not use it, as it is not used in the regular procedure of cementing, either. Finally, we controlled the findings on cement penetration by sawing the bones off at the measured depths and taking photographs of the sawed-off surface.

For this study, we used 3 femoral heads which had been removed during total hip arthroplasty. All patients consented to the use of the redundant femoral heads. We prepared these femoral heads on the day of the resection. One femoral head was used to measure the radio-density range of pure PMMA cement and of cement-penetrated trabecular bone, as well as to validate the measured percentage of penetrated cement by comparing it to photographs of the femoral head slices sawed off at the required depth. The other two femoral heads were used as cadaver models for measuring cement penetration depth after cementing a tibia prosthesis into each of them, and one of these two femoral heads was used again for examining the influence of metal tibia prosthesis on the CT images.

The CT slices were analyzed with Osirix® (version 3.2.1 32-bit). OsiriX® is an image processing software dedicated to DICOM images produced by a CT scan and has been specifically designed for navigation and visualization of multimodality and multidimensional images. The photographs of the sawed-off slices were analysed with Adobe Photoshop® CS2 (version 9.0), a graphics editing program that can select an area of an image and sample it for future use.

HU ranges of trabecular tibia bone

To measure the radio-density range of trabecular tibia bone, we used CT images of 4 patients who had undergone a diagnostic CT scan of the knee. The radio-density range of the area 1 to 6 mm beneath the lowest point of the tibia plateau was defined as the clinically relevant area of trabecular tibia bone. The HU value of this area was measured in transversal and coronal slices.

HU ranges of PMMA cement

To measure the radio-density range of pure cement, we used a slice of one of the femoral heads. From the middle of the cut surface of this slice, 1.0 cubic centimetre of trabecular bone was removed and the hole was filled with cement. Several CT scans were made (Figure 1). Three areas were selected for measurement in transversal slices. In the resulting CT images, radio-density measurements taken in the pure cemented cubic centimetre were defined as the true radio-density range of cement.

HU ranges of cement-penetrated trabecular bone

To measure the radio-density range of cement-penetrated trabecular bone, another slice of one of the femoral heads was used. The cement was pressurised on top of the cut surface of the slice to achieve good cement penetration into the trabecular bone. Several CT scans were made of the cemented slice. In the resulting CT images, radio-density measurements taken in the transversal slice 3 to 6 millimetres beneath the cut surface were defined as the radio-density range of cement-penetrated trabecular bone.

Cement penetration at various depths

The tops of two of the femoral heads were sawed off in such a way that the tibial prostheses would fit easily onto the cut surface. The cut surface was prepared for insertion of the smallest NexGen® tibia prostheses (Zimmer®, Warsaw, Indiana, USA), using the NexGen® implantation tools. To cement the tibia prosthesis, the PMMA cement was only applied to the underside of the tibia component and not to the keel. Good compression was achieved by thrusting the tibia prosthesis into the femoral head with a tibial impactor, in line with the way a TKA is usually performed during surgery.

Spiral CT scans were taken of both femoral heads, scanning parallel to the cut surface of the femoral head. The spiral CT scanner (Philips® Gemini GXL 16 slice) produced 0.8 mm slices. The slices were analyzed with Osirix®. Osirix® calculated the mean HU value of the selected areas as well as the standard deviations (SDs) of the mean HU values in the selected areas. These SDs provided an indication of the homogeneity of the scanned material in the selected areas and were identified as the homogeneity values of the selected areas.

By measuring the amount of cement in the cross-sections of every 0.8 mm slice below the underside of the tibial tray, we calculated the penetration depth of the cement in percentages of the trabecular bone surfaces.

Influence of metal tibia prosthesis on the CT images

To assess the influence of metal tibia prosthesis on the CT images, CT scans were made of the femoral head with a tibia prosthesis *in situ* and once again after removal of the tibia prosthesis. Measurements were taken in the transversal slices parallel to the tibial tray. To measure the cement distribution in trabecular bone with the prosthesis *in situ* and without the prosthesis, three areas were selected, two beside and one posterior to the prosthesis (Figure 2).

Automatic ROI marking

We defined ranges of HU values which enable automatic ROI marking in the CT slices. These ranges were defined to be the mean HU plus and minus twice the mean homogeneity value plus the SD of the mean homogeneity value.

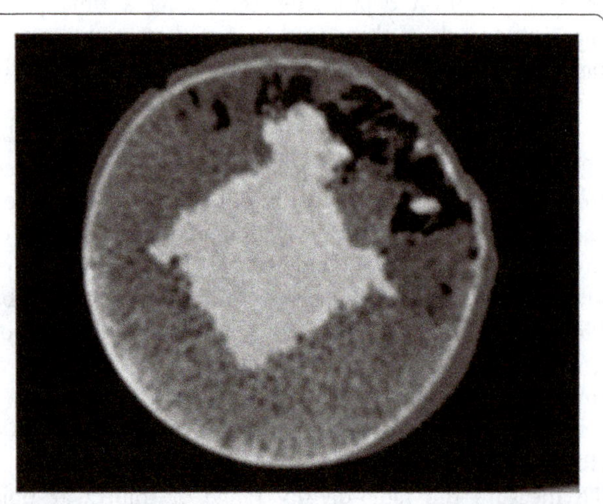

Figure 1 CT scan of the pure cemented cubic centimetre.

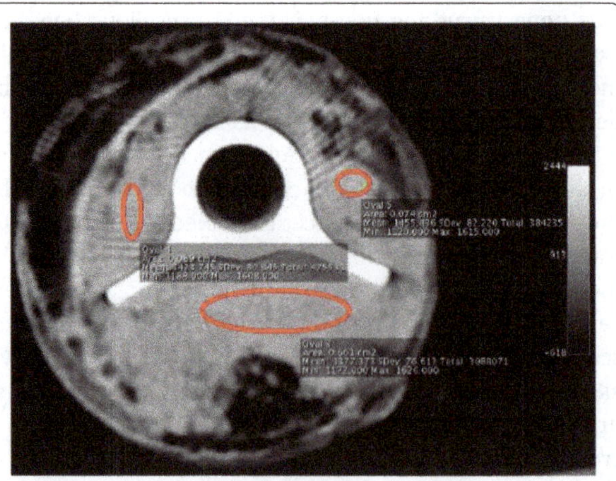

Figure 2 CT scan of a femoral head 3 mm beneath the cemented tibial tray. Three areas were selected, two beside the prosthesis and one posterior to the prosthesis.

Validation with photographs

After the radio-density ranges of interest (ROI) were defined, they were used to measure the percentage penetrated cement in the total scanned surface in transversal slices 3 to 6 mm beneath the cut surface. A femur head was cut into halves, both cut surfaces were pressurised with cement and a tantalum bead of 0.5 mm was placed 3 mm beneath the cut surface to facilitate orientation in the CT scans. CT scans were taken of both halves, and the total surface of the transversal slices was measured with Osirix®. Then the radio-density ROI of cement-penetrated trabecular bone was marked to be able to measure the surface of the cement-penetrated trabecular bone area. Next, the radio-density ROI of cement-penetrated trabecular bone was indicated as a percentage of the total scanned surface.

After the CT scans were made, we controlled the findings by means of photographs. A transversal slice was sawed off each half of the femoral head at 3 mm below the cut surfaces, just above the tantalum beads. Both slices were photographed, and the photographs were analysed with Adobe Photoshop® CS2. First the pixels of the total slices were measured, then the colour range of the cement was marked and all pixels in this range were measured. Next, the surface of the cement area was calculated as a percentage of the total slice. The percentages measured in the photographs of the slices were compared with the percentages measured in the corresponding transversal CT slices.

Statistical analysis

Analyses were performed using SPSS® Statistics for Windows Version 21, Chicago, IL, USA. Differences between the mean percentages of penetrated cement measured in the photographs of the femoral head slices and the percentages measured in the corresponding transversal CT slices were analyzed using the independent t-tests (Student *T*-test). P-values less than 0.05 were considered significant.

Results

HU ranges of trabecular tibia bone

In the diagnostic CT scans of four patients, the selected areas in the transversal slices had a mean value of 163 HU (SD 12), with a mean homogeneity value of 152 HU (SD 14). In the coronal slices, the selected areas had a mean value of 162 HU (SD 24), with a mean homogeneity value of 123 HU (SD 16).

HU ranges of PMMA cement

The mean radio-density value in the selected areas of pure cement was 1328 HU (SD 27), with a mean homogeneity value of 66 HU (SD 12).

HU ranges of cement-penetrated trabecular bone

The mean radio-density value of cement-penetrated trabecular bone in the selected areas was 1363 HU (SD 30), with a mean homogeneity value of 71 HU (SD 17).

Cement penetration underneath the tibia prosthesis

The mean value of the selected areas was 1384 HU (SD 53), with a mean homogeneity of 81 HU (SD 30).

Influence of metal tibia prosthesis on the CT images

Table 1 shows the results of the CT scan measurements of the femoral head with and without the removable tibia prosthesis and of the CT scan measurements of the femoral head with the attached tibia prosthesis. The results indicate that there was no significant difference in mean HU values when measuring with or without the tibia prosthesis.

Automatic ROI marking

Table 2 shows the HU ranges for automatic ROI marking.

CT slices compared with photographs of the transversal slices

Table 3 shows the mean percentages of penetrated cement measured in three different photographs of the femoral head slices at 3 mm beneath the cut surface. Table 3 also shows the percentages measured in the corresponding transversal CT slices, defined by means of the tantalum beads, and the slices 0.8 mm beneath the corresponding transversal CT slices. The percentages of measured cement-penetrated trabecular bone in the CT slices of the specimen were within the range of percentages that could be expected based on the measurements with the photographs ($p = 0.04$).

Discussion

The objective of this study was to assess whether CT images can be used to accurately measure the percentage of penetrated cement in the total scanned surface underneath a tibia prosthesis, and to develop and validate a measuring technique that can be used *in vivo* after cementing a total knee arthroplasty. The results showed that trabecular bone and cement-penetrated trabecular bone had no overlap in quantitative scale of radio density, indicating that this method of measuring cement penetration may be useful in a clinical setting. In addition, there was no significant difference in quantitative radio-density values when measuring with or without the metal prosthesis, indicating that modern CT imaging technology no longer has the disadvantage of turning metal elements into artefacts that confound the interpretation of the images.

Our findings confirm the assumptions of other studies which used CT-scans for femoral implants and defined

Table 1 HU values of selected areas measured in CT scans with and without prosthesis

CT slice	Femur head with removable prosthesis		Femur head without removable prosthesis		Femur head with attached prosthesis	
	HU value of selected area	Homogeneity value	HU value of selected area	Homogeneity value	HU value of selected area	Homogeneity value
1	1377	77	1424	64	1422	129
	1423	81	1350	97	1296	81
	1455	82	1334	76	1402	91
2	1299	122	1395	65	1431	144
	1367	125	1349	89	1433	161
	1262	133	1421	59	1338	53
3	1366	109	1405	39	1534	102
	1372	80	1400	89	1497	104
	1436	116	1386	72	1352	56
4	1304	82	1428	116	1436	143
	1377	93	1478	96	1518	120
	1534	75	1335	97		
5	1413	107	1406	66	1479	159
	1315	120	1340	63	1495	160
	1568	72	1422	69		
Mean (SD)	1391 (84)	98 (21)	1392 (42)	77 (20)	1433 (72)	116 (38)

the Hounsfield Units for (cancellous) bone, PMMA and prosthesis in the same region as we found with our study [10,14].

Our results showed no overlap in the radio-density ROIs of trabecular bone, cement-penetrated trabecular bone and the prostheses. This indicates that when the radio-density ROI of cement-penetrated trabecular bone was registered, there was no trabecular bone or prosthesis in the areas under investigation. Thus it is possible to see the differences between trabecular bone, cement-penetrated trabecular bone or prosthesis in every CT-slice underneath the tibia prosthesis. This enables clinicians to get a good impression of the three-dimensional extent of cement penetration into the trabecular bone after cementing the tibia component of a TKA.

A comparison between the CT slices and the corresponding optical pictures showed different percentages of penetrated cement of the total surfaces of the transversal slices (Table 3). Nevertheless, the percentages of measured cement-penetrated trabecular bone in the CT slices of the specimen were within the range of percentages that could be expected based on the measurements with the photographs ($p = 0.04$). While the percentages of penetrated cement measured in the corresponding CT slices were higher than the percentages of penetrated cement measured in the photographs, the percentages of penetrated cement in the CT slices 0.8 mm beneath the corresponding CT slices were slightly lower, both 0.6%, than the percentages of penetrated cement measured in the photographs. The difference in percentage of penetrated cement of the total surface can be explained by the fact that the corresponding CT slices did not exactly correspond with the cut surface of the transversal slices. The corresponding CT slices were defined using the tantalum beads as an orientation point, but the CT scans made 0.8 mm slices, implying a possible fault margin of maximally 0.8 mm, which must have resulted in a different cement percentage of the surface. The CT slice of the area slightly above the cut surface of the slice will show a higher percentage of

Table 2 HU ranges for automatic ROI marking for several materials

ROI of	Range in HU
Trabecular tibia bone	−192 to 516
Penetrated cement	1062 to 1706
Cortical bone	1386 to 1864
Prosthesis	> 2475

Table 3 Penetrated cement in CT slices and photographs as a percentage of the total transversal slice 3 mm beneath the cut surface

	Penetrated cement in photographs	Penetrated cement in corresponding CT slices	Penetrated cement in CT slice 0.8 mm beneath the corresponding slice
Slice 1	35.4%	39.7%	34.8%
Slice 2	31.3%	34.7%	30.7%
Mean (SD)	33.35% (2.9)	37.2% (3.5)	32.75% (2.9)

penetrated cement, because the cement in that area met with less resistance and could penetrate to a greater extent.

Limitations

A limitation of this study was that we used human femoral heads instead of the proximal part of a tibia. The femoral heads were much easier to acquire and we could use them on the same day after the resection during surgery of a total hip arthroplasty. Moreover, there are no big differences between the HU values of cancellous bone in tibia and femoral heads. According to Scheerlinck et al. [14] the HU value of cancellous bone is on average 30 HU (SD 350 HU). Since this is in line with our findings, we consider our results to be relevant for measuring cement penetration in the proximal part of a tibia.

Another limitation was that our findings showed an overlap in the radio-density ROI of cement-penetrated trabecular bone and the radio-density ROI of cortical bone. However, this overlap had only a small influence on the measured percentages of penetrated cement, because only the thin edge on the transversal CT slices consists of cortical bone. Furthermore, all transversal slices had almost the same percentage of cortical bone, and, consequently, the final effect of this overlap in radio-density ROIs was the same in all slices. Therefore we do not expect this to affect the clinical use of the proposed method.

A third limitation is that we compared the cement area to the total scanned surface, without subtracting the metal. However, this did not influence our measurements, since the prosthesis constituted nearly the same percentage of the cross-sectional surface over the measured depth of 3 to 6 mm.

A fourth limitation is that we did not examine the radio-density ROI directly beside the prosthesis. Still, the CT technique we used showed nearly no effect of the metal prosthesis on the surrounding bone/cement. In addition, there was no significant difference in quantitative radio-density values when measuring with or without the metal prosthesis, indicating that modern CT imaging technology no longer has the disadvantage of turning metal elements into artefacts that confound the interpretation of the images.

A final limitation of our study is that with this CT technique, it is impossible to differentiate between bulk cement, like filled bony defects or cysts, and trabecular bone that is interlocked with cement. When cement is pressurized into trabecular bone, the cement fills up the space between the trabecals, which enlarges the density and improves the homogeneity. As a result, the homogeneity value of cement-penetrated trabecular bone is almost the same as the homogeneity value of pure cement. With this result we can make the assumption that the density of cement-penetrated trabecular bone equals the density of pure cement. To differentiate between them, we would have to use micro-CT, which cannot be used *in vivo*. We therefore accepted this drawback as a limitation, since this study aimed to develop and validate a measuring technique that can be used *in vivo* in clinical practice.

Suggestions for further research

In this study we established that CT imaging can be used to measure the amount of cement at different depths beneath the cutting surface of the femoral head and to calculate the percentage of cement penetrated into the cancellous bone versus the percentage of cancellous bone without penetrated cement. We presented this percentage at a depth of 3 mm beneath the cutting surface, but the same technique can be used to establish the percentage at a depth of 5 mm. Further research might focus on the optimal percentage of cement-penetrated bone that is required at these depths to prevent loosening of the TKA.

Conclusions

In conclusion, the trabecular cement penetration in TKA can be measured reliably by means of transversal CT slices in combination with the automatically marked radio-density ROI of cement-penetrated trabecular bone and Osirix® computer software. The metal prostheses had no significant effect on the measured radio-density values in the CT images, and there was no overlap between the automatically marked radio-density ROIs of trabecular bone and cement-penetrated trabecular bone. The percentages of cement penetration measured in the CT slices were within the range of percentages that could be expected based on the measurements in the optical pictures. This reproducible technique is, until now, the only way to measure the three-dimensional extent of cement penetration into the trabecular bone after cementing the tibia component of a TKA. Moreover, this technique will make it easier to compare the results of different cementing methods in TKA.

Abbreviations

TKA: Total knee arthroplasty; CT: Computed tomography; HU: Hounsfield unit; PMMA: Polymethylmetacrylate; SD: Standard deviation; ROI: Range of interest.

Competing interests

The authors declare that they have no competing interests.

Authors' contributions

All authors made substantive intellectual contributions to this research study. HV, LR and PP conceptualized the primary research questions and constructed the study design. LR performed the implantations of the prosthesis and LR and WV assessed the CT scans. HV and LR are responsible for writing this article. All authors read and approved the final manuscript.

Author details

[1]Department of Orthopaedics, Reinier de Graaf Groep, Reinier de Graafweg 3, 2625 AD Delft, The Netherlands. [2]Department of Nuclear Medicine, Reinier de Graaf Groep, Reinier de Graafweg 3, 2625 AD Delft, The Netherlands.

References

1. Lutz MJ, Pincus PF, Whitehouse SL, Halliday BR: **The effect of cement gun and cement syringe use on the tibial cement mantle in total knee arthroplasty.** *J Arthroplast* 2009, **24**(3):461–467.
2. Marx R, Qunaibi M, Wirtz DC, Niethard FU, Mumme T: **Surface pretreatment for prolonged survival of cemented tibial prosthesis components: full- vs. surface-cementation technique.** *Biomed Eng Online* 2005, **4**:61.
3. Bauze AJ, Costi JJ, Stavrou P, Rankin WA, Hearn TC, Krishnan J, Slavotinek JP: **Cement penetration and stiffness of the cement-bone composite in the proximal tibia in a porcine model.** *J Orthop Surg* 2004, **12**(2):194–198.
4. Peters CL, Craig MA, Mohr RA, Bachus KN: **Tibial component fixation with cement: full- versus surface-cementation techniques.** *Clin Orthop Relat Res* 2003, **409**:158–168.
5. Gebert De Uhlenbrock A, Puschel V, Puschel K, Morlock MM, Bishop NE: **Influence of time *in-situ* and implant type on fixation strength of cemented tibial trays - a post mortem retrieval analysis.** *Clinical Biomechanics* 2012, **27**(9):929–935.
6. Cawley DT, Kelly N, McGarry JP, Shannon FJ: **Cementing techniques for the tibial component in primary total knee replacement.** *Bone Joint J* 2013, **95-B**(3):295–300.
7. Vanlommel J, Luyckx JP, Labey L, Innocenti B, De Corte R, Bellemans J: **Cementing the tibial component in total knee arthroplasty: which technique is the best?** *J Arthroplast* 2011, **26**(3):492–496.
8. Hofmann AA, Goldberg TD, Tanner AM, Cook TM: **Surface cementation of stemmed tibial components in primary total knee arthroplasty: minimum 5-year follow-up.** *J Arthroplast* 2006, **21**(3):353–357.
9. Walker PS, Soudry M, Ewald FC, McVickar H: **Control of cement penetration in total knee arthroplasty.** *Clin Orthop Relat Res* 1984, **185**:155–164.
10. Efe T, Figiel J, Sibbert D, Fuchs-Winkelmann S, Tibesku CO, Timmesfeld N, Paletta JR, Skwara A: **Revision of tibial TKA components: bone loss is independent of cementing type and technique: an *in vitro* cadaver study.** *BMC Musculoskelet Disord* 2011, **12**:6.
11. Goodheart JR, Miller MA, Mann KA: ***In vivo* loss of cement-bone interlock reduces fixation strength in total knee arthroplasties.** *J Ortho Res Official Publ Ortho Res Soc* 2014, **32**(8):1052–1060.
12. Liu PT, Pavlicek WP, Peter MB, Spangehl MJ, Roberts CC, Paden RG: **Metal artifact reduction image reconstruction algorithm for CT of implanted metal orthopedic devices: a work in progress.** *Skelet Radiol* 2009, **38**(8):797–802.
13. Mann KA, Miller MA, Pray CL, Verdonschot N, Janssen D: **A new approach to quantify trabecular resorption adjacent to cemented knee arthroplasty.** *J Biomech* 2012, **45**(4):711–715.
14. Scheerlinck T, de Mey J, Deklerck R: ***In vitro* analysis of the cement mantle of femoral hip implants: development and validation of a CT-scan based measurement tool.** *J Ortho Res Official Publ Ortho Res Soc* 2005, **23**(4):698–704.

8

Immune reconstitution inflammatory syndrome due to *Mycobacterium avium* complex successfully followed up using ^{18}F-fluorodeoxyglucose positron emission tomography-computed tomography in a patient with human immunodeficiency virus infection

Ho Namkoong[1,2], Hiroshi Fujiwara[3], Makoto Ishii[1*], Kazuma Yagi[1], Mizuha Haraguchi[1], Masako Matsusaka[1], Shoji Suzuki[1], Takanori Asakura[1], Takahiro Asami[1], Fumitake Saito[1], Koichi Fukunaga[1], Sadatomo Tasaka[1], Tomoko Betsuyaku[1] and Naoki Hasegawa[3]

Abstract

Background: In human immunodeficiency virus (HIV)-infected patients, immune reconstitution inflammatory syndrome (IRIS) due to nontuberculous mycobacteria (NTM) infection is one of the most difficult types of IRIS to manage. ^{18}F-fluorodeoxyglucose positron emission tomography/computed tomography (^{18}F-FDG PET/CT) has been suggested as a useful tool for evaluating the inflammatory status of HIV-infected patients. We present the first case of *Mycobacterium avium* complex (MAC)-associated IRIS (MAC-IRIS) that was successfully followed up using ^{18}F-FDG PET/CT.

Case presentation: A 44-year-old homosexual Japanese man was referred to our hospital with fever and dyspnea. He was diagnosed with *Pneumocystis jiroveci* pneumonia and found to be HIV positive. After the initiation of combined antiretroviral therapy (cART), the patient's mediastinal and bilateral hilar lymphadenopathy gradually enlarged, and bilateral infiltrates appeared in the upper lung fields. ^{18}F-FDG PET/CT was performed five months after the initiation of cART and showed intense accumulation of fluorodeoxyglucose (FDG) corresponding to the lesions of infiltration as well as the mediastinal and bilateral hilar lymphadenopathy. A bronchial wash culture and pathology findings led to a diagnosis of MAC-IRIS. Anti-mycobacterial chemotherapy with rifampicin, ethambutol, clarithromycin, and levofloxacin was started. One year after the chemotherapy was initiated, there was a significant reduction in FDG uptake in the area of the lesions except in the mediastinal lymph node. This implied incomplete resolution of the MAC-IRIS-related inflammation. Anti-mycobacterial chemotherapy was continued because of the residual lesion. To date, the patient has not experienced a recurrence of MAC-IRIS, a period of nine months.

(Continued on next page)

* Correspondence: ishii@z6.keio.jp
[1]Division of Pulmonary Medicine, Department of Medicine, Keio University School of Medicine, 35 Shinanomachi, Shinjuku-ku, Tokyo 160-8582, Japan
Full list of author information is available at the end of the article

(Continued from previous page)

Conclusion: We present a case of MAC-IRIS in an HIV-infected patient whose disease activity was successfully followed up using ^{18}F-FDG PET/CT. Our data suggest that ^{18}F-FDG PET/CT is useful for evaluating the disease activity of NTM-IRIS and assessing the appropriate duration of anti-mycobacterial chemotherapy for NTM-IRIS in HIV-infected patients.

Keywords: Immune reconstitution inflammatory syndrome, Human immunodeficiency virus, Nontuberculous mycobacteria, *Mycobacterium avium* complex, ^{18}F-fluorodeoxyglucose positron emission tomography/computed tomography

Background

Combined antiretroviral therapy (cART) targeting the human immunodeficiency virus (HIV) has dramatically improved the prognosis of HIV-infected patients by suppressing HIV and restoring the disrupted host immune system [1]. During host immune recovery after the initiation of cART, a subset of HIV-infected patients experience a paradoxical worsening of coexisting infections or the appearance of new diseases; this has been named the immune reconstitution inflammatory syndrome (IRIS). Since IRIS, a fatal complication, occurs in 13 % of HIV-infected patients, the clinical importance of these patients has increased in the cART era [2]. IRIS is associated with a variety of medical conditions including cytomegalovirus retinitis, cryptococcal meningitis, tuberculosis (TB), progressive multifocal leukoencephalopathy, and herpes zoster infection [2]. Among these IRIS conditions, nontuberculous mycobacteria (NTM)-associated IRIS (NTM-IRIS) is one of the most difficult diseases to manage since it often results in a poor prognosis, even if intensive anti-NTM chemotherapy is initiated [3]. A detailed clinical characterization of NTM-IRIS should be performed to establish an appropriate management strategy for NTM-IRIS; however, only a few reports have described detailed clinical findings, and radiological findings are lacking [4].

Recently, ^{18}F-fluorodeoxyglucose (FDG) positron emission tomography/computed tomography (^{18}F-FDG PET/CT) has been used for diagnosing fever of unknown origin and acquired immunodeficiency syndrome (AIDS)- and non-AIDS-related cancers in HIV-infected patients [5–7]. In addition, the methodology has been suggested as a potential tool for evaluating the responsiveness of TB infection to anti-tuberculous therapy in HIV-infected patients [8]. However, there have been no case reports of patients with NTM-IRIS whose disease activity was assessed using ^{18}F-FDG PET/CT. Herein, we report a case of an HIV-infected patient with *Mycobacterium avium* complex (MAC)-associated IRIS (MAC-IRIS) that was successfully followed up using ^{18}F-FDG PET/CT.

Case presentation

A 44-year-old homosexual Japanese man was referred to our hospital with fever and dyspnea. *Pneumocystis jiroveci* pneumonia (PCP) was diagnosed using a sputum smear, and the patient was found to be positive for HIV. At the time of the HIV/AIDS diagnosis, the patient's CD4-positive T cell count was 11 cells/μL, and his HIV-RNA viral load was 2.0×10^6 copies/mL. The patient was an ex-smoker (5 pack-years) and social drinker. Two months after the successful treatment of PCP, chest radiograph findings returned to almost normal (Fig. 1a), and cART was started with emtricitabine/tenofovir (200 mg/300 mg daily), darunavir (400 mg daily), and ritonavir (100 mg daily). Due to the low CD4-positive T cell count, sulfamethoxazole/trimethoprim (400 mg/80 mg daily) and azithromycin (1000 mg weekly) were prophylactically prescribed.

Five months after the initiation of the cART, a chest radiograph displayed bilateral infiltrates of the upper lung fields and bilateral hilar lymphadenopathy (Fig. 1b). Consistently, a high-resolution computed tomography (CT) scan revealed bilateral infiltrates of the upper lobe of the lungs and mediastinal and bilateral hilar lymphadenopathy (Fig. 2a–2d). However, the patient did not have any symptoms such as fever, general fatigue, or respiratory symptoms (including cough and purulent sputum). For further radiological investigation, ^{18}F-FDG PET/CT was performed. It showed intense accumulation of FDG corresponding to the lesions of the infiltrates as well as the mediastinal and bilateral hilar lymphadenopathy (maximum standardized uptake value: 18.42; Fig. 2e and 2f). The differential diagnosis of the lung infiltrates and lymphadenopathy at that time included NTM-IRIS, TB-IRIS, sarcoidosis, malignant lymphoma, fungal infection, and Kaposi's sarcoma.

The patient was admitted to the Keio University Hospital for further investigations. At the time of admission, vital signs and physiological examinations were normal except for a bilateral deep cervical lymphadenopathy. The results of blood tests are shown in Table 1. The patient's white blood cell count (2900/μL) and hemoglobin levels (12.2 g/dL) were low, while alkaline phosphatase levels (403 IU/L) were high. The concentrations of C-reactive protein (0.13 mg/dL), anti-glycopeptidolipid core IgA antibody (<0.1 U/mL), angiotensin-converting enzyme (16.2 IU/mL), and soluble interleukin-2

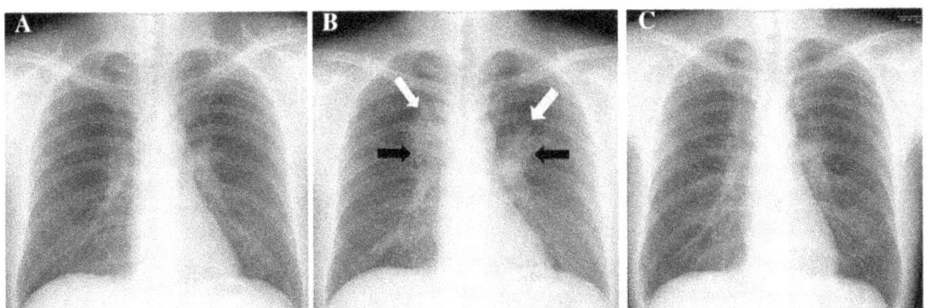

Fig. 1 Serial changes on chest radiograph. **a** Chest radiograph taken at the time of starting combined antiretroviral therapy (cART), showing almost normal findings. **b** Chest radiograph taken five months after starting cART, showing infiltrates in the bilateral upper lung fields (white arrow) and bilateral hilar lymphadenopathy (black arrow). **c** Chest radiograph taken one year after starting anti-mycobacterial chemotherapy, showing slight hilar lymphadenopathy

receptor (482 U/mL) were unremarkable. The CD4-positive T cell count had risen to 125 cells/μL, while the HIV-RNA viral load had decreased to undetectable levels. A smear was negative for acid-fast bacilli. Blood and sputum cultures were negative for bacteria and mycobacteria. We performed an endobronchial biopsy of the endobronchial mass and a bronchial wash of the left upper lobe bronchus (Fig. 3a, 3b). Histological examination of the biopsy specimen revealed granulomatous change but was negative for malignancy, human herpes virus-8, and fungi such as *Aspergillus* species and *Cryptococcus* species. Caseating granuloma, the typical histological finding of mycobacteria (including *Mycobacterium tuberculosis* and NTM), was not identified in the specimen. Although the smear test was negative for mycobacteria, a bronchial wash culture that was performed later was positive for MAC. Accordingly, the patient was diagnosed with MAC-IRIS, and anti-MAC chemotherapy with rifampicin (450 mg daily), ethambutol (750 mg daily), clarithromycin (800 mg daily), and levofloxacin (500 mg daily) was started. Since we could not exclude the possibility of TB or TB-IRIS, we added isoniazid (300 mg per day) to the chemotherapy regimen. We also changed the cART regimen from darunavir and ritonavir to raltegravir to avoid a potential drug interaction.

We did not consider using concomitant non-steroidal anti-inflammatory drugs or steroids for two reasons: 1) the patient was able to continue anti-mycobacterial chemotherapy without remarkable side effects and 2) his chest radiograph findings showed a gradual improvement in the bilateral upper lung field and the hilar lymphadenopathy. One year after the introduction of the anti-mycobacterial chemotherapy, chest radiograph and high-resolution CT findings showed slight hilar lymphadenopathy (Figs. 1c, 2g, and 2h). To evaluate disease activity more precisely, ^{18}F-FDG PET-CT was performed. It showed a marked reduction in FDG uptake, but accumulation of FDG was still seen in a right lower paratracheal lymph node (station #4R; maximum standardized uptake value: 6.24), implying incomplete resolution of the NTM-IRIS-associated inflammation. Based on these findings, we continued anti-mycobacterial chemotherapy for an additional nine months to the present date. The patient has not experienced any further recurrence of NTM-IRIS as assessed based on his symptoms and chest radiographs.

Conclusion

MAC infection often causes disseminated disease in patients with AIDS. On the other hand, MAC can also present as IRIS after the initiation of cART in HIV-infected patients. MAC-IRIS occurs in about 3.5 % of HIV-infected patients treated with cART, and 20 % of MAC-IRIS is fatal [2]. No case reports have evaluated the long-term radiological findings of MAC-IRIS.

To our knowledge, this is the first case report of an HIV-infected patient with MAC-IRIS whose disease activity was followed up and evaluated using ^{18}F-FDG PET/CT. Although there are no established guidelines for the management of NTM-IRIS, several approaches have been suggested, such as the interruption of cART and the initiation of anti-NTM chemotherapy in combination with or without non-steroidal anti-inflammatory drugs or steroids [3]. However, since the interruption of cART can exacerbate the immunosuppressed status in HIV-infected patients, it is preferable to avoid choosing the interruption of cART, if possible. In particular, the interruption of cART can result drug-resistant HIV. In the current case, we chose only anti-NTM chemotherapy to avoid these risks.

It is important to evaluate whether anti-MAC chemotherapy for MAC-IRIS has been successful in clinical settings. Clinicians can use ^{18}F-FDG PET/CT to assess the accumulation of FDG as well as to determine the size of a lesion to determine disease activity. Previous studies that assessed TB disease activity in an HIV-infected patient showed that ^{18}F-FDG PET/CT had a

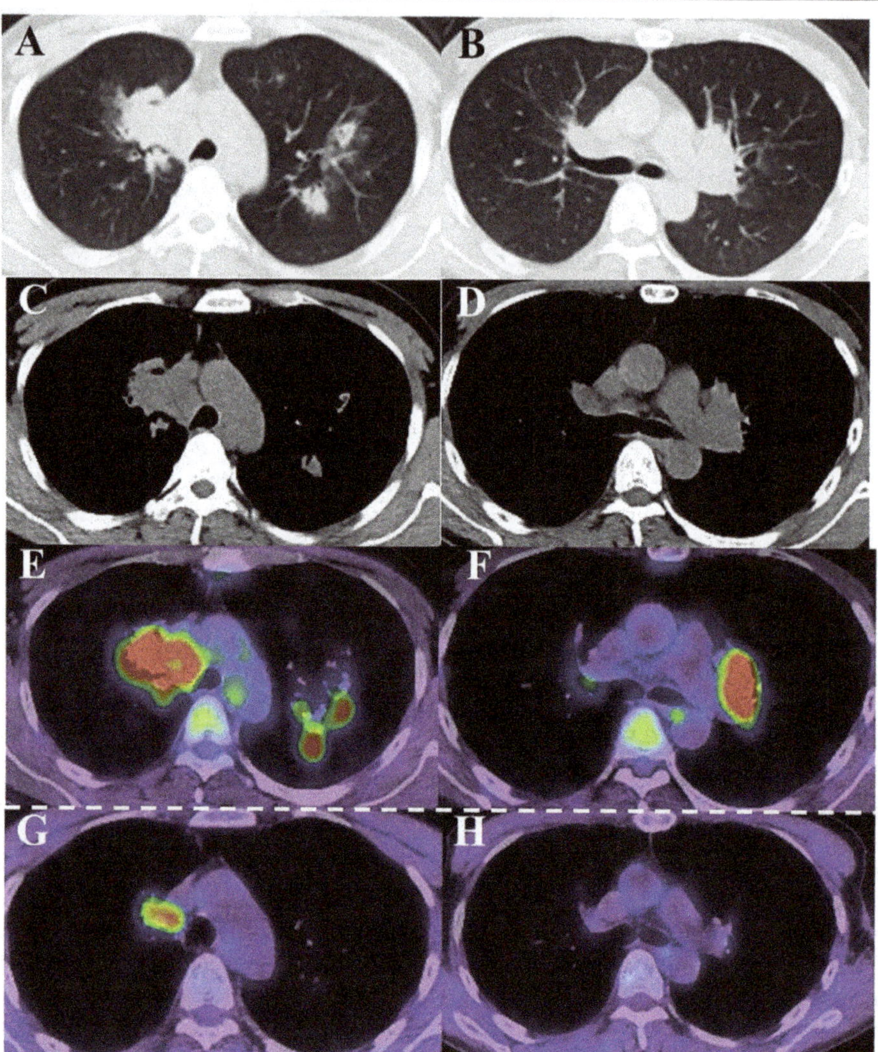

Fig. 2 Chest computed tomography and ^{18}F-fluorodeoxyglucose positron emission tomography-computed tomography findings. **a–d** A computed tomography scan performed five months after starting cART showed bilateral infiltrates in the upper lobes of the lungs and mediastinal and bilateral hilar lymphadenopathy. **e, f** The ^{18}F-fluorodeoxyglucosepositron emission tomography-computed tomography (^{18}F-FDG PET/CT) scan performed five months after starting cART showed intense accumulation of fluorodeoxyglucose (FDG) around the infiltrates and the mediastinal and bilateral hilar lymphadenopathy (maximum standardized uptake value: 18.42). **g, h** The ^{18}F-fluorodeoxyglucose positron emission tomography-computed tomography (^{18}F-FDG PET/CT) scan performed one year after starting anti-mycobacterial chemotherapy showed a decreased uptake of FDG when compared to the scan performed five months after starting combined antiretroviral therapy (cART). Moreover, a reduction in FDG uptake was observed in the area of the lesions with the exception of a right-lower paratracheal lymph node (station #4R; maximum standardized uptake value: 6.24)

high sensitivity and specificity in distinguishing TB-infected HIV patients who responded to anti-mycobacterial chemotherapy from those who did not [8, 9]. Since a high FDG accumulation has also been reported in the lesions of patients with non-HIV MAC infections, it is reasonable to consider utilizing ^{18}F-FDG PET/CT in MAC-infected HIV patients [10].

The usefulness of serological inflammatory markers for evaluating the disease activity of mycobacterium-associated IRIS in HIV-infected patients remains controversial. In fact, C-reactive protein levels, white blood cell counts, and erythrocyte sedimentation rates were not elevated in the present case.

The optimal duration of anti-mycobacterial chemotherapy in regards to the disease activity of NTM-IRIS remains unknown [11]. In particular, patients with MAC-IRIS tend to relapse frequently after treatments such as anti-mycobacterial chemotherapy or steroids [3]. ^{18}F-FDG PET/CT imaging may help determine the appropriate duration of anti-mycobacterial chemotherapy. In the present case, considering the residual inflammation observed in ^{18}F-FDG PET/CT, we continued the

Table 1 Laboratory findings on admission

Complete blood count	
White blood cells	2900/μL
Band cells + segmented cells	63.8 %
Lymphocytes	24.9 %
Monocytes	7.7 %
Eosinophil granulocytes	3.2 %
Basophil granulocytes	0.4 %
Hemoglobin	12.2 g/dL
Mean corpuscular volume	77/fL
Platelets	16.9×10^4/μL
Biochemistry	
Total protein	6.4 g/dL
Albumin	4.2 g/dL
Total bilirubin	0.3 mg/dL
Aspartate transaminase	18 IU/L
Alanine transaminase	13 IU/L
Lactate dehydrogenase	184 IU/L
Urea nitrogen	8.9 mg/dL
Creatinine	0.68 mg/dL
Sodium	137.7 mEq/L
Potassium	3.8 mEq/L
Chloride	104 mEq/L
Alkaline phosphatase	403 IU/L
Serological studies	
C-reactive protein	0.13 mg/dL
β-D-glucan	4.4 pg/mL
Aspergillus antigen	0.1 COI
Cryptococcus antigen	0.0 COI
QuantiFERON® TB Gold test	Negative
Anti-glycopeptidolipid core IgA antibody	<0.1 U/mL
Angiotensin-converting enzyme	16.2 IU/mL
Soluble interleukin-2 receptor	482 U/mL
CD4 positive T cells	125 counts/μL
HIV RNA viral load	<20 copies/mL

anti-mycobacterial therapy. According to the study by Demura et al., a maximum standardized uptake value greater than 4.0 is generally compatible with highly active mycobacterial granuloma lesions. Since the maximum standardized uptake value was still 6.24 one year after introducing anti-mycobacterial chemotherapy, it was continued [12]. This treatment strategy could contribute to preventing the patient's relapse with MAC-IRIS.

The use of ^{18}F-FDG PET/CT for assessing disease activity of MAC in HIV-infected patients has several limitations. First, the possibility of malignancy should be considered, since there has been an increase in both

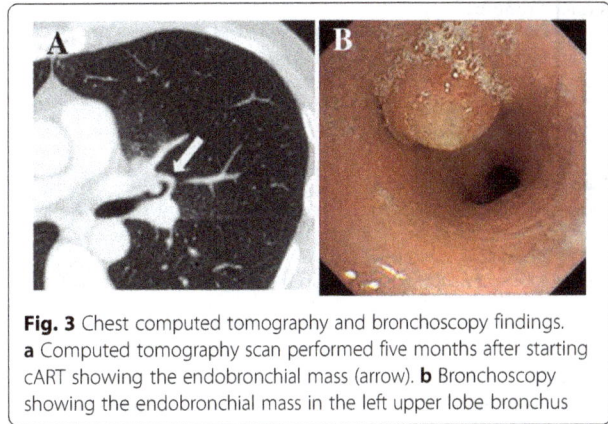

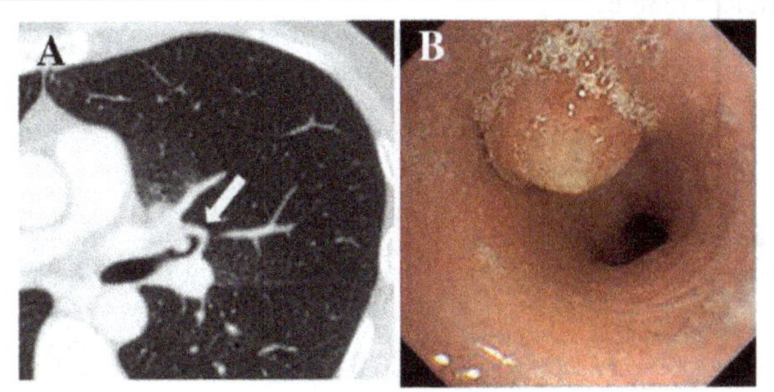

Fig. 3 Chest computed tomography and bronchoscopy findings. **a** Computed tomography scan performed five months after starting cART showing the endobronchial mass (arrow). **b** Bronchoscopy showing the endobronchial mass in the left upper lobe bronchus

AIDS- and non-AIDS-related cancers in HIV-infected patients. The maximum standardized uptake of FDG cannot differentiate malignancy from other inflammatory diseases [13]. Therefore, pathology and culture results remain important for an accurate diagnosis. In the case presented herein, sputum and gastric fluid samples were negative for acid-fast bacteria, except for the positive culture from the bronchial wash fluid, although the culture tests were repeated several times. We speculate that there was only a small amount of MAC in the lesion. Thus, the culture of the bronchial wash fluid is essential for the diagnosis of MAC-associated lung disease. FDG uptake can have false positive results in an HIV patient with poor virus control, because areas of HIV replication in lymphoid tissue can contribute to FDG accumulation in the tissue [14]. Therefore, assessment of FDG accumulation should be undertaken with great care, particularly in cases of HIV with uncontrolled HIV RNA levels.

In conclusion, ^{18}F-FDG PET/CT can be useful for evaluating NTM-IRIS disease activity and assessing the appropriate duration of anti-mycobacterial chemotherapy in HIV-infected patients with NTM-IRIS.

Consent

Written informed consent was obtained from the patient for publication of this case report and any accompanying images. A copy of the written consent is available for review by this journal.

Abbreviations

AIDS: Acquired immunodeficiency syndrome; cART: Combined antiretroviral therapy; CT: Computed tomography; FDG: Fluorodeoxyglucose; HIV: Human immunodeficiency virus; IRIS: Immune reconstitution inflammatory syndrome; MAC: *Mycobacterium avium* complex; NTM: Nontuberculous mycobacteria; PCP: *Pneumocystis jiroveci* pneumonia; TB: Tuberculosis; ^{18}F-FDG PET/CT: ^{18}F-fluorodeoxyglucose positron emission tomography/computed tomography.

Competing interests

The authors state that they have no conflicts of interest.

Authors' contributions

HN drafted the manuscript. HN, HF, KY, MH, MM, FS, KF, TB, and NH contributed to the diagnosis and treatment. HN, HF, and NH obtained the patient's written informed consent. NH conceived the study. MI, SS, TA, ST, and TB reviewed the manuscript. All the authors read and approved the final version of the manuscript.

Author details

[1]Division of Pulmonary Medicine, Department of Medicine, Keio University School of Medicine, 35 Shinanomachi, Shinjuku-ku, Tokyo 160-8582, Japan. [2]Japan Society for the Promotion of Science, Tokyo, Japan. [3]Center for Infectious Diseases and Infection Control, Keio University School of Medicine, Tokyo, Japan.

References

1. Sterne JA, Hernán MA, Ledergerber B, Tilling K, Weber R, Sendi P, et al. Long-term effectiveness of potent antiretroviral therapy in preventing AIDS and death: a prospective cohort study. Lancet. 2005;366:378–84.
2. Müller M, Wandel S, Colebunders R, Attia S, Furrer H, Egger M, et al. Immune reconstitution inflammatory syndrome in patients starting antiretroviral therapy for HIV infection: a systematic review and meta-analysis. Lancet Infect Dis. 2010;10:251–61.
3. Phillips P, Bonner S, Gataric N, Bai T, Wilcox P, Hogg R, et al. Nontuberculous mycobacterial immune reconstitution syndrome in HIV-infected patients: spectrum of disease and long-term follow-up. Clin Infect Dis. 2005;15:1483–97.
4. Buckingham SJ, Haddow LJ, Shaw PJ, Miller RF. Immune reconstitution inflammatory syndrome in HIV-infected patients with mycobacterial infections starting highly active anti-retroviral therapy. Clin Radiol. 2004;59:505–13.
5. Castaigne C, Tondeur M, de Wit S, Hildebrand M, Clumeck N, Dusart M. Clinical value of FDG-PET/CT for the diagnosis of human immunodeficiency virus-associated fever of unknown origin: a retrospective study. Nucl Med Commun. 2009;30:41–7.
6. Just PA, Fieschi C, Baillet G, Galicier L, Oksenhendler E, Moretti JL. 18 F-fluorodeoxyglucose positron emission tomography/computed tomography in AIDS-related Burkitt lymphoma. AIDS Patient Care STDS. 2008;22:695–700.
7. Sathekge M, Maes A, Kgomo M, Pottel H, Stolz A, Van De Wiele C. FDG uptake in lymph-nodes of HIV+ and tuberculosis patients: implications for cancer staging. Q J Nucl Med Mol Imaging. 2010;54:698–703.
8. Sathekge M, Maes A, D'Asseler Y, Vorster M, Gongxeka H, Van de Wiele C. Tuberculous lymphadenitis: FDG PET and CT findings in responsive and nonresponsive disease. Eur J Nucl Med Mol Imaging. 2012;39:1184–90.
9. Vorster M, Sathekge MM, Bomanji J. Advances in imaging of tuberculosis: the role of ^{18}F-FDG PET and PET/CT. Curr Opin Pulm Med. 2014;20:287–93.
10. Kawate E, Yamazaki M, Kohno T, Fujimori S, Takahashi H. Two cases with solitary pulmonary nodule due to non-tuberculous mycobacterial infection showing intense 18 F-fluorodeoxyglucose uptake on positron emission tomography scan. Geriatr Gerontol Int. 2010;10:251–4.
11. Masur H, Brooks JT, Benson CA, Holmes KK, Pau AK, Kaplan JE. Prevention and treatment of opportunistic infections in HIV-infected adults and adolescents: Updated Guidelines from the Centers for Disease Control and Prevention, National Institutes of Health, and HIV Medicine Association of the Infectious Diseases Society of America. Clin Infect Dis. 2014;58:1308–11.
12. Demura Y, Tsuchida T, Uesaka D, Umeda Y, Morikawa M, Ameshima S, et al. Usefulness of 18 F-fluorodeoxyglucose positron emission tomography for diagnosing disease activity and monitoring therapeutic response in patients with pulmonary mycobacteriosis. Eur J Nucl Med Mol Imaging. 2009;36:632–9.
13. Sathekge M, Maes A, Van de Wiele C. FDG-PET imaging in HIV infection and tuberculosis. Semin Nucl Med. 2013;43:349–66.
14. Brust D, Polis M, Davey R, Hahn B, Bacharach S, Whatley M, et al. Fluorodeoxyglucose imaging in healthy subjects with HIV infection: impact of disease stage and therapy on pattern of nodal activation. AIDS. 2006;20:495–503.

Osteoporosis imaging: effects of bone preservation on MDCT-based trabecular bone microstructure parameters and finite element models

Thomas Baum[1*], Eduardo Grande Garcia[1,2], Rainer Burgkart[2], Olga Gordijenko[1], Hans Liebl[1], Pia M. Jungmann[1], Michael Gruber[3], Tina Zahel[1], Ernst J. Rummeny[1], Simone Waldt[1] and Jan S. Bauer[4]

Abstract

Background: Osteoporosis is defined as a skeletal disorder characterized by compromised bone strength due to a reduction of bone mass and deterioration of bone microstructure predisposing an individual to an increased risk of fracture. Trabecular bone microstructure analysis and finite element models (FEM) have shown to improve the prediction of bone strength beyond bone mineral density (BMD) measurements. These computational methods have been developed and validated in specimens preserved in formalin solution or by freezing. However, little is known about the effects of preservation on trabecular bone microstructure and FEM. The purpose of this observational study was to investigate the effects of preservation on trabecular bone microstructure and FEM in human vertebrae.

Methods: Four thoracic vertebrae were harvested from each of three fresh human cadavers ($n = 12$). Multi-detector computed tomography (MDCT) images were obtained at baseline, 3 and 6 month follow-up. In the intervals between MDCT imaging, two vertebrae from each donor were formalin-fixed and frozen, respectively. BMD, trabecular bone microstructure parameters (histomorphometry and fractal dimension), and FEM-based apparent compressive modulus (ACM) were determined in the MDCT images and validated by mechanical testing to failure of the vertebrae after 6 months.

Results: Changes of BMD, trabecular bone microstructure parameters, and FEM-based ACM in formalin-fixed and frozen vertebrae over 6 months ranged between 1.0–5.6 % and 1.3–6.1 %, respectively, and were not statistically significant ($p > 0.05$). BMD, trabecular bone microstructure parameters, and FEM-based ACM as assessed at baseline, 3 and 6 month follow-up correlated significantly with mechanically determined failure load ($r = 0.89$–0.99; $p < 0.05$). The correlation coefficients r were not significantly different for the two preservation methods ($p > 0.05$).

Conclusions: Formalin fixation and freezing up to six months showed no significant effects on trabecular bone microstructure and FEM-based ACM in human vertebrae and may both be used in corresponding in-vitro experiments in the context of osteoporosis.

Keywords: Osteoporosis, Bone preservation, Trabecular bone microstructure, Finite element model

* Correspondence: thbaum@gmx.de
[1]Institut für Radiologie, Klinikum rechts der Isar, Technische Universität München, Ismaninger Str. 22, 81675 München, Germany
Full list of author information is available at the end of the article

Background

Osteoporosis is defined as a skeletal disorder characterized by compromised bone strength due to a reduction of bone mass and deterioration of bone microstructure predisposing an individual to an increased risk of fracture [1]. Osteoporotic vertebral and hip fractures are associated with an increased mortality [2]. Due to the aging population, the prevalence of osteoporosis and consecutively the incidence of osteoporotic fractures is expected to increase [3]. Therefore, osteoporosis is classified as public health problem.

The World Health Organisation (WHO) based the diagnosis of osteoporosis on the measurement of bone mineral density (BMD) at the spine and hip using dual-energy X-ray absorptiometry (DXA) [4]. Alternatively, BMD can be assessed by using quantitative computed tomography (QCT). QCT allows for the assessment of volumetric BMD (vBMD), in contrast to DXA assessing areal BMD (aBMD) [5]. Importantly, BMD values often underestimate fracture risk, since osteoporotic fractures frequently occur in patients with non-pathological BMD values [6, 7]. Therefore, considerable research effort has been undertaken to improve fracture risk prediction by using high-resolution imaging techniques including high-resolution peripheral quantitative computed tomography (hr-pQCT), multi-detector computed tomography (MDCT), and magnetic resonance imaging (MRI) [8]. Trabecular bone microstructure parameters and finite element models (FEM) have been computed in the acquired images which significantly improved prediction of bone strength beyond BMD [9]. These computational methods have been developed in human specimens in-vitro and validated with mechanical bone strength measurements as gold standard.

After harvesting, the specimens are usually preserved in formalin solution or are frozen until imaging and mechanical testing is performed. Previous studies have reported that human cortical and trabecular bone samples showed no significant differences in their mechanical properties and tissue parameters (including mineral and lipid content and composition) after freezing or formalin fixation up to several weeks [10, 11]. However, weakened viscoelastic and plastic properties of bovine, murine, and human bone by formalin fixation up to six months were demonstrated as compared to freezing [12–14]. Lochmüller et al. reported that DXA-based BMD measurements in human cadavers within 48 h of death and after 10 months of formalin fixation were not significantly different [15].

Little is known about the effects of preservation on trabecular bone microstructure and FEM in human bone specimens. Therefore, the purpose of our study was to investigate the effects of preservation (formalin fixation and freezing) on trabecular bone microstructure and FEM in intact, human vertebrae as determined by MDCT imaging at baseline, 3 and 6 month follow-up and validated by mechanical testing to failure of the vertebrae after 6 months.

Methods

Specimens

Donors with a history of pathological bone changes other than osteoporosis (i.e., bone metastases, hematological, or metabolic bone disorders) were excluded at the outset. Four thoracic vertebrae between the thoracic vertebra 5 and 12 were harvested from each of three fresh human cadavers ($n = 12$). The donors consisted of one osteoporotic woman aged 74 years and two non-osteoporotic men aged 46 and 62 years, respectively. They had dedicated their body for educational and research purposes to the local Institute of Anatomy in compliance with local institutional and legislative requirements. The study protocol was reviewed and approved by the local Institutional Review Boards (Ethikkommission der Fakultaet fuer Medizin der Technischen Universitaet Muenchen). The surrounding muscle, fat tissue, and intervertebral discs were completely removed from the vertebrae. Each vertebra was embedded in resin (Rencast Isocyanat and Polyol, Huntsman Group, Bad Säckingen, Germany) up to 2 mm above respectively below their vertebral endplates for the purpose of mechanical testing. The resin fixation was performed with parallel alignment of the upper and lower endplate of the vertebrae with the outer surface of the resin chock to guarantee strict axial loading conditions of the vertebrae during the uniaxial mechanical test.

MDCT imaging was performed at baseline, 3 and 6 month follow-up. In the intervals between the MDCT acquisitions, two vertebrae from each donor were stored in a 3.5 % formalin solution, while the other two vertebrae were stored in sealed plastic bags in a freezer at −40 °C. The vertebrae in the freezer were defrosted for 18 h at 20 °C before 3 and 6 month follow-up MDCT imaging, respectively. All vertebrae were degassed in sodium chloride solution at least 3 h before MDCT imaging to prevent air artifacts. The vertebrae were sealed in vacuum plastic boxes filled with sodium chloride solution during MDCT imaging.

Imaging

MDCT images of the vertebrae at baseline, 3 and 6 month follow-up were acquired by using a clinical whole-body 256-row CT scanner (iCT, Philips Medical Care, Best, Netherlands). Scan parameters were a tube voltage of 120 kVp, a tube load of 585 mAs, an image matrix of 1024 × 1024 pixels, and a field of view of 150 mm. Transverse sections were reconstructed with a high-resolution bone kernel (YE). The interpolated voxel size was of 146 × 146 × 300 μm^3, while the real spatial resolution, as determined at ρ50 of the modulation-transfer-function, was 250 × 250 × 600 μm^3. A dedicated calibration phantom (Mindways Osteoporosis Phantom, San Francisco, CA, USA) was placed in the scanner mat beneath the vertebrae.

Assessment of BMD and trabecular bone microstructure

MDCT images obtained at baseline, 3 and 6 month follow-up were transferred to a remote LINUX workstation and loaded into an in-house developed program based on IDL (Interactive Data Language, Research Systems, Bolder, CO, USA). Firstly, the 15 most central slices displaying the vertebra equidistant to its endplates were identified. Then, 15 circular regions of interest (ROIs) were manually placed in the ventral half of the vertebral body in the selected slices of the MDCT images similar to QCT-based BMD measurements [5]. The circular ROIs had a diameter of 10 mm (Fig. 1). ROIs' pixel attenuations in [HU; Hounsfield Units] were converted into BMD values in [mg/cm^3 calcium hydroxyapatite] by using the calibration phantom. Afterwards, MDCT images were binarized to calculate trabecular bone microstructure parameters. An optimized global threshold was applied to all MDCT images. Similar to previous studies, 200 mg/cm^3 calcium hydroxyapatite was identified as optimized global threshold [16, 17]. Four morphometric parameters were calculated in the ROIs in analogy to standard histomorphometry using the mean intercept length method [18]: bone volume divided by total volume (BV/TV), trabecular number (TbN; [mm^{-1}]), trabecular separation (TbSp; [mm]), and trabecular thickness (TbTh; [mm]). Parameters were labeled as apparent (app.) values, since given the limited spatial resolution they cannot depict the true trabecular microstructure. Furthermore, fractal dimension (FD) as texture measurement of the trabecular bone microstructure was determined in the MDCT images using a box counting algorithm as previously described [16]. The reproducibility error expressed as the root mean square error coefficient of variation amounted to 1.2 % for BMD and ranged between 0.5 % and 2.0 % as outlined in a previous study [16].

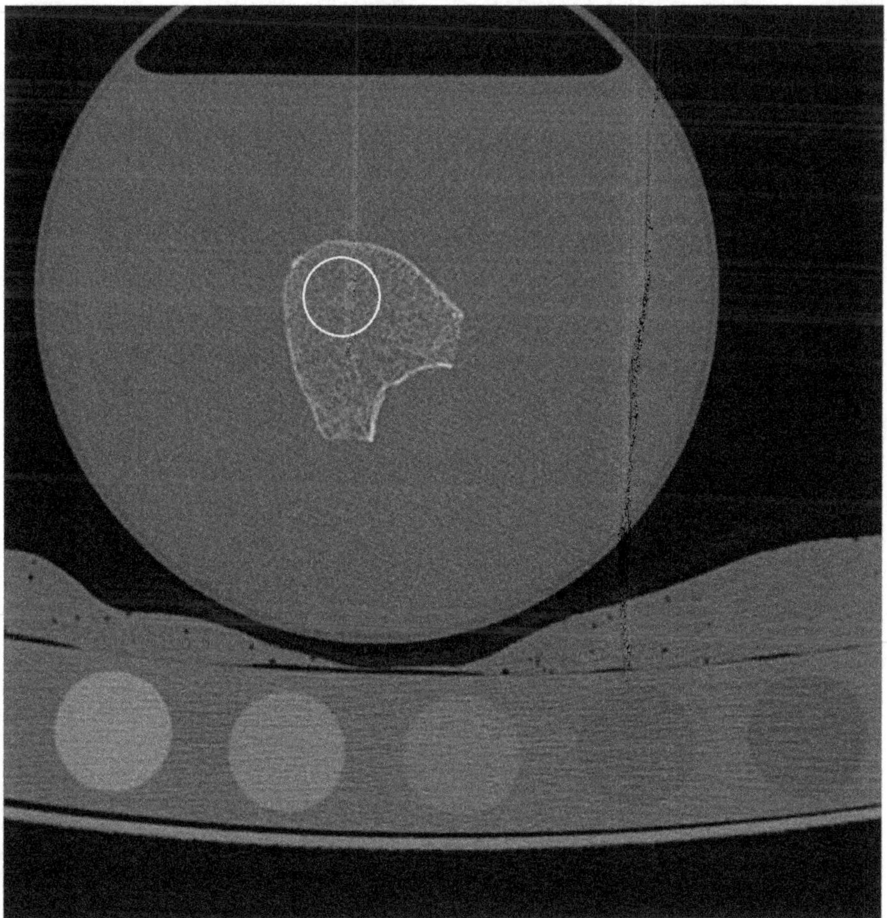

Fig. 1 Representative MDCT image of a vertebra: a circular region of interest (white) was placed in the ventral half of the vertebral body in the 15 most central slices equidistant to its endplates. The calibration phantom was positioned below the plastic box containing the vertebrae

FEM

Finite element models (FEM) were computed in the baseline, 3 and 6 month follow-up MDCT images to assess apparent compressive modulus (ACM) of each vertebral body in the superior-inferior direction. Three-dimensional models of the vertebrae were created from the MDCT images by identifying the contour of the vertebrae. The in-plane MDCT resolution was selected as mesh refinement. The uniform hexahedral meshes were generated by using ANSYS Workbench (ANSYS, Canonsburg, PA, USA). The material properties of each element were assigned by using a mapping procedure. Firstly, the elements' values in [HU] were converted into BMD values ρ_{BMD} in [g/cm^3 calcium hydroxyapatite] by using the calibration phantom. Secondly, the elements' information (position and ρ_{BMD}) were saved in a text file. Thirdly, a subroutine written in APDL (ANSYS Parametric Design Language) was used to read the text file and assign the material properties to each element (Fig. 2). The equation $\rho_{ash} = 1.22\ \rho_{BMD} + 0.0526\ g/cm3$ was used for the conversion of ρ_{BMD} into ρ_{ash} [19, 20]. The isotropic elastic modulus E in [N/mm^2] was determined for each element by using the established relationships between E and ρ_{ash} as reported previously [21–23]: $E = 33900\rho_{ash}^{2.20}$; $\rho_{ash} \le 0.27$, $E = 5307\rho_{ash} + 469$; $0.27 < \rho_{ash} < 0.6$, and $E = 10200\ \rho_{ash}^{2.01}$; $\rho_{ash} \ge 0.6$. Each element was assigned a Poisson's ratio of $\nu = 0.3$ [23]. Finally, the apparent compressive modulus (ACM) of the FEMs in [N/mm^2] was obtained by applying a displacement force on one vertebral endplate and fixing the opposite one.

Mechanical testing

After 6 month follow-up MDCT imaging, the resin embedded vertebrae were fixed in a mechanical testing system (Wolpert Werkstoffprüfmaschinen AG, Schaffhausen, Switzerland). The mechanical testing was performed similar to previous studies [16, 24, 25]. Firstly, ten preconditioning cycles with uniaxial tension-compression up

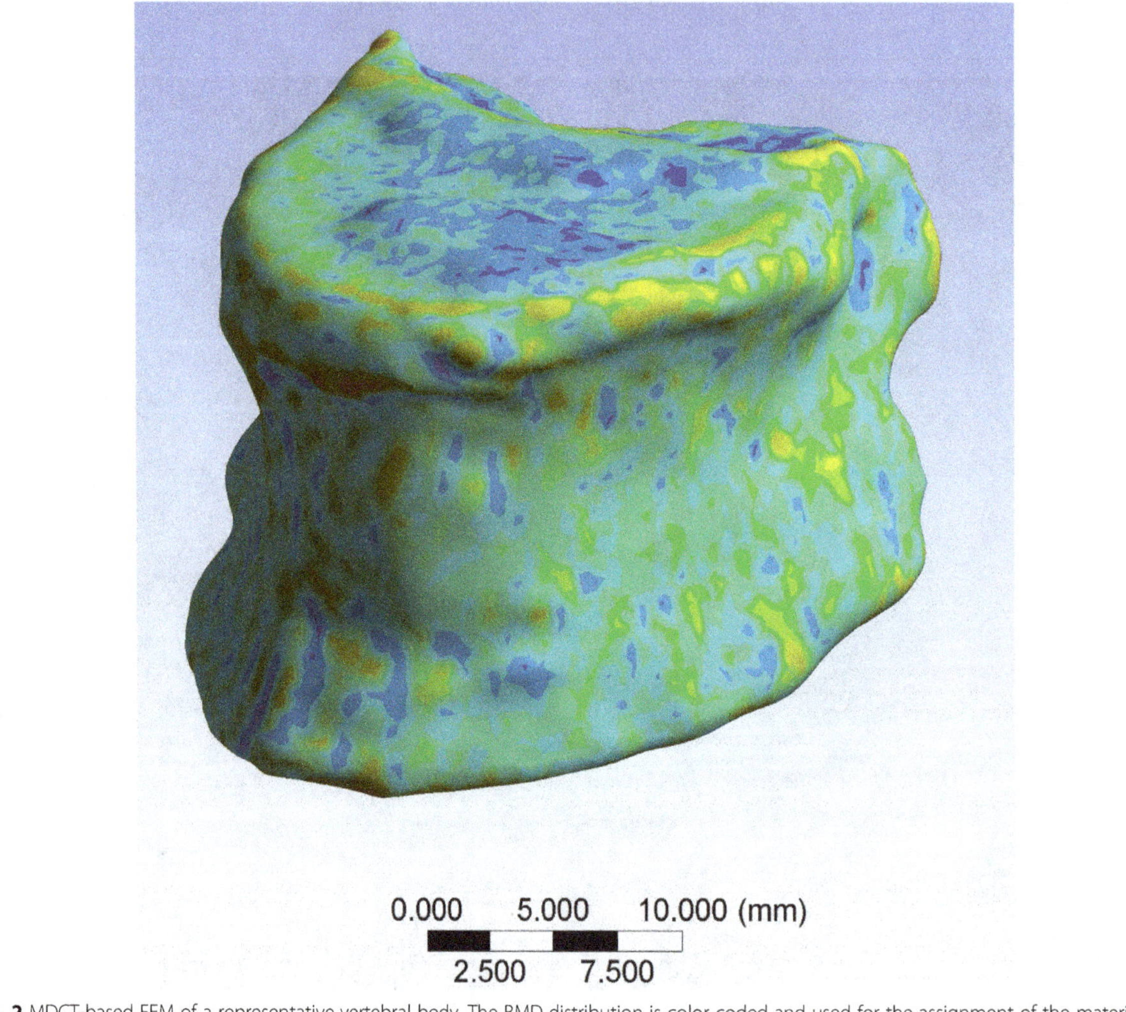

Fig. 2 MDCT-based FEM of a representative vertebral body. The BMD distribution is color-coded and used for the assignment of the material properties for each element of the FEM

to a load between 10 N and 400 N with a rate of 5 mm/min were applied. Then, a monotonic, uniaxial compression was performed at the same rate. The load–displacement curve was recorded and vertebral failure load (FL) was defined as the first peak of the load–displacement curve with a subsequent drop of >10 %.

Statistical analysis

The statistical analyses were performed with SPSS (SPSS, Chicago, IL, USA). All tests were done using a two-sided 0.05 level of significance. Mean and standard deviation (SD) of FEM-based ACM, BMD, and trabecular bone microstructure parameters were calculated at each time point separately for the formalin-fixed and frozen vertebrae. The Kolmogorov-Smirnov test showed for most parameters a significant difference from a normal distribution ($p < 0.05$). Therefore, changes of FEM-based ACM, BMD, and trabecular bone microstructure parameters over 6 months were assessed by using the Friedmann test separately for the formalin-fixed and frozen vertebrae. The root-mean-square coefficients of variation (RMSCV) in [%] were calculated to express the changes of each parameter over time [26]. Correlations between FEM-based ACM, BMD, and trabecular bone microstructure parameters with FL were evaluated with the Spearman's rank correlation coefficient (r). Significant differences between correlation coefficients were assessed by using the Fisher Z transformation.

Results

Failure load values of all specimens are shown in Table 1. Mean ± SD of FEM-based ACM, BMD, and trabecular bone microstructure parameters of the formalin-fixed and frozen vertebrae at baseline, 3 and 6 month follow-up are listed in Table 2. Changes of the computed parameters expressed as RMSCV ranged between 1.0–5.6 % and 1.3–6.1 % in formalin-fixed and frozen vertebrae, respectively (Table 2). Neither formalin fixation nor freezing significantly changed the computed parameters over six months ($p > 0.05$; Table 2).

Table 1 Failure load values in [N] for each specimen

ID	Preservation	Failure load
Donor 1 vertebra 1	frozen	3181
Donor 1 vertebra 2	formalin	3991
Donor 1 vertebra 3	frozen	3719
Donor 1 vertebra 4	formalin	4147
Donor 2 vertebra 1	frozen	1212
Donor 2 vertebra 2	formalin	1912
Donor 2 vertebra 3	frozen	1704
Donor 2 vertebra 4	formalin	1853
Donor 3 vertebra 1	frozen	1951
Donor 3 vertebra 2	formalin	1990
Donor 3 vertebra 3	frozen	2513
Donor 3 vertebra 4	formalin	3141

FEM-based ACM, BMD, and trabecular bone microstructure parameters at baseline, 3 and 6 month follow-up showed significant correlations with FL for both, formalin-fixed and frozen vertebrae ($p < 0.05$; Table 3). Correlations coefficients r ranged between 0.89 and 0.99, and were not significantly different for the two preservation methods as compared by using the Fisher Z transformation ($p > 0.05$).

Discussion

Human bone specimens have been frequently used to assess mechanical features of new orthopedic implants and to validate new computational methods for the improvement of fracture risk prediction in the context of osteoporosis. Fresh bone specimens would represent the best conditions to guarantee the original structural and mechanical properties. However, the availability of fresh specimens is limited and the setup of many studies requires some type of preservation of the bone tissue due to time constraints. Freezing has the advantages of not significant altering the mechanical properties of human bone specimens [11, 14]. The disadvantage of freezing is the risk of infection of investigators working on bone specimens from a variety of pathogens including HIV and the hepatitis virus [27]. Therefore, bone specimens are often embalmed in formalin solution to minimize the risk of infection. Furthermore, bone specimens available from pathology dissections include high numbers of patients with severe diseases. In contrast, specimens from courses of macroscopic dissections are usually embalmed in formalin solution and could be used to constitute more representative study samples [15]. These cadaver bodies are generally stored for one year or more after they are embalmed. However, formalin fixation may alter the mechanical properties, BMD, and trabecular bone microstructure of the specimens which are particularly important in the context of osteoporosis.

Controversial findings have been reported with regard to the changes of the mechanical properties due to formalin fixation. Haaren et al. reported that long-term preservation by freezing or formalin fixation up to one year did not alter the mechanical properties of cortical bone in goats [28]. In contrast, Wilke et al. reported that formalin fixation strongly influences the mechanical properties of calf spines [29]. Consistently, further studies reported weakened viscoelastic and plastic properties of bovine, murine, and human bone by formalin fixation up to six months as compared to freezing [12–14].

Changes of DXA-based BMD measurements at the lumbar spine and proximal femur due to formalin fixation were assessed by Lochmüller et al. in seven intact

Table 2 Mean ± SD of FEM-based ACM, BMD, and trabecular bone microstructure parameters of the formalin-fixed and frozen vertebrae at baseline, 3 and 6 month follow-up. Changes of the computed parameters over 6 months are expressed as root-mean-square coefficients of variation (RMSCV) and were not significant ($p > 0.05$) as assessed by using the Friedmann test

	Preservation	Baseline	3 month follow-up	6 month follow-up	RMSCV [%]	p-value
FEM-based ACM [N/mm^2]	frozen ($n = 6$)	498 ± 214	500 ± 197	504 ± 187	4.0	0.846
FEM-based ACM [N/mm^2]	formalin ($n = 6$)	494 ± 164	480 ± 152	494 ± 162	2.9	0.513
BMD [mg/cm^3]	frozen ($n = 6$)	125 ± 34	125 ± 35	124 ± 36	1.3	0.565
BMD [mg/cm^3]	formalin ($n = 6$)	128 ± 34	129 ± 34	129 ± 34	1.0	0.467
app. BV/TV	frozen ($n = 6$)	0.266 ± 0.121	0.274 ± 0.108	0.277 ± 0.110	5.4	0.311
app. BV/TV	formalin ($n = 6$)	0.269 ± 0.199	0.261 ± 0.123	0.263 ± 0.114	4.0	0.119
app. TbN [mm^{-1}]	frozen ($n = 6$)	0.860 ± 0.270	0.864 ± 0.206	0.894 ± 0.248	4.4	0.311
app. TbN [mm^{-1}]	formalin ($n = 6$)	0.835 ± 0.255	0.832 ± 0.211	0.847 ± 0.264	4.6	0.846
app. TbSp [mm]	frozen ($n = 6$)	0.990 ± 0.479	0.923 ± 0.367	0.910 ± 0.398	6.1	0.223
app. TbSp [mm]	formalin ($n = 6$)	1.048 ± 0.555	1.035 ± 0.507	1.047 ± 0.559	5.6	0.846
app. TbTh [mm]	frozen ($n = 6$)	0.295 ± 0.050	0.307 ± 0.053	0.301 ± 0.041	3.0	0.119
app. TbTh [mm]	formalin ($n = 6$)	0.308 ± 0.056	0.298 ± 0.069	0.297 ± 0.052	4.0	0.135
FD	frozen ($n = 6$)	1.453 ± 0.145	1.472 ± 0.114	1.484 ± 0.139	2.0	0.311
FD	formalin ($n = 6$)	1.471 ± 0.151	1.470 ± 0.134	1.459 ± 0.159	2.6	0.607

FEM finite element model, *ACM* apparent compressive modulus, *BMD* bone mineral density, *app. BV/TV* apparent bone volume divided by total volume, *app. TbN* apparent trabecular number, *app. TbSp* apparent trabecular separation, *app. TbTh* apparent trabecular thickness, *FD* fractal dimension

human cadavers [15]. They measured BMD within 48 h of death and after 10 months of formalin fixation, and observed no significant deviation in BMD values. Edmondston et al. investigated the correlation of DXA-based BMD and mechanically determined failure load in ten fresh and ten formalin-fixed sheep lumbar spines [30]. The slopes of the regression for BMD and failure load of both groups were not significantly different.

In the line of these studies, we investigated the effects of preservation on QCT-based BMD and advanced computational methods of osteoporosis research, i.e., trabecular bone microstructure parameters and FEM. In

Table 3 Spearman's rank correlation coefficients (r with respective p-value) of FEM-based ACM, BMD, and trabecular bone microstructure parameters of the formalin-fixed and frozen vertebrae at baseline, 3 and 6 month follow-up with failure load (FL) as determined after six months. Correlation coefficients were not significantly different for the two preservation methods as compared by using the Fisher Z transformation ($p > 0.05$)

		FL [N]		
	Preservation	Baseline	3 month follow-up	6 month follow-up
FEM-based ACM [N/mm^2]	frozen ($n = 6$)	0.94 ($p = 0.005$)	0.99 ($p < 0.001$)	0.99 ($p < 0.001$)
FEM-based ACM [N/mm^2]	formalin ($n = 6$)	0.94 ($p = 0.005$)	0.94 ($p = 0.005$)	0.94 ($p = 0.005$)
BMD [mg/cm^3]	frozen ($n = 6$)	0.99 ($p < 0.001$)	0.99 ($p < 0.001$)	0.99 ($p < 0.001$)
BMD [mg/cm^3]	formalin ($n = 6$)	0.89 ($p = 0.019$)	0.93 ($p = 0.008$)	0.89 ($p = 0.019$)
app. BV/TV	frozen ($n = 6$)	0.94 ($p = 0.005$)	0.93 ($p = 0.008$)	0.89 ($p = 0.019$)
app. BV/TV	formalin ($n = 6$)	0.94 ($p = 0.005$)	0.89 ($p = 0.019$)	0.89 ($p = 0.019$)
app. TbN [mm^{-1}]	frozen ($n = 6$)	0.94 ($p = 0.005$)	0.89 ($p = 0.019$)	0.89 ($p = 0.019$)
app. TbN [mm^{-1}]	formalin ($n = 6$)	0.94 ($p = 0.005$)	0.89 ($p = 0.019$)	0.89 ($p = 0.019$)
app. TbSp [mm]	frozen ($n = 6$)	−0.94 ($p = 0.005$)	−0.89 ($p = 0.019$)	−0.89 ($p = 0.019$)
app. TbSp [mm]	formalin ($n = 6$)	−0.94 ($p = 0.005$)	−0.89 ($p = 0.019$)	−0.89 ($p = 0.019$)
app. TbTh [mm]	frozen ($n = 6$)	0.94 ($p = 0.005$)	0.99 ($p < 0.001$)	0.94 ($p = 0.005$)
app. TbTh [mm]	formalin ($n = 6$)	0.94 ($p = 0.005$)	0.94 ($p = 0.005$)	0.89 ($p = 0.019$)
FD	frozen ($n = 6$)	0.94 ($p = 0.005$)	0.94 ($p = 0.005$)	0.93 ($p = 0.008$)
FD	formalin ($n = 6$)	0.89 ($p = 0.019$)	0.89 ($p = 0.019$)	0.89 ($p = 0.019$)

FEM finite element model, *ACM* apparent compressive modulus, *BMD* bone mineral density, *app. BV/TV* apparent bone volume divided by total volume, *app. TbN* apparent trabecular number, *app. TbSp* apparent trabecular separation, *app. TbTh* apparent trabecular thickness, *FD* fractal dimension

consistency with Lochmüller et al., we observed no significant changes of QCT-based BMD over six months for both formalin-fixed and frozen vertebrae [15]. Furthermore, we demonstrated for the first time that trabecular bone microstructure parameters and FEM-based ACM are not significantly altered due to formalin fixation or freezing over six months. Furthermore, the computed parameters correlated well with mechanically determined bone strength independent of the preservation method. These findings are consistent with the association of BMD and failure load in fresh and formalin-fixed sheep lumbar spines as reported by Edmondston et al. [30].

The strength of our study was use of intact, human vertebrae, since this is the most important in-vitro scenario in the context of osteoporosis research. Previous studies have been often limited by investigating trabecular or cortical bone samples only which were sometimes not even harvested from human donors [13, 28, 30]. The limitation of our study was the relatively small sample size, i.e., all the vertebrae were harvested from three donors only.

Conclusions

Formalin fixation and freezing up to six months showed not significant effects on QCT-based BMD, trabecular bone microstructure, and FEM in intact, human vertebrae. Therefore, both preservation methods may be used in corresponding in-vitro experiments in the context of osteoporosis.

Competing interests

The authors declare that they have no competing interests.

Authors' contributions

Study conception and design: TB, RB, JSB. Acquisition of data: TB, EGG, RB, OG, HL, PMJ, MG, TZ, EJR, SW, JSB. Analysis and interpretation of data: TB, EGG, RB, OG, HL, PMJ, MG, TZ, EJR, SW, JSB. Drafting of Article: TB. Review/revision: TB, EGG, RB, OG, HL, PMJ, MG, TZ, EJR, SW, JSB. Final Approval: TB, EGG, RB, OG, HL, PMJ, MG, TZ, EJR, SW, JSB. All authors read and approved the final manuscript.

Acknowledgements

This work was supported by grants of the Deutsche Forschungsgemeinschaft (DFG BA 4085/2-1 and BA 4906/1-1), by the Commission for Clinical Research, Technische Universität München (TUM), TUM School of Medicine, Munich, Germany (Project No. 8762152), and by the Technische Universität München within the funding program Open Access Publishing.

Author details

[1]Institut für Radiologie, Klinikum rechts der Isar, Technische Universität München, Ismaninger Str. 22, 81675 München, Germany. [2]Klinik für Orthopädie, Abteilung für Biomechanik, Klinikum rechts der Isar, Technische Universität München, Ismaninger Str. 22, 81675 München, Germany. [3]Universitätsklinik für Radiologie und Nuklearmedizin, Abteilung für Neuroradiologie und Muskuloskeletale Radiologie, Medizinischen Universität Wien, Währinger Gürtel 18-20, 1090 Wien, Austria. [4]Abteilung für Neuroradiologie, Klinikum rechts der Isar, Technische Universität München, Ismaninger Str. 22, 81675 München, Germany.

References

1. NIH. NIH Consensus Development Panel on Osteoporosis Prevention, Diagnosis, and Therapy, March 7–29, 2000: highlights of the conference. South Med J. 2001;94:569–73.
2. Ioannidis G, Papaioannou A, Hopman WM, Akhtar-Danesh N, Anastassiades T, Pickard L, et al. Relation between fractures and mortality: results from the Canadian Multicentre Osteoporosis Study. CMAJ. 2009;181:265–71.
3. Burge R, Dawson-Hughes B, Solomon DH, Wong JB, King A, Tosteson A. Incidence and economic burden of osteoporosis-related fractures in the United States, 2005–2025. J Bone Miner Res. 2007;22:465–75.
4. WHO Study Group. Assessment of fracture risk and its application to screening for postmenopausal osteoporosis. Report of a WHO Study Group. World Health Organ Tech Rep Ser. 1994;843:1–129.
5. Adams JE. Quantitative computed tomography. Eur J Radiol. 2009;71:415–24.
6. Schuit SC, van der Klift M, Weel AE, de Laet CE, Burger H, Seeman E, et al. Fracture incidence and association with bone mineral density in elderly men and women: the Rotterdam Study. Bone. 2004;34:195–202.
7. Siris ES, Chen YT, Abbott TA, Barrett-Connor E, Miller PD, Wehren LE, et al. Bone mineral density thresholds for pharmacological intervention to prevent fractures. Arch Intern Med. 2004;164:1108–12.
8. Link TM. Osteoporosis imaging: state of the art and advanced imaging. Radiology. 2012;263:3–17.
9. Baum T, Karampinos DC, Liebl H, Rummeny EJ, Waldt S, Bauer JS. High-resolution bone imaging for osteoporosis diagnostics and therapy monitoring using clinical MDCT and MRI. Curr Med Chem. 2013;20:4844–52.
10. Boskey AL, Cohen ML, Bullough PG. Hard tissue biochemistry: a comparison of fresh-frozen and formalin-fixed tissue samples. Calcif Tissue Int. 1982;34:328–31.
11. Ohman C, Dall'Ara E, Baleani M, Van Sint JS, Viceconti M. The effects of embalming using a 4 % formalin solution on the compressive mechanical properties of human cortical bone. Clin Biomech (Bristol, Avon). 2008;23:1294–8.
12. Unger S, Blauth M, Schmoelz W. Effects of three different preservation methods on the mechanical properties of human and bovine cortical bone. Bone. 2010;47:1048–53.
13. Nazarian A, Hermannsson BJ, Muller J, Zurakowski D, Snyder BD. Effects of tissue preservation on murine bone mechanical properties. J Biomech. 2009;42:82–6.
14. Linde F, Sorensen HC. The effect of different storage methods on the mechanical properties of trabecular bone. J Biomech. 1993;26:1249–52.
15. Lochmuller EM, Krefting N, Burklein D, Eckstein F. Effect of fixation, soft-tissues, and scan projection on bone mineral measurements with dual energy X-ray absorptiometry (DXA). Calcif Tissue Int. 2001;68:140–5.
16. Baum T, Grabeldinger M, Rath C, Grande GE, Burgkart R, Patsch JM, et al. Trabecular bone structure analysis of the spine using clinical MDCT: can it predict vertebral bone strength? J Bone Miner Metab. 2014;32:56–64.
17. Baum T, Carballido-Gamio J, Huber MB, Muller D, Monetti R, Rath C, et al. Automated 3D trabecular bone structure analysis of the proximal femur–prediction of biomechanical strength by CT and DXA. Osteoporos Int. 2010;21:1553–64.
18. Parfitt AM, Drezner MK, Glorieux FH, Kanis JA, Malluche H, Meunier PJ, et al. Bone histomorphometry: standardization of nomenclature, symbols, and units. Report of the ASBMR Histomorphometry Nomenclature Committee. J Bone Miner Res. 1987;2:595–610.
19. Keyak JH, Falkinstein Y. Comparison of in situ and in vitro CT scan-based finite element model predictions of proximal femoral fracture load. Med Eng Phys. 2003;25:781–7.
20. Les CM, Keyak JH, Stover SM, Taylor KT, Kaneps AJ. Estimation of material properties in the equine metacarpus with use of quantitative computed tomography. J Orthop Res. 1994;12:822–33.
21. Crawford RP, Cann CE, Keaveny TM. Finite element models predict in vitro vertebral body compressive strength better than quantitative computed tomography. Bone. 2003;33:744–50.
22. Keller TS. Predicting the compressive mechanical behavior of bone. J Biomech. 1994;27:1159–68.
23. Kopperdahl DL, Morgan EF, Keaveny TM. Quantitative computed tomography estimates of the mechanical properties of human vertebral trabecular bone. J Orthop Res. 2002;20:801–5.
24. Chevalier Y, Charlebois M, Pahra D, Varga P, Heini P, Schneider E, et al. A patient-specific finite element methodology to predict damage accumulation in vertebral bodies under axial compression, sagittal flexion and combined loads. Comput Methods Biomech Biomed Engin. 2008;11:477–87.

25. Dall'Ara E, Pahr D, Varga P, Kainberger F, Zysset P. QCT-based finite element models predict human vertebral strength in vitro significantly better than simulated DEXA. Osteoporos Int. 2012;23:563–72.
26. Gluer CC, Blake G, Lu Y, Blunt BA, Jergas M, Genant HK. Accurate assessment of precision errors: how to measure the reproducibility of bone densitometry techniques. Osteoporos Int. 1995;5:262–70.
27. Duma SM, Rudd RW, Crandall JR. A protocol system for testing biohazardous materials in an impact biomechanics research facility. Am Ind Hyg Assoc J. 1999;60:629–34.
28. van Haaren EH, van der Zwaard BC, van der Veen AJ, Heyligers IC, Wuisman PI, Smit TH. Effect of long-term preservation on the mechanical properties of cortical bone in goats. Acta Orthop. 2008;79:708–16.
29. Wilke HJ, Krischak S, Claes LE. Formalin fixation strongly influences biomechanical properties of the spine. J Biomech. 1996;29:1629–31.
30. Edmondston SJ, Singer KP, Day RE, Breidahl PD, Price RI. Formalin fixation effects on vertebral bone density and failure mechanics: an in-vitro study of human and sheep vertebrae. Clin Biomech (Bristol, Avon). 1994;9:175–9.

10

Correlation of clinical and physical-technical image quality in chest CT: a human cadaver study applied on iterative reconstruction

An De Crop[1*], Peter Smeets[2], Tom Van Hoof[1], Merel Vergauwen[2], Tom Dewaele[2], Mathias Van Borsel[2], Eric Achten[2], Koenraad Verstraete[2], Katharina D'Herde[1], Hubert Thierens[1] and Klaus Bacher[1]

Abstract

Background: The first aim of this study was to evaluate the correlation between clinical and physical-technical image quality applied to different strengths of iterative reconstruction in chest CT images using Thiel cadaver acquisitions and Catphan images. The second aim was to determine the potential dose reduction of iterative reconstruction compared to conventional filtered back projection based on different clinical and physical-technical image quality parameters.

Methods: Clinical image quality was assessed using three Thiel embalmed human cadavers. A Catphan phantom was used to assess physical-technical image quality parameters such as noise, contrast-detail and contrast-to-noise ratio (CNR).
Both Catphan and chest Thiel CT images were acquired on a multislice CT scanner at 120 kVp and 0.9 pitch. Six different refmAs settings were applied (12, 30, 60, 90, 120 and 150refmAs) and each scan was reconstructed using filtered back projection (FBP) and iterative reconstruction (SAFIRE) algorithms (1,3 and 5 strengths) using a sharp kernel, resulting in 24 image series. Four radiologists assessed the clinical image quality, using a visual grading analysis (VGA) technique based on the European Quality Criteria for Chest CT.

Results: Correlation coefficients between clinical and physical-technical image quality varied from 0.88 to 0.92, depending on the selected physical-technical parameter. Depending on the strength of SAFIRE, the potential dose reduction based on noise, CNR and the inverse image quality figure (IQF_{inv}) varied from 14.0 to 67.8 %, 16.0 to 71.5 % and 22.7 to 50.6 % respectively. Potential dose reduction based on clinical image quality varied from 27 to 37.4 %, depending on the strength of SAFIRE.

Conclusion: Our results demonstrate that noise assessments in a uniform phantom overestimate the potential dose reduction for the SAFIRE IR algorithm. Since the IQF_{inv} based dose reduction is quite consistent with the clinical based dose reduction, an optimised contrast-detail phantom could improve the use of contrast-detail analysis for image quality assessment in chest CT imaging. In conclusion, one should be cautious to evaluate the performance of CT equipment taking into account only physical-technical parameters as noise and CNR, as this might give an incomplete representation of the actual clinical image quality performance.

Keywords: Chest CT, Image quality, Iterative reconstruction, Human cadaver study, Visual grading analysis

* Correspondence: An.decrop@ugent.be
[1]Department of Basic Medical Sciences, Ghent University, Proeftuinstraat 86, B-9000 Ghent, Belgium
Full list of author information is available at the end of the article

Background

The number of CT examinations has increased rapidly over the last few years, resulting in a substantial increase in radiation dose of the population in the Western world [1]. It has been estimated that these CT examinations may be responsible for approximately 2 % of all incident cancer cases in the United States [2]. Consequently, a lot of efforts have been made over the last decade to reduce the radiation dose for the patient by introducing new techniques such as automatic tube current modulation, adaptive collimation and iterative reconstruction [3–6]. If new dose reduction techniques are implemented, the impact on the image quality has to be investigated.

Medical physicists assess the image quality in CT using technical phantoms, evaluating parameters as noise, modulation transfer function (MTF), contrast-to-noise ratio (CNR) and/or contrast-detail. However, as these phantom models are not related to patient anatomy, it is unclear whether this methodology is appropriate to evaluate the clinical image quality. Particularly for noise, this can be problematic, since noise measurements in a uniform phantom don't account for the complex relationship between anatomical variability and image quality [7]. To be able to compare the performance of different CT scanners or to evaluate dose optimisation tools, it is of critical importance that physical-technical image quality based dose optimisation performance is related to the clinical image quality based dose optimisation performance.

Clinical image quality is typically assessed by applying a visual grading analysis (VGA) [8] or a receiver operating characteristics (ROC) [9] study setup in a patient population. However, these patient studies are rather difficult to implement since either large numbers of patient images must be available or one patient has to be exposed to different dose settings, which should be avoided from ethical point of view. As an alternative, clinical images of an anthropomorphic phantom can be acquired. Compared to physical-technical phantoms, these phantoms approximate better the clinical reality with respect to anatomical features [10].

In present study, patient image quality of chest CT was assessed by means of human cadavers, conserved using the Thiel embalming technique [11]. In contrast to the classical formol embalming technique, the Thiel embalming method results in excellent preservation of the flexibility and plasticity of organs and tissues [11, 12]. As a result, lungs can be inflated during image acquisition to simulate the anatomy of a chest CT [13]. Consequently, these Thiel embalmed cadavers are an excellent model to investigate the link between clinical and physical-technical image quality. This link was already established in conventional chest radiography [13]. However, with respect to CT imaging, the correlation between clinical and physical-technical image quality was not yet examined.

The first aim of this study was to evaluate the correlation between clinical and physical-technical image quality applied to different strengths of iterative reconstruction in chest CT images using Thiel cadaver acquisitions and Catphan images. The second aim was to determine the potential dose reduction of iterative reconstruction compared to conventional filtered back projection based on different clinical and physical-technical image quality parameters.

Methods

Thiel embalmed cadavers

The use of human cadavers is in compliance with the Helsinki Declaration and fulfilled the requirements of the ethical committee of our institution (Ghent University, B67020095736). The cadavers were obtained from body donations to the department of Anatomy of Ghent University.

Three human cadavers (2 male, 1 female) were embalmed using the methodology of Prof. Em. Walther Thiel, Anatomisches Institut Karl-Franzens-Universität, Graz, Austria [12].

Hereby, 4-chloro-3-methylenphenol as well as various salts are used for fixation and boric acid is added for disinfection. Furthermore, ethylene glycol is used for preservation of tissue plasticity, while the concentration of formalin is kept to the strict minimum (0.8 %) [11]. In contrast to standard formalin-embalmed human cadavers, this technique results in well preserved organs and tissues concerning colour, consistency, natural flexibility and natural plasticity. As a result, lung tissue is preserved completely which makes it possible to ventilate the lungs by performing a tracheotomy in combination with balloon ventilation. After ventilating the lungs, chest CT acquisitions can be acquired for subjective image quality analysis. In the cadavers used in this study, the lungs showed signs of pulmonary oedema and pulmonary parenchymal consolidation. Equivalency of patient and Thiel thoracic CT images is displayed in Fig. 1.

Catphan phantom

To evaluate the physical-technical image quality the Catphan@504 phantom (The Phantom laboratory, Salem, New York, USA) was used. The phantom consists of several modules to evaluate high and low contrast resolution, CNR and noise (Fig. 2). In the low contrast module there are three areas with different contrast levels: 1, 0.5 and 0.3 %. Each contrast level contains targets with decreasing diameters (15, 9, 8, 7, 6, 5, 4, 3 and 2 mm). The CT number linearity and CT number accuracy module contains targets made from teflon, delrin, acrylic, polystyrene, low density polyethylene (LDPE), polymethylpentene (PMP) and air. The image uniformity module is made from a uniform material. The material's CT number is designed to

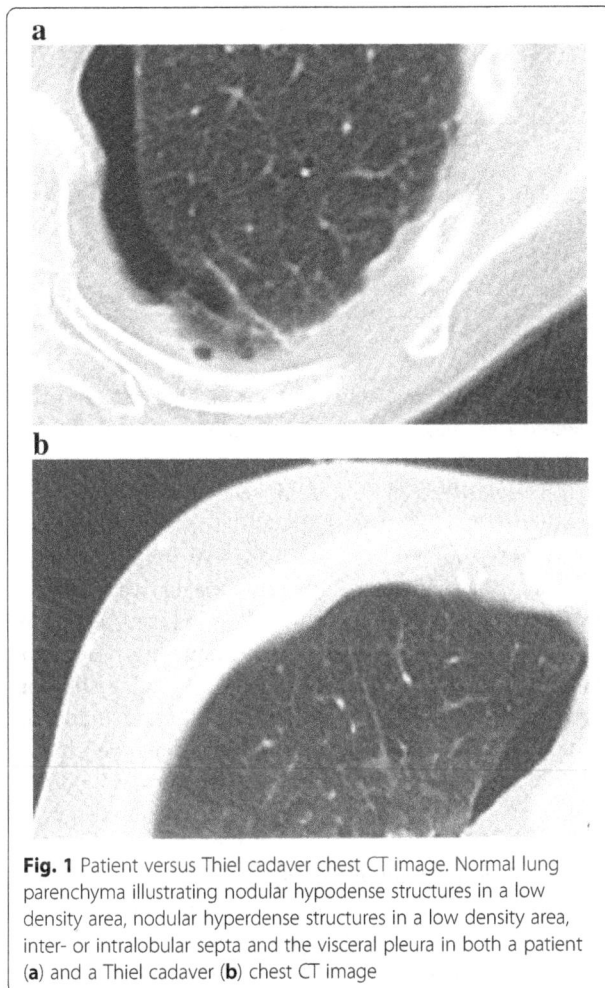

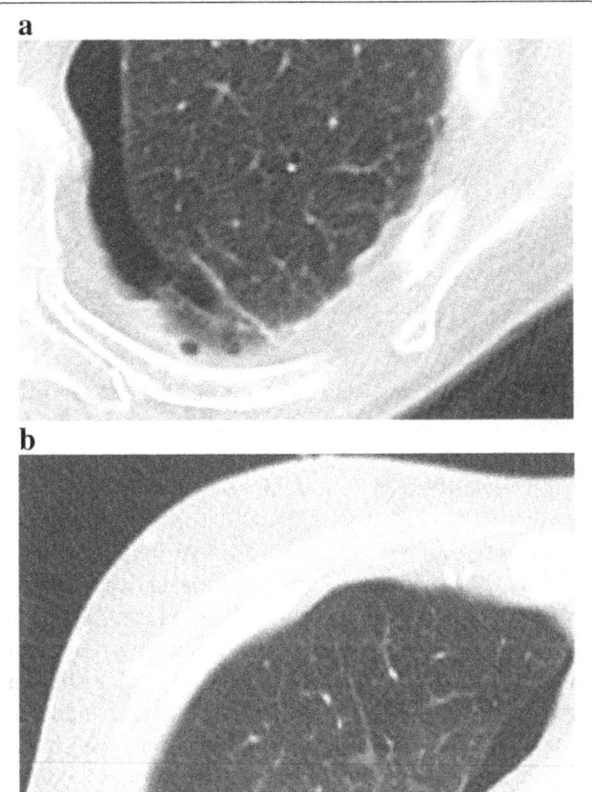

Fig. 1 Patient versus Thiel cadaver chest CT image. Normal lung parenchyma illustrating nodular hypodense structures in a low density area, nodular hyperdense structures in a low density area, inter- or intralobular septa and the visceral pleura in both a patient (**a**) and a Thiel cadaver (**b**) chest CT image

be within 2 % (20 HU) of water's density at standard scanning protocols.

Image acquisition

All images in this study were acquired with a Somatom Definition Flash CT scanner (Siemens Healthcare, Erlangen, Germany). The CT scanner is equipped with the dual source technology, CARE Dose4D, CARE kV, and Sinogram Affirmed Iterative Reconstruction (SAFIRE).

Chest CT scans of the lung ventilated Thiel embalmed cadavers were acquired using CARE Dose4D at different reference mAs values (12, 30, 60, 90, 120 and 150 refmAs), resulting in a mean $CTDI_{vol}$ of 0.84, 2.05, 4.08, 6.18, 8.35 and 11.59 mGy respectively. The 90 refmAs setting is clinically applied in our institution. Other scan parameters were 120 kVp and pitch 0.9. Each data set was reconstructed at 3 mm using filtered back projection (FBP) with a sharp kernel (B70). To compare the FBP and the SAFIRE technique, all six data sets were also reconstructed using different strengths of IR (1,3 and 5 iteration steps). Similarly to the FBP reconstructed images, IR images were reconstructed using a sharp kernel (I70-1, I70-3, I70-5), resulting in a total of 24 image series (6 refmAs settings with each 4 reconstruction settings).

Afterwards Catphan images were acquired without CARE Dose4D at a mAs value corresponding to the mean mAs value over the different slices in the Thiel cadaver acquired at the six different refmAs settings, resulting in a CTDIvol of 0.84, 2.11, 4.19, 6.37, 8.82 and 12.23 mGy respectively. The same reconstruction settings as for the Thiel embalmed cadavers were used. All scanning and reconstruction parameters and the investigated phantoms and image quality parameters are listed in Table 1.

Image quality analysis

After acquisition, all data were sent to a PACS Workstation (GE Centricity PACS version 2.0 CRS5 SP2) for image quality assessment. Images were displayed on a 30-inch, 3-megapixel high-contrast color monitor (Barco MDCC 6130DL, Kortrijk, Belgium). The monitor was calibrated to comply with the DICOM Part 3.14 Greyscale Standard Display Function, using calibration software

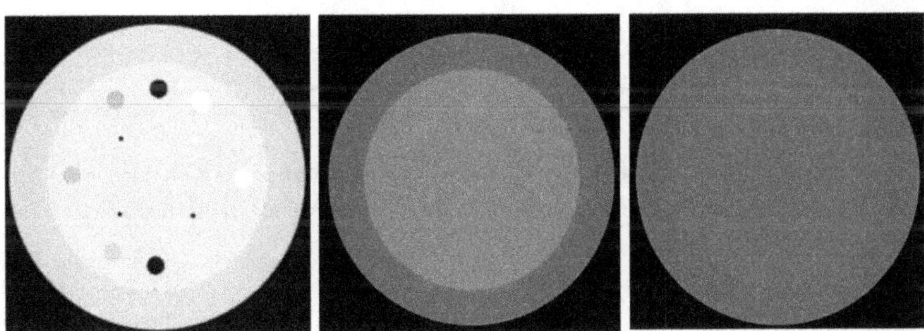

Fig. 2 Catphan@504 phantom. The figure represents a CT image of the Catphan phantom. On the left, the CT number linearity and CT number accuracy module, which includes samples of teflon and acrylic used to calculate the CNR. In the middle, the low contrast module containing targets with different contrast levels: 1, 0.5 and 0.3 %. Each contrast level has 9 targets with different diameters: 15, 9, 8, 7, 6, 5, 4, 3, 2 mm. On the right the image uniformity module

Table 1 Scanning and reconstruction parameters, investigated phantoms and image quality parameters used in this study

Fixed scan parameters	$CTDI_{(vol)}$ Thiel/ Catphan	Reconstruction parameters for each $CTDI_{(vol)}$	Scanned objects	Investigated image quality parameters	
				Thiel	Catphan
120 kVp	0.84 / 0.84	B70	Thiel cadavers (3)	VGAS	Noise
0.9 pitch	2.11 / 2.05	I70/1	Catphan phantom		IQF_{inv}
3 mm reconstruction thickness	4.19 / 4.08	I70/3			CNR
	6.37 / 6.18	I70/5			
	8.82 / 8.35				
	12.23 / 11.59				

provided by the manufacturer (MediCal Pro, BARCO, Kortrijk, Belgium) [14]. Maximum luminance of all monitors was adjusted to 400 cd/m^2 and ambient lighting levels were below 50 lux as recommended by AAPM TG 18 [15].

Scoring of Thiel images

Four experienced radiologists (PS: 25 years of experience; TDW, MVB and MV: 6 years of experience) assessed the chest CT scans and scored the image quality using criteria based on the European Guidelines on Quality Criteria for Computed Tomography [16]. The criteria are listed in Table 2. All criteria were evaluated in a predefined image area and a predefined image slice. For all three Thiel bodies, each stack was viewed individually and each structure was rated on a scale from 1 to 4 according to Table 3. An absolute VGA score (VGAS) for each reader was calculated as:

$$VGAS = \frac{\sum_{s=1}^{S}\sum_{t=1}^{T} G_{abs,s,t}}{S*T}$$

[17]

were $G_{abs,s,t}$ is the rating for a particular structure (s) and Thiel body (t). S and T are the number of structures and Thiel body's, respectively 9 and 3. The latter scoring reflected the image quality of the individual images without using a reference image [18].

All series were evaluated by the radiologists using Viewdex [19], a Java-based DICOM-compatible software tool for presentation and evaluation of images, without influencing the image quality. All images were blinded for acquisition and reconstruction parameters. The readers were allowed to adjust the image brightness and contrast and to magnify the images to full resolution. Viewdex defines a random order for each individual reader and all stacks were interpreted independently.

Before starting the study, a training session was organised to familiarise the readers with the scoring methodology.

Scoring of the Catphan phantom

Six medical physicists identified the minimally visible target diameter at three different contrast levels. The inverse image quality figure (IQFinv) was introduced for quantitative comparison of the contrast-detail images [20]. The inverse image quality figure is defined as

$$IQFinv = \frac{100}{\sum_{i=1}^{n} C_i D_{i,th}}$$

where $D_{i,th}$ denotes the threshold diameter for contrast i in mm and C_i denotes the contrast value. The higher the

Table 2 Image quality criteria for chest CT

Criterion no.	Description:
1	Visually sharp reproduction of a nodular hypodense structure in a high density area such as an alveolus in consolidated lung parenchyma
2	Visually sharp reproduction of a nodular hypodense structure in a low density area such as normal lung parenchyma
3	Visually sharp reproduction of a nodular hyperdense structure in a low density area such as a vessel in aerated lung parenchyma
4	Visually sharp reproduction of an inter- or intralobular septum
5	Visually sharp reproduction of the bronchial wall
6	Visually sharp reproduction of the lung fissure
7	Visually sharp reproduction of a peripheral pulmonary artery branch
8	Visually sharp reproduction of fibrous strands
9	Visually sharp reproduction of the parietal and or visceral pleura

Table 3 Rating used to evaluate the clinical images

Rating	The structure in the image is:
1	Not visible
2	Poorly reproduced
3	Adequately reproduced
4	Very well reproduced

IQFinv, the better the low-contrast visibility. The IQFinv was calculated for all analysed images and averaged over the six readers.

The contrast to noise ratio relative to acrylic (soft tissue equivalent material) for teflon (bone equivalent material) was defined as:

$$CNR = \frac{(ROI_t - ROI_a)}{SD_a}$$

where ROI_t is the mean attenuation for teflon, ROI_a the mean attenuation for acrylic and SD_a the mean noise for acrylic. CT attenuation values and mean noise (in Hounsfield units) for teflon and acrylic were obtained by manually placing a circular region of interest (ROI) of 200 pixels in the target materials. CNR's were calculated in four consecutive slices of the Catphan CT number linearity and CT number accuracy module.

The image noise was evaluated using a circular ROI of 230 × 230 pixels in 11 following slices in the Catphan uniformity module.

Statistical analysis

To determine the influence of different exposure and reconstruction settings, data were analysed using the Friedman test, a signed rank, non-parametric test used when comparing more than two related samples.

Inter-observer agreement for VGAS and IQF_{inv} values was determined by calculating the intraclass correlation coefficient. An intraclass correlation coefficient greater than 0.9 was considered to suggest an excellent inter-observer agreement [21].

After analysis of different fitting curves, a power function was selected as the best possible fit. Power functions are plotted for VGAS, noise, IQF_{inv} and CNR as a function of the mAs value. These curves are used to calculate the potential dose reduction when changing from a filtered back projection kernel (B70) at the clinically applied 90 refmAs to an iterative reconstruction kernel while maintaining the same value for noise, contrast-detail or CNR. To obtain a significant dose reduction, the two curves that are used, should differ significantly. This was examined by means of a Wilcoxon test, a signed rank, non-parametric test used when comparing two related samples. For this, all different readings (4, 11, 6, and 4 for VGAS, noise, IQFinv and CNR) for the six different mAs settings are considered which result in 24, 66, 36 and 24 data points for VGAS, noise, IQF_{inv} and CNR respectively.

A 95 % confidence interval was used for all statistical measures. All calculations were performed using the SPSS software tool (IBM SPSS statistics 22, IBM corp., NY, USA).

Results

Excellent inter-observer agreement among the participating radiologists and among medical physicists was found by means of an intraclass correlation coefficient of 0.919 ($p < 0.001$) and 0.951 ($p < 0.001$) for the VGAS and IQF_{inv} parameters respectively. As a result, in the further analysis, scores averaged over the readers were used.

To evaluate the correlation between clinical and physical-technical image quality, regression curves were plotted for noise, CNR and IQF_{inv} as a function of VGA scores for the different refmAs settings (Fig. 3). Good correlation was found between noise and VGAS, 0.90, $p < 0.001$. A correlation coefficient of 0.88, $p < 0.001$ was obtained for CNR and VGAS. Contrast-detail (IQF_{inv}) and VGAS resulted in a correlation coefficient of 0.92, $p < 0.001$.

To examine the influence of the iterative reconstruction strengths, the reconstruction settings mentioned in the materials and methods were applied to the Thiel images at 90 ref mAs. Catphan images acquired at mAs settings corresponding to 90 ref mAs were selected. A significant effect of the IR strengths was found for both the physical-technical and clinical image quality parameters ($p < 0.05$) except for IQF_{inv} ($p = 0.706$).

For both clinical and physical-technical image quality parameters as a function of the mAs value, a power function fit was applied for all types of kernels (noise and CNR $r^2 > 0.9$, VGAS and IQF_{inv} $r^2 > 0.8$, $p < 0.05$). As expected, for all 4 different types of reconstruction kernel , a significant effect of mAs settings was confirmed by means of a Friedman test for noise and contrast detail ($p < 0.001$) and for CNR ($p < 0.05$). Correspondingly, this influence was also found for VGAS ($p < 0.05$).

A significant difference was found between the curve of the B70 kernel and the curve of each strength of iterative reconstruction for all clinical and physical-technical image quality parameters, except for VGAS B70-I70/1.

The power function for VGAS, noise, CNR and IQF_{inv} as a function of refmAs settings is shown in Figs. 4, 5, 6 and 7. These curves were used to calculate the potential dose reduction when changing from a filtered back projection kernel at the clinically applied 90 refmAs to an iterative reconstruction kernel while maintaining the same value for noise, CNR or contrast-detail. In general, higher strengths of SAFIRE result in higher potential dose reduction. The potential dose reduction based on noise and CNR and IQF_{inv} varied from 14.0 to 37.8 %,16.0

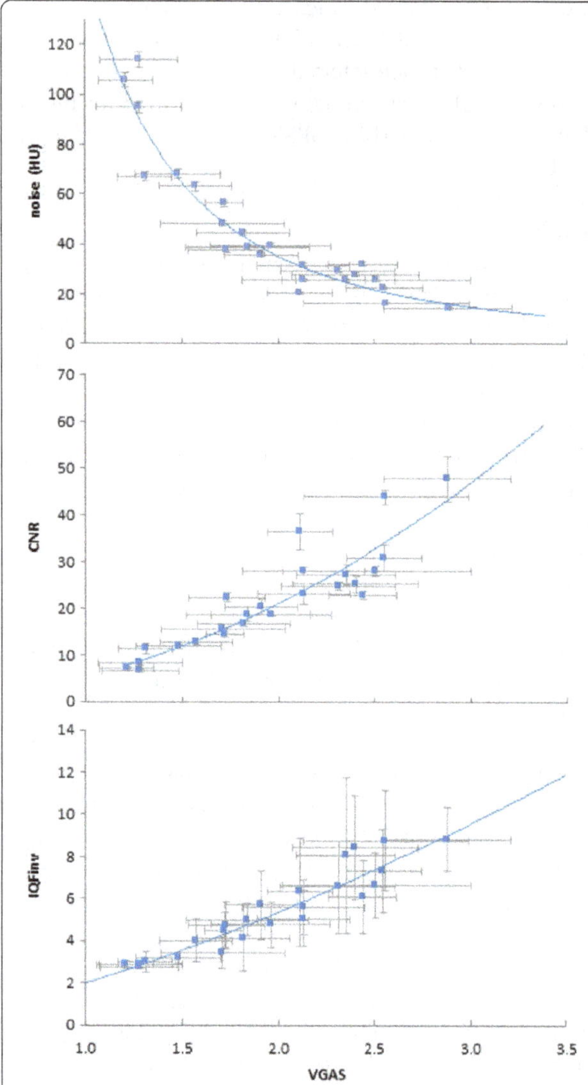

Fig. 3 Mean noise, CNR and IQF_{inv} versus mean VGAS. The error bars in the x direction represent the standard deviation between the scores of the different radiologists. For noise, the error bars in the y direction represent the standard deviation between noise measurements in 11 following slices in the Catphan uniformity module. For CNR, the error bars in the y direction represent the standard deviation between CNR measurements in four consecutive slices of the Catphan CT number linearity and CT number accuracy module. For IQF_{inv}, the error bars in the y direction represent the standard deviation between the six readers of the contrast-detail module in the Catphan phantom. Regression lines were plotted resulting in an r^2 of 0.90, 0.88 and 0.92, $p < 0.001$, for noise, CNR and IQF_{inv} respectively

to 71.5 % and 22.7 to 50.6 % respectively, depending on the strength of iterative reconstruction. Potential dose reduction based on clinical image quality varied from 27 to 37.4 % depending on the strength of iterative reconstruction. Consequently, the potential dose reduction is strongly dependent on the selected clinical or physical-technical parameter. From the physical-technical image quality parameters, dose reductions based on IQF_{inv}

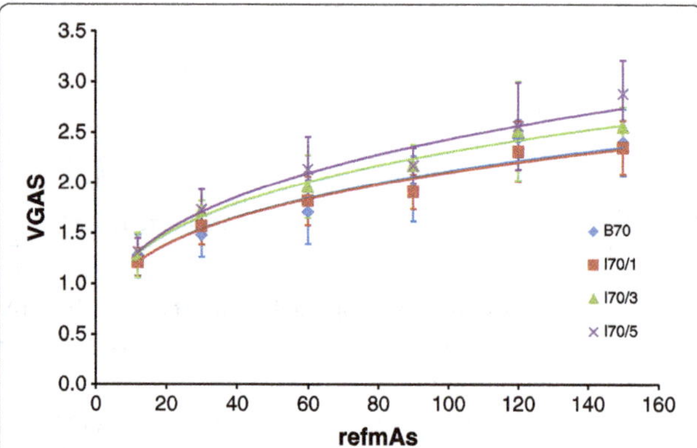

Fig. 4 Mean VGAS versus refmAs for B70, I70/1, I30/3 and I70/5. The error bars in the y direction represent the standard deviation between the scores of the different readers. Power functions were plotted and for all kernels an $r^2 > 0.8$ was obtained, $p < 0.05$

correspond best with dose reductions based on VGAS The results are summarized in Table 4.

Discussion

Methods for patient dose evaluation are easily available but techniques for objective clinical image quality optimisation are far more complicated. VGA and ROC studies are commonly used to assess clinical image quality [22]. In VGA studies, a relative or absolute scoring is performed based on the visibility of normal anatomical structures [8]. The task for observers in a ROC study is to detect whether a patient's image contains a pathological structure or not [9]. However, these studies are difficult to implement in routine practice since they imply a significant additional workload for the radiologists and large patient data groups must be available. Therefore, the latter methods are not feasible within a routine quality assurance programme.

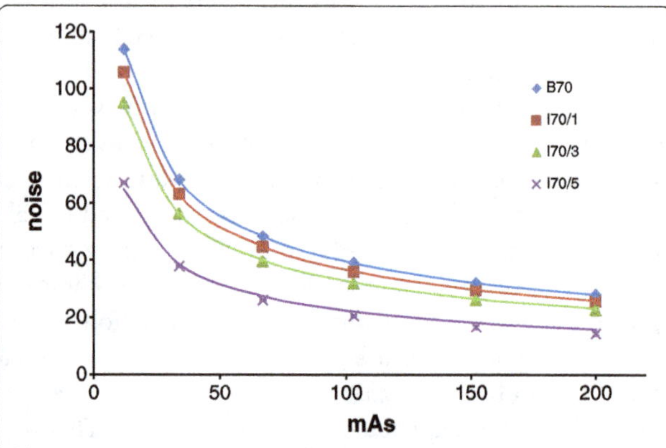

Fig. 5 Mean noise versus mAs for B70, I70/1, I70/3 and I70/5. The error bars in the y direction represent the standard deviation between noise measurements in 11 following slices in the Catphan uniformity module. $\frac{a}{\sqrt{mAs}}$ regression curves were added

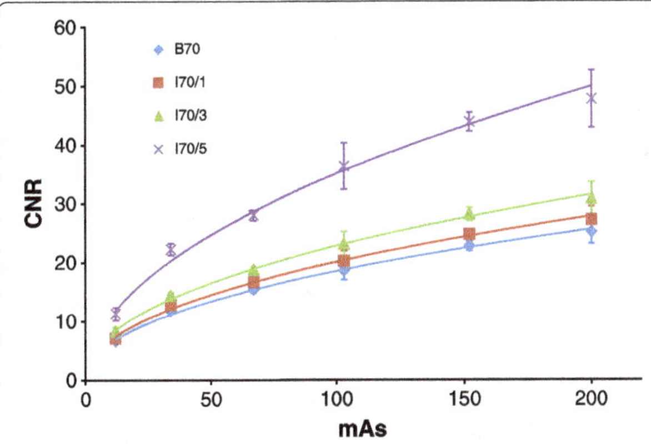

Fig. 6 Mean CNR versus mAs for B70, I70/1, I70/3 and I70/5. The error bars in the y direction represent the standard deviation between CNR measurements in four consecutive slices of the Catphan CT number linearity and CT number accuracy module. Power functions were plotted and for all kernels an $r^2 > 0.9$ was obtained, $p < 0.05$

A more practical approach to assess the image quality is the use of physical-technical phantoms, such as the Catphan phantom, where physical-technical parameters such as noise, CNR, MTF and contrast-detail can be analysed. Such physical-technical phantoms have been widely used for the objective analysis of the image quality performance of CT systems [23]. Catphan studies are easily implemented in a quality assurance programme since no patient data are required and images can be analysed by the medical physics expert. However, the disadvantage of the Catphan phantom is the uniform background. Actual patient images are clearly not uniform and contain detailed anatomical features and textures. These background anatomical textures can influence image quality, both because the presence of anatomical texture affects observer performance and quantum noise [7].

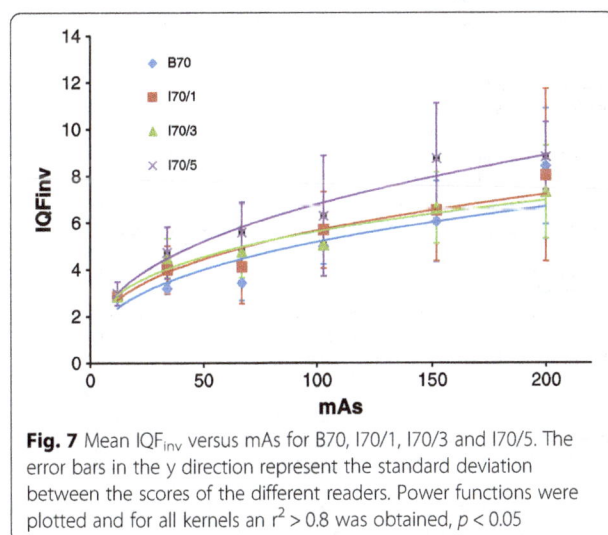

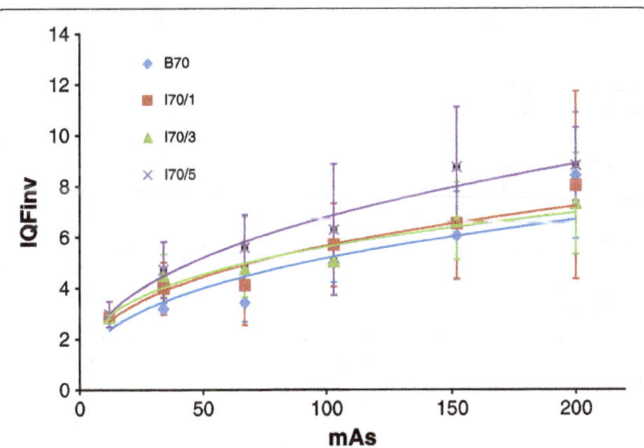

Fig. 7 Mean IQF_{inv} versus mAs for B70, I70/1, I70/3 and I70/5. The error bars in the y direction represent the standard deviation between the scores of the different readers. Power functions were plotted and for all kernels an $r^2 > 0.8$ was obtained, $p < 0.05$

Table 4 Potential dose reduction for different clinical and physical image quality parameters and different iterations steps

	Potential dose reduction (p-value)			
Reconstruction kernel	VGAS	Noise	IQF_{inv}	CNR_{teflon}
I70/1	0 % (0.887)	14.0 % (<0.001)	22.7 % (0.034)	16.0 % (<0.001)
I70/3	27.0 % (0.021)	31.4 % (<0.001)	23.0 % (0.031)	35.8% (<0.001)
I70/5	37.4 % (0.001)	67.8 % (<0.001)	50.6 % (<0.001)	71.5 % (<0.001)

In present study, a VGA and Catphan study was set up to assess the relationship between physical-technical and clinical image quality in chest CT examinations, using Thiel embalmed cadavers and the Catphan@504 phantom. In contrast to conventional embalming procedures using formalin for conservation, this new technique results in a very well preservation of the lung structures [11, 12]. To approximate as good as possible the normal patient anatomy, Thiel bodies were ventilated during image acquisition [13]. After assessment of different thoracic regions by experienced radiologists, it was confirmed that Thiel bodies can be applied to assess clinical image quality using VGA and ROC studies.

Recently, there is growing interest in developing and utilising model observers to accurately predict human observer performance for image system optimization and comparison. A model observer is a mathematical model that can be used to predict human detection performance for some specific imaging tasks [24]. A variety of models, which differ in how much information about signal and noise are used and whether certain properties of the human visual system responses are incorporated, have been proposed and applied to medical image research [24, 25]. However, up till now, phantom images and simulated lesions are used to assess these models. How much real lesions and anatomical backgrounds affect model observer performance remains under investigation [26]. Possibly, the concept of Thiel embalmed cadavers could be used to help validate model observer applications.

Although good correlation was found between physical-technical image quality parameters (noise, CNR and contrast-detail) and clinically observed quality as scored by radiologists (VGAS), the potential dose reduction based on the physical-technical image quality parameters noise and CNR, is much higher compared to the potential dose reduction based on the clinical image quality. This overestimate of the dose reduction can be explained because the uniform phantom does not account for the complex relationship between anatomical variability and image quality. On the contrary, the potential dose reduction based on IQF_{inv} is more consistent with the potential dose reduction based on VGAS. However the measurements are very crude using the Catphan phantom as only three contrast levels are present. Optimisation of a contrast-detail phantom for CT is necessary and could give added value to the concept of contrast-detail analysis in CT image quality studies similar to the use of contrast-detail phantoms in mammography and conventional radiology [27, 28].

While this study illustrates that noise measurements in uniform backgrounds are not ideal to assess the effect of iterative reconstruction, a large part of the literature is still based on this technique. Mieville et al. [29] used the Catphan phantom to assess noise, CT number accuracy, noise power spectrum and MTF at varying CTDI values for both FBP images and IR images. Milim Kim et al. [30] used the phantom of the American College of Radiology, a solid water phantom with 5 imbedded test objects to evaluate image noise, SNR and CNR. No comparisons were made between the possible dose reduction based on the different parameters. Ghetti et al. [31, 32] assessed image noise in a uniform water phantom. Since noise reduction in these studies are based on uniform phantoms, it is questionable if these results are applicable in clinical practice. The nonlinear nature of IR methods has also introduced significant challenges to the characterization of spatial resolution performance. In this framework, Li et al. introduced a concept of task specific measurements of the spatial resolution by locally measuring the point spread function for a given feature of interest at a given radiation dose level in an anthropomorphic phantom [33].

Other studies performed clinical image quality assessment on patient data, which automatically limits the amount of dose settings that can be used. Exact calculation of the potential dose reduction without loss of image quality is thereby impossible. Prakash et al. [34] scanned 54 patients at a mean effective dose of 12.2 mSv reconstructed with FBP and 98 patients at a mean effective dose of 8.9 mSv reconstructed with an iterative reconstruction technique (30 % ASIR, GE) resulting in a mean dose reduction of 27.6 %. All chest CT examinations were scored diagnostically acceptable. Pontana et al. [35] scanned 80 patients two times with constant CT parameters except for the refmAs which was decreased by 30 %. High dose chest CT images were reconstructed with FBP, low dose chest CT images were reconstructed with an iterative reconstruction technique (IRIS algorithm, Siemens). There was no significant difference in objective noise, CNR, SNR and overall subjective image quality between the two groups. In both studies, physical-technical as well as clinical image quality was assessed. However, no further correlation analysis was made between the physical-technical and clinical image quality. Since only two dose settings were examined, the dose reduction based on clinical and physical-technical image quality was identical. Consequently, the maximum potential dose reduction without loss of image quality, could not be assessed and no conclusions can be made about the discrepancy in potential dose reduction when using physical-technical parameters rather than clinical image quality assessment.

There are several limitations of our study. Firstly, the available Thiel cadavers all had a BMI between 20 and 25. It is possible that the correlation between clinical and physical-technical image quality and the effect of iterative reconstruction can be influenced by patient size. Secondly, clinical image quality was assessed on unenhanced CT images. Possibly the correlation and potential dose reduction can be affected when contrast agents are used. Thirdly, clinical image quality was assessed by a subjective overall quality score and not by means of detection of pathology. Detection of lesions by means of a receiver operating characteristic (ROC) analysis could give a more precise assessment of image quality for a specific clinical application.

Conclusions

In summary, our results demonstrate that noise assessments in a uniform phantom overestimate the potential dose reduction for the SAFIRE IR algorithm. Since the IQF_{inv} based dose reduction is quite consistent with the clinical based dose reduction, an optimised contrast-detail phantom could improve the use of contrast-detail analysis for image quality assessment in chest CT imaging. In conclusion, one should be cautious to evaluate the performance of CT equipment taking into account only physical-technical parameters as noise and CNR, as this might give an incomplete representation of the actual clinical image quality performance.

Competing interests

The authors declare that they have no competing interests.

Authors' contributions

The following authors participated in the design of the research: ADC, PS, KB and HT. The following authors participated in the collection of the data, reading of the clinical and physical-technical images: ADC, PS, MV, MVB, KV, EA, KD, TVH and TD. The following authors participated in the analysis and interpretation of the data: ADC, KB, and HT. All authors have participated in the drafting and revision of the manuscript and have approved it.

Author details

[1]Department of Basic Medical Sciences, Ghent University, Proeftuinstraat 86, B-9000 Ghent, Belgium. [2]Department of Radiology, Ghent University Hospital, De Pintelaan 185, B-9000 Ghent, Belgium.

References

1. ICRP. Publication 87: Managing patient dose in computed tomography. 2000.
2. Brenner DJ, Hall EJ. Computed tomography - an increasing source of radiation exposure. N Engl J Med. 2007;357:2277–84.

3. Deak PD et al. Effects of adaptive section collimation on patient radiation dose in multisection spiral CT. Radiology. 2009;252(1):140–7.
4. Lee T-Y, Chhem RK. Impact of new technologies on dose reduction in CT. Eur J Radiol. 2010;76:28–35.
5. Kalra MK et al. Strategies for CT radiation dose optimization. Radiology. 2004;230(3):619–28.
6. Kubo T et al. Radiation dose reduction in chest CT: a review. AJR Am J Roentgenol. 2008;190(2):335–43.
7. Solomon J, Samei E. Quantum noise properties of CT images with anatomical textured backgrounds across reconstruction algorithms: FBP and SAFIRE. Med Phys. 2014;41(9):12.
8. Mieville FA et al. Paediatric cardiac CT examinations: impact of the iterative reconstruction method ASIR on image quality - preliminary findings. Pediatr Radiol. 2011;41(9):1154–64.
9. Martinsen AC et al. Iterative reconstruction reduces abdominal CT dose. Eur J Radiol. 2012;81(7):1483–7.
10. Veldkamp W, Kroft L, Geleijns J. Dose and perceived image quality in chest radiography. Eur J Radiol. 2009;72:209–17.
11. Thiel W. Die Konservierung ganzer Leichen in natürlichen Farben. Ann Anat. 1992;174:185–95.
12. Thiel W. Ergänzung für die Konservierung ganze Leichen nach W. Thiel. Ann Anat. 2002;184:267–9.
13. De Crop A et al. Correlation of contrast-detail analysis and clinical image quality assessment in chest radiography with a human cadaver study. Radiology. 2012;262(1):298–304.
14. AAPM report no.39, Specification and acceptance testing of computed tomography scanners. AAPM, 1993.
15. Samei E et al. Assessment of display performance for medical imaging systems: executive summary of AAPM TG18 report. Med Phys. 2005;32(4):1205–25.
16. Commission of the European Communities, European guidelines on quality criteria for computed tomography (EUR 16262). 1999.
17. Commission of the European Communities. CEC quality criteria for diagnostic radiographic images and patient exposure trial. (EUR 12952 EN). 1990.
18. Sund P et al. Comparison of visual grading analysis and determination of detective quantum efficiency for evaluation system performance in digital chest radiography. Eur Radiol. 2004;14:48–58.
19. Borjesson S et al. A software tool for increased efficiency in observer performance studies in radiology. Radiat Prot Dosim. 2005;114(1–3):45–52.
20. Thijssen M, Bijkerk K, van der Burgth R. Manual Contrast-Detail Phantom CDRAD type 2.0. Project Quality Assurance in Radiology, Department of Radiology, University Hospital Nijmegen, St. Radboud, The Netherlands. 1998.
21. Viner M et al. Liver SULmean at FDG PET/CT: Interreader Agreement and Impact of Placement of Volume of Interest. Radiology. 2013;267(2):596–601.
22. Bath M. Evaluating imaging systems: practical applications. Radiat Prot Dosimetry. 2010;139(1–3):26–36.
23.]Baker ME et al. Contrast-to-noise ratio and low-contrast object resolution on full- and low-dose MDCT: SAFIRE versus filtered back projection in a low-contrast object phantom and in the liver. Am J Roentgenol. 2012;199(1):8–18.
24. Barrett HH et al. Model observers for assessment of image quality. Proc Natl Acad Sci U S A. 1993;90(21):9758–65.
25. Richard S, Siewerdsen JH. Comparison of model and human observer performance for detection and discrimination tasks using dual-energy x-ray images. Med Phys. 2008;35(11):5043–53.
26. Zhang Y et al. Correlation between human and model observer performance for discrimination task in CT. Phys Med Biol. 2014;59(13):3389–404.
27. Yip M et al. Validation of a simulated dose reduction methodology using digital mammography CDMAM images and mastectomy images. Digital Mammography. 2010;6136:78–85.
28. Veldkamp W et al. Contrast-detail evaluation and dose assessment of eight digital chest radiography systems in clinical practice. Eur Radiol. 2006;16:333–41.
29. Mieville FA et al. Iterative reconstruction methods in two different MDCT scanners: physical metrics and 4-alternative forced-choice detectability experiments - a phantom approach. Phys Med. 2013;29(1):99–110.
30. Kim M et al. Adaptive iterative dose reduction algorithm in CT: effect on image quality compared with filtered back projection in body phantoms of different sizes. Korean J Radiol. 2014;15(2):195–204.
31. Ghetti C, Ortenzia O, Serreli G. CT iterative reconstruction in image space: a phantom study. Phys Med. 2012;28(2):161–5.
32. Ghetti C et al. Physical characterization of a new CT iterative reconstruction method operating in sinogram space. J Appl Clin Med Phys. 2013;14(4):263–71.
33. Li K et al. Statistical model based iterative reconstruction (MBIR) in clinical CT systems. Part II. Experimental assessment of spatial resolution performance. Med Phys. 2014;41(7):12.
34. Prakash P et al. Radiation dose reduction with chest computed tomography using adaptive statistical iterative reconstruction technique: initial experience. J Comput Assist Tomogr. 2010;34(1):40–5.
35. Pontana F et al. Chest computed tomography using iterative reconstruction vs filtered back projection (Part 2): image quality of low-dose CT examinations in 80 patients. Eur Radiol. 2011;21(3):636–43.

11

Vision-based markerless registration using stereo vision and an augmented reality surgical navigation system

Hideyuki Suenaga[1*], Huy Hoang Tran[2], Hongen Liao[3,4], Ken Masamune[2,5], Takeyoshi Dohi[6], Kazuto Hoshi[1] and Tsuyoshi Takato[1]

Abstract

Background: This study evaluated the use of an augmented reality navigation system that provides a markerless registration system using stereo vision in oral and maxillofacial surgery.

Method: A feasibility study was performed on a subject, wherein a stereo camera was used for tracking and markerless registration. The computed tomography data obtained from the volunteer was used to create an integral videography image and a 3-dimensional rapid prototype model of the jaw. The overlay of the subject's anatomic site and its 3D-IV image were displayed in real space using a 3D-AR display. Extraction of characteristic points and teeth matching were done using parallax images from two stereo cameras for patient-image registration.

Results: Accurate registration of the volunteer's anatomy with IV stereoscopic images via image matching was done using the fully automated markerless system, which recognized the incisal edges of the teeth and captured information pertaining to their position with an average target registration error of < 1 mm. These 3D-CT images were then displayed in real space with high accuracy using AR. Even when the viewing position was changed, the 3D images could be observed as if they were floating in real space without using special glasses.

Conclusion: Teeth were successfully used for registration via 3D image (contour) matching. This system, without using references or fiducial markers, displayed 3D-CT images in real space with high accuracy. The system provided real-time markerless registration and 3D image matching via stereo vision, which, combined with AR, could have significant clinical applications.

Keywords: Augmented reality, Integral videography, Markerless registration, Stereo vision, Three-dimensional image

Background

Augmented reality (AR) involves the co-display of a virtual image and a real-time image so that the user is able to utilize and interact with the components of both images simultaneously [1]. This image-based navigation facilitates *in situ* visualization during surgical procedures [2] because visual cues obtained from a preoperative radiological virtual image can enhance visualization of surgical anatomy [3], thus improving preoperative planning and supporting the surgeon's skill by simplifying the anatomical approach to complex procedures [4]. In recent years, the technical application of AR has been studied in the context of various clinical applications. Examples of recent research which has sought to determine how the application of AR may lead to improvements in medical outcomes have included a study examining the use of AR to improve the precision of minimally invasive laparoscopic surgeries [3]; comparison between planned and actual needle locations in MRI-guided lumbar spinal injection procedures [5]; and studies examining the application of AR for image-guided neurosurgery for brain tumors [6], for the overlay of preoperative radiological 3-dimensional (3D) models onto the intraoperative laparoscopic videos [7]; and to facilitate vessel localization in neurovascular surgery [8]. AR also has potential as an aid to surgical

* Correspondence: suenaga-tky@umin.ac.jp
[1]Department of Oral-Maxillofacial Surgery, Dentistry and Orthodontics, The University of Tokyo Hospital, 7-3-1 Hongo, Bunkyo ku, Tokyo 113 8656, Japan
Full list of author information is available at the end of the article

teaching [4]. Furthermore, CT-free navigation systems, which do not rely on the acquisition of pre-procedure image acquisition but instead intra-operatively recognize the position and orientation of defined patient features, are also being evaluated [9, 10]. AR has the potential to increase the surgeon's visual awareness of high-risk surgical targets [7] and to improve the surgeon's intuitive grasp of the structures within the operational fields [11].

Similarly, there are an increasing number of studies examining the potential use of image-guided systems for oral and maxillofacial surgeries (OMS) [12, 13]. Patient or image registration (overlay) is key to associating the surgical field with its virtual counterpart [14, 15]. The disadvantages of the current navigation systems used in OMS include bulky optical trackers and lower accuracy of electromagnetic trackers in locating surgical instruments, invasive and error-prone image registration procedures, and an additional reference marker to track patient movement [16]. In addition, errors related to position, angle, distance, vibration of the optical tracker, the reference frame and probe tip of the equipment are high. With anatomical landmark-based registration, each observer is only prone to human error based on personal preference of anatomical landmarks in the surgical field [17, 18]. Moreover, frequent hand-eye transformation, which corrects the displacement between the probe tip and the image reference frame, is required for constant comparisons between the surgical field and the displayed image. Furthermore, images in real space are projected using a 3D display via binocular stereopsis, with the disadvantage that the observed video does not change with changes in viewing position since only relative depth is recognized. Thus, accurate 3D positioning cannot be reproduced without incurring motion parallax. Head mounted displays and head-mounted operating microscopes with stereoscopic vision have been used many times for AR visualization in the medical field. However, such video see through devices have two views that present only horizontal parallax, instead of the full parallax. Projector-based AR visualization is appropriate for large operative field overlays; however, it lacks depth perception. As described in our previous study, we have developed an autostereoscopic 3-D image overlay using a translucent mirror [15]. The integral videography (IV) principle applied in this study differs from binocular stereopsis, and allows both binocular parallaxes for depth perception and motion parallax, wherein depth cues are recognized even if the observer is in motion [15, 19–21]. Results from our previous research have shown that the 3D AR system using integral videographic images is a highly effective and accurate tool for surgical navigation in OMS [22].

To overcome the challenges of image-guided OMS, we developed a more simplified AR navigation system that provides automatic markerless image registration using real-time autostereoscopic 3D (IV) imaging and stereo vision for dental surgery. Patient-image registration achieved by patient tracking via contour matching has been previously described [14]. The current study evaluated the feasibility of using a combination of AR and stereo vision technologies to project IV images obtained from preoperative CT data onto the actual surgical site during real time and automatic markerless registration, respectively, in a clinical setting; this feasibility study was performed on a volunteer. Therefore, this study proposes use of this simplified image-guided AR technology for superimposing a region-specific 3D image of the jaw bone on the actual surgical site in real time. This technology can aid surgical treatment of structures that are in spatial positions but not directly observable.

Methods

The apparatus for the entire system was comprised of 3D stereo camera and the 3D-IV imaging system, as shown in Fig. 1a. We used two computer systems; one to track the surgical procedure using stereo vision and the other to generate 3D-IV images for a projected overlay. The study was conducted in accordance with Good Clinical Practice (GCP) guidelines and the Declaration of Helsinki, and the study protocol was approved by the medical ethics committee of the Graduate School of Medicine of the University of Tokyo, Japan. Written informed consent was provided by the volunteer prior to study initiation.

Generation of 3D-IV images

The 3D-IV images to be projected onto the surgical site were generated from CT images of the jaw bones using an Aquilion ONE™ (Toshiba, Tokyo, Japan) 320-row area detector CT scanner and from images of the teeth using a Rexcan DS2 3D scanner (Solutionix, Seoul, Korea). Conditions for the area detector CT (ADCT) scan were: tube voltage, 120 kV; tube current, 270 mA; and slice thickness, 0.5 mm. Thus, the IV image generated from the preoperative CT data was a "real" 3D representation of the jaws. Next, 3D surface models of the upper and lower jawbones were generated using Mimics® Version 16 (Materialise, Leuven, Belgium) and Geomagic Control (Geomagic, Cary, NC, USA) medical image-processing software. Similarly, the 3D scanned images of a dental plaster model were recorded onto a CT image using the Rexcan DS2 3D scanner. Briefly, the IV image of the 3D CT was constructed as an assembly of reconstructed light sources. The complete 3D-IV image was displayed directly onto the surgical site using a half-silvered mirror (Fig. 1a), which makes it appear that the 3D image is inside the patient's body, and could be viewed directly without special glasses. Technical details

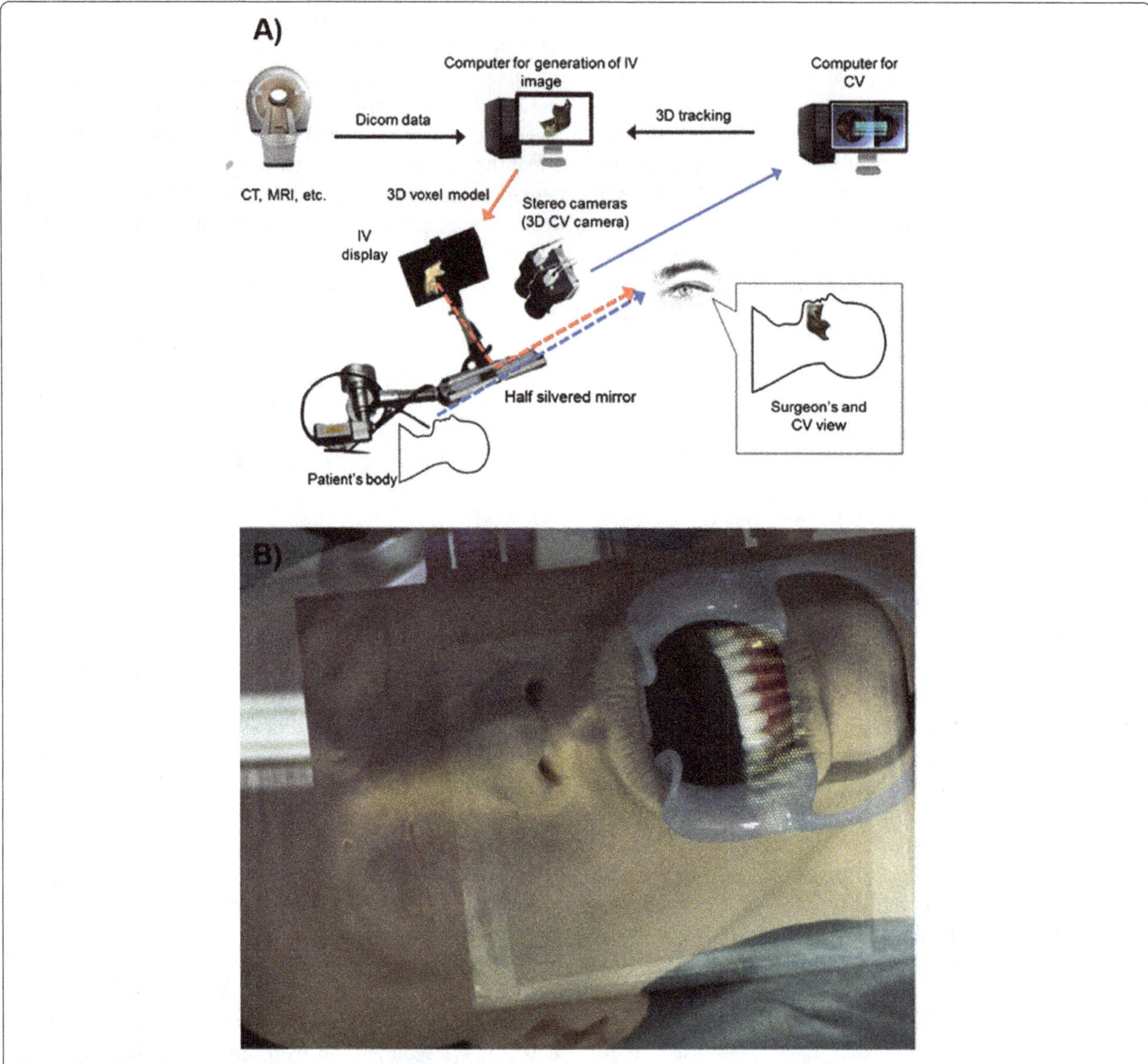

Fig. 1 The physical setup of the system. **a** The configuration of the markerless surgical navigation system based on stereo vision and augmented reality, and **b** a 3D rapid prototyping model

for the generation of the 3D-IV images have been described in previous publications [15, 19, 20, 22, 23]. Each point, shown in a 3D space, was reconstructed at the same position as the actual object by the convergence of rays from the pixels of the element images on the computer display after they pass through the lenses in a microconvex lens array. The surgeon can see any point on the display from various directions, as though it were fixed in 3D space. Each point appears as a different light source. The system was able to render IV images at a rate of 5 frames per second. For the IV image to be displayed in the correct position, the coordinates of the preoperative model obtained from CT data are registered intraoperatively with the contour derived from the 3D scanner image of the subject in real space. The triangle mesh model of the teeth is created using the marching cubes algorithm and is rendered by OpenGL.

Rapid prototyping model

With the 3D-IV images generated, a feasibility study was conducted on a phantom head using a 3D rapid prototyping (RP) model of the mandible using Alaris™ 30U RP technology (Objet Geometries, Rehovot, Israel) based on CT data of the subject (Fig. 1b). Technical details of the registration of the RP model have been described in previous publications, with registration errors reported to be between 0.27 and 0.33 mm [18]. The mean overall error of the 3D image overlay in the current study was 0.71 mm, which met clinical requirements [15].

Patient tracking

"Patient tracking" refers to tracking of the 3D contours of the teeth (incisal margins). The incisal margins were tracked, with the right and left images obtained through the stereo camera in real time; spatial positions of the teeth were obtained by matching the right and left images for 3D-contour reconstruction. The reconstructed 3D image was then compared with the actual image from the subject using the stereo camera.

Specifications for the tracking system included an Intel® Core™ i7 3.33 GHz processor combined with an NVIDIA® GeForce® GTX 285 GPU and an EO-0813CCD 2 charge-coupled device stereo camera (Edmund Optics Inc., Barrington, NJ, USA). The camera had a maximum frame rate of 60 frames per second with an image resolution of 1280 × 1024 pixels.

Image-based calibration of IV display

The 3D-IV images were calibrated using a calibration model with known geometry that included: a) visualization of the calibration model with five feature points in the IV frame; b) display of the 3D image of the calibration model; c) stereo image capture of the 3D image with the stereo camera through the half silvered mirror; and d), matching of parallax images (right and left images) from the stereo camera to obtain a final 3D-IV image. Similarly, the final calibrated 3D-IV images of the subject's jaw that appeared to be floating in real space were projected into the correct position based on the coordinates of the image obtained from preoperative CT data and the real object from the subject using HALCON software Version 11 (MVTec Software GmbH, Munich, Germany) and Open CV, the Open Source Computer Vision Library.

Patient-image registration

Typically, fixed external anatomic landmarks on the patient and imaging data define the accuracy of imaging system [24] whereby anatomic landmarks identified on the surface of the organ can be correlated with accuracy to the predefined landmarks in the computer's coordinate system. In the current study, the natural landmarks (incisal margins) were tracked with the stereo camera instead of manual identification. The 3D position of this natural landmark was accurately determined using the right and left images (parallax images) captured by the stereo camera [25]. Thereafter, the preoperative 3D-CT image was integrated with images from the subject using 3D image-matching technology (stereo vision). The detected feature point of a tooth (actual image) was then correlated with the corresponding feature point of a tooth on the 3D CT image. This means that mutually corresponding feature points in both the images (i.e., 3D-CT image and actual image of a tooth) were matched. Matching of the 3D-CT image and volunteer position was based on the correlation of ≥ 200 feature points on the incisal margin. Because of the high contrast between the teeth and the oral cavity, the 3-D contour of the front teeth is easily extracted using template matching and edge extraction. An image template is first manually selected using the left camera image and then matched to the corresponding right camera image to select the regions of interest (ROI). 2-D edges of the front teeth are then extracted with subpixel accuracy within the detected ROIs, and the extracted teeth edges are stereo-matched using epipolar constraint searching. Sub-pixel estimation is the process of estimating the value of a geometric quantity to better than pixel accuracy, even though the data was originally sampled on an integer pixel quantized space. Frequency based shift calculated methods using phase correlation (PC) have been widely used because of its accuracy and low complexity for shift motion due to translation, rotation or scale changes between images. The PC method for images alignment relies mainly on the shift property of the Fourier transform to estimate the translation between two images. The epipolar line is the straight line of intersection of the epipolar plane with the image plane. It is the image in one camera of a ray through the optical centre and image point in the other camera. All epipolar lines intersect at the epipole. This epipolar line is an extremely important constraint in the stereo matching step. Epipolar constraint searching aims to establish a mapping between points in the left image and lines in the right image and vice versa so that "the correct match must lie on the epipolar line". 11 × 11 area is defined as the patch size of 11 × 11 pixel. A normalized cross correlation coefficient describes the similarity between two patches and can be used for solving correspondence problems between images. The basic steps involves (i) extracting a reference patch from the reference image; the conjugate position of this reference patch in the search image is determined, (ii) defining a search area and specific sampling positions (search patches) for correlation, within the search image, (iii) computing the correlation value (with respect to the reference patch) at each of the defined sample position, and (iv) finding the sample position with the maximum correlation value, which indicates the search patch with highest similarity to the reference patch. If multiple edge points appear on the epipolar line, the one with the closest normalized cross correlation value (calculated in an 11 × 11 area centered at the candidate edge point) is chosen for the match. Full details of the algorithms used for matching have been previously described [15]. An HDC-Z10000 3D video camera (Panasonic Co, Ltd, Tokyo, Japan) was used to document the procedure. Although we adapted the steps from published literature

[15, 25], the novelty of our method is that this is the first study in which dentomaxillofacial 3D computed tomography (CT) data (both maxillary and mandibular jaws along with teeth) generated by a 3D IV image display system using augmented reality (AR) navigation system that provides a markerless registration system using stereo vision in oral and maxillofacial surgery were superimposed on a human volunteer. Previous studies were made on phantom models. We focused on investigating the property of the intraoral environment of human. Patient movement was a challenge that needed to be addressed when applying the method on a human subject in real clinical setting. The challenge of patient movement was overcome by the use of a custom designed stereo camera which tracked the patient movement and updated the image registration on real time without manual involvement.

Evaluation of recognition time and positioning error

Because registration and tracking were performed using the stereo camera, the measurement error of the stereo camera system was considered a major source of registration error. Since it was considered impractical to evaluate the accuracy of each stage of the registration process, the accuracy of the final 3D-IV image was used to confirm the accuracy of this novel system. Error calculation was conducted as per our previous study, based on the alignment of 14 points on the surface of the teeth with the actual 3D-IV images using the stereo camera [23]. Because these points were not used at any stage of the registration process, the accuracy of this experiment can be considered as a target registration error (TRE). Each point was measured 20 times in the stereoscopic model and 3D-IV images to determine average value, standard deviation (SD) and 3D differences for the target position [1]. Calculations were performed according to Fitzpatrick and West [26].

The accuracy of the cameras was based on the following equations:

$$XYdirection\ :\ \Delta_x = \Delta_y = \frac{z}{f}\Delta_d$$

$$Zdirection\ :\ \Delta_z = \frac{z^2}{fb}\Delta_d$$

where, z is the distance from the camera to the object (~500 mm), f is the focal length of the cameras (12 mm), b is the distance between the cameras (120 mm) and Δ_d represents half of a pixel's size on the sensor (2.325 μm).

Results

The calibrated images of the setup based on five feature points and the resulting 3D-IV image were displayed in real space as shown in Fig. 2a and 2b, respectively, which were then recognized and matched by our automatic measurement method using the stereo camera (Fig. 2c); extraction of characteristic points is shown in Fig. 3a. Registration of the 3D-IV and subject images was performed, wherein the contours were automatically detected, their outline generated and both were matched using the stereo camera (Fig. 3b). The 3D reconstruction of the teeth contours in the stereo camera after image matching is shown in Fig. 3c. By automatically detecting the feature points of the teeth, complete automatic registration was possible (Fig. 3b and 3c). Therefore, this system allowed real-time patient-image registration through tracking of teeth contours and image matching with the pre-operative model. The 3D-CT images of the mandible and maxilla in real space obtained using AR technology are shown in Fig. 4a and 4b (Additional files 1 and 2). Furthermore, CT data were displayed in real space as high-accuracy stereoscopic images with the teeth as landmarks for capturing information regarding the position of structures, thus negating the need for markers. The mandibular canal, tooth root and impacted third molar could also be visualized in the 3D-IV image (Fig. 4c; Additional file 3). The actual accuracy of the camera system was computed to be 0.096 mm along the XY axis and 0.403 mm along the Z axis (depth); the accuracy limit in positioning was theoretically calculated to be 0.425 mm. The error component in each direction is shown in Fig. 5. The mean (SD) error between the IV image and object was 0.28 (0.21) mm along the X axis, 0.25 (0.17) mm along the Y axis and 0.36 (0.33) mm along the Z axis.

The current study evaluated the feasibility of using a combination of AR and stereo vision technologies to project IV images obtained from preoperative CT data onto the actual surgical site during real time and automatic markerless registration, respectively, in a clinical setting on a volunteer. The existing methods using this type of system is so far done on phantom models. Here we have successfully done the markerless registration of patient image on a patient volunteer in a clinical setup for the first time. So there is no other similar study for comparison.

Discussion

Dental surgery requires highly precise operations, with surgical targets often hidden by surrounding structures that must remain undamaged during the procedure. The use of AR system may provide a solution to address challenges presented in routine surgical practice.

The current study strategically simplified and improved the application of AR in OMS. The study used region-specific 3D-CT images displayed in real space with high accuracy and depth perception by using

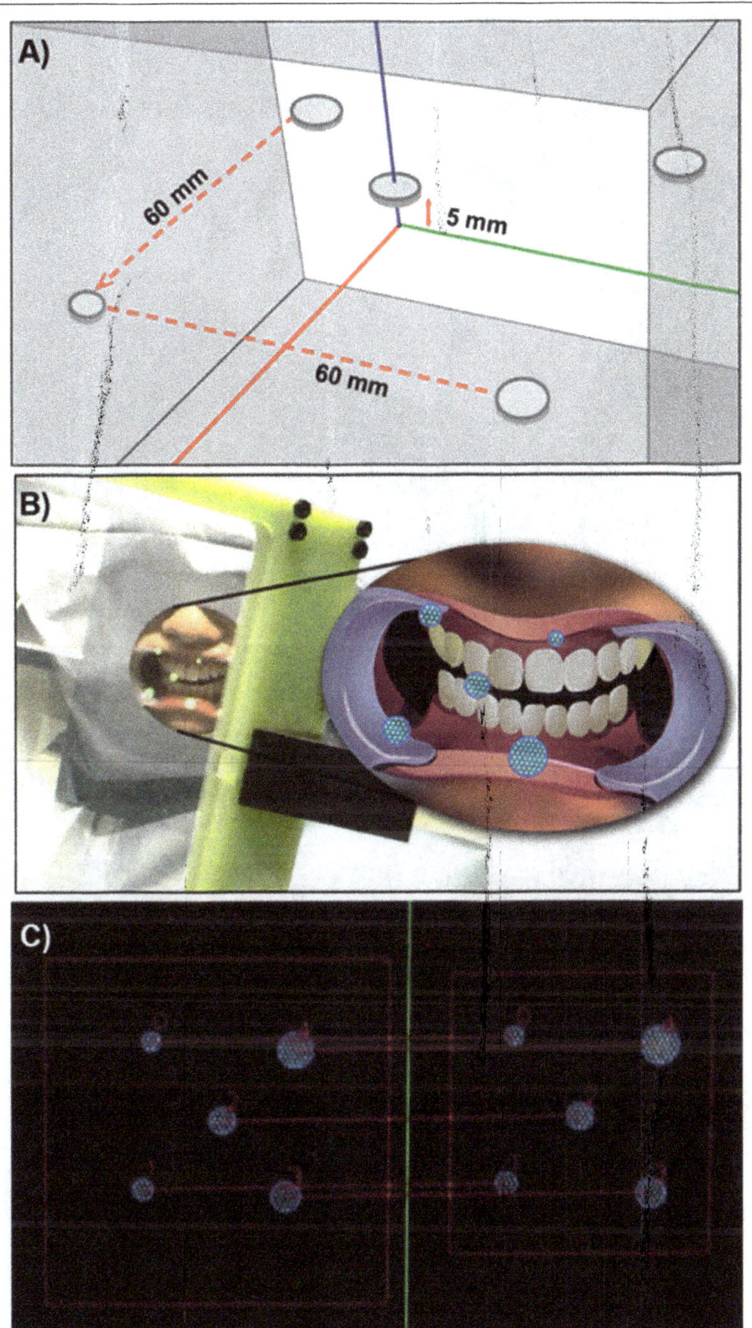

Fig. 2 Calibration of the integral videography (IV) display. This includes **a** five feature points for calibration, **b** The IV image displayed in real space, and **c** recognition results for the calibrated IV images (matching of left and right images via stereo vision)

markerless registration through stereo vision. The study also used 320-row ADCT to provide a larger number of detector rows, and a single rotation of the gantry obtains 320 slices of CT images for a 16 cm volume area without a helical scan. Traditional methods of registration include an external registration frame or marker frames with a screw, [13, 24, 27] which are fraught with errors and also restrict the operating space. Furthermore, registrations for soft tissues are associated with low accuracy [28]. Zhu and colleagues [29] used an occlusal splint for registration in mandibular angle oblique-split osteotomy with good results; however, the system could not be used in edentulous patients and the markers were limited to the lower half of the face. A study using markerless registration showed variations between three different methods based on anatomic landmarks such as

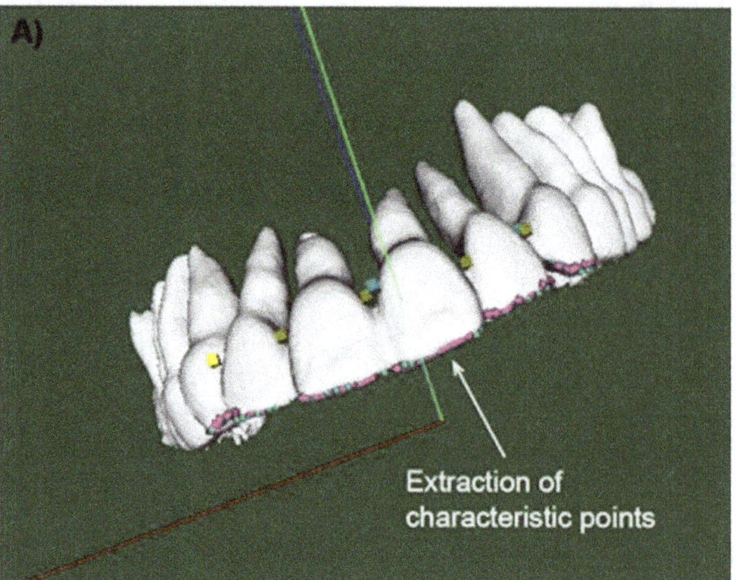

Stereo vision images

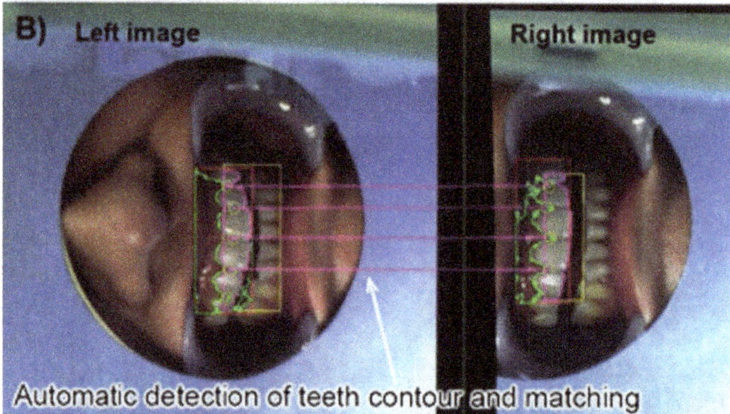

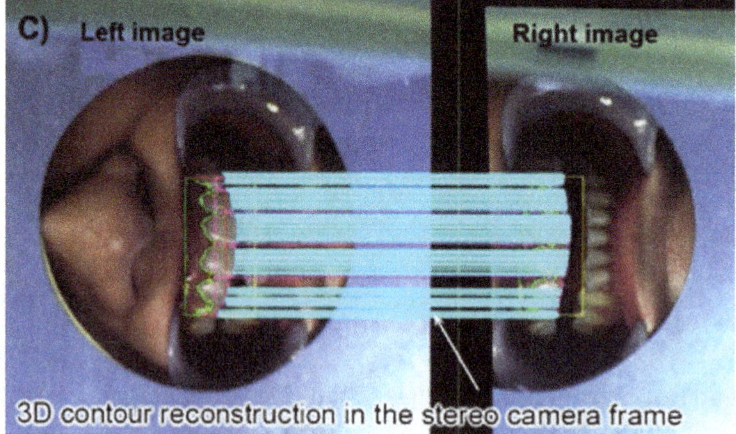

Fig. 3 Automatic registration of the 3D-CT image and volunteer's position. This included **a** extraction of characteristic points, **b** automatic detection of teeth contour and matching of right and left images via stereo vision, and **c** 3D contour reconstruction in the stereo camera frame

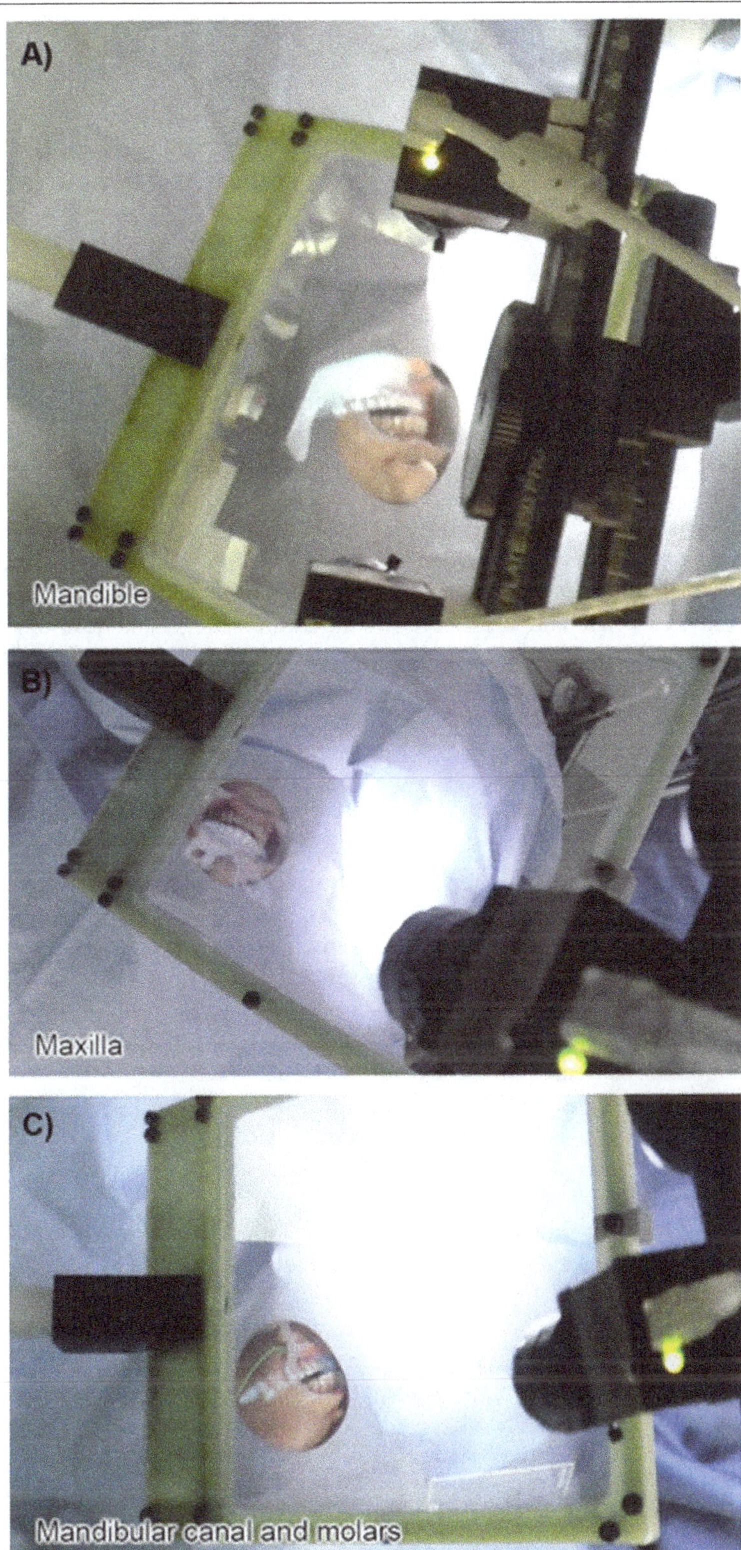

Fig. 4 The IV images are overlaid on the surgical site. This included the **a** mandible, **b** maxilla overlaid on the surgical site, and **c** visualization of the mandibular canal, tooth root, and impacted third molar

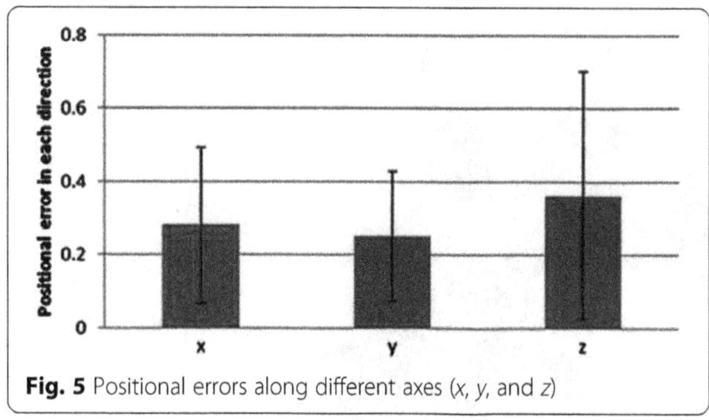

Fig. 5 Positional errors along different axes (*x*, *y*, and *z*)

the zygoma, sinus posterior wall, molar alveolar, premolar alveolar, lateral nasal aperture and the infraorbital areas that were used during navigational surgery of the maxillary sinus [30]. The results of that study showed that although the use of skin adhesive markers and anatomic landmarks was noninvasive and practical, it had limited accuracy and was restricted to craniofacial surgery. In the current study, complete automatic registration was possible because of the use of the anatomic features of teeth; they are the only hard tissues externally exposed, which makes them useful targets for registration based on 3D image matching via stereo vision. We believe that the registration procedure used in the present study can be used in the anterior teeth as well as molars (both jaws), thus including the entire oral surgery site; the only requirement being registration of the teeth. The introduction of stereo cameras into the IV image-overlay system eliminated the use of an external optical tracker.

During navigation in image-guided surgery, since the surgeon cannot simultaneously look at the screen and the operative site, this limitation can cause surgical errors [24]. In the current study using AR and stereo vision technologies, the IV image could be accurately aligned with the preoperative patient model, as observed from both directions. An added benefit was the facility to observe 3D images when changing the viewing position from horizontal to vertical on the subject similarly to real space without the need for special glasses. Because the 3D-AR display in this system obviated the need to avert the operator's eyes from the surgical field or change focus, necessary information could be read in real-time during surgery.

In a comparative study of two navigation systems using frames for registration, the accuracy varied from 0.5 to 4 mm [27]. The average registration error in the current system approximated the theoretical value and was reported as 0.63 ± 0.23 mm, which was much lower than that reported in the other studies [31, 32]. The measurement resolution capacity of the stereo camera system in the current study was 0.1 mm along the XY axis and 0.4 mm along the Z axis. A comparative tracking error analysis of five different optical tracking systems showed that their position-measuring accuracy, ranging from 0.1 to 0.4 mm [33], was considered highly acceptable, whereas the position-measuring accuracy in the current study was theoretically calculated as 0.425 mm using the stereo camera [34]. Because our extraction algorithm was accurate up to the sub-pixel level, planar coordinates of a 3D point could be computed accurately to within 0.1 mm, which was superior to that of an optical tracking system. However, as both registration and tracking were carried out using a stereo camera set, measurement error was one of the major sources of registration errors. It was anticipated that the TRE for the proximal'-characteristic features' used for registration would be less than that in the region more distal. The pre-and intra-operative contours of each part (anterior or left and right molars) could be easily extracted using the method shown in this study, and the pair near the surgical site should be used for patient-image registration. Thus, the location of the surgical site should determine the selection of anterior teeth or molar tracking for patient-image registration. The potential for error increases with increases in the number of steps in a procedure. Therefore, the possibility of segmentation errors in CT data and registration errors related to incorporating digital dental models in CT data cannot be completely ruled out. In the field of oral surgery, the complexity of the anatomical structures involved often makes it difficult to visualize the operating field site. Ability to grasp the 3D relationships between such structures through direct visualization promises to greatly facilitate surgical procedures. Furthermore, the actual clinical accuracy in terms of clinical outcomes will require assessment of this procedure in surgery-specific randomized controlled trials.

Conclusion

In conclusion, this system, without the use of references and fiducial markers, displayed 3D-CT images in real space with high accuracy. The system provided real-time markerless registration and 3D image matching using stereo vision, which, combined with AR, could have significant clinical applications. The entire registration process took less than three seconds to complete and the time for computation was acceptable. To improve accuracy and processing speed, future research should aim to improve the resolution of cameras, create finer displays and increase the computational power of the computer systems. Depth resolution could be improved using a camera with a smaller pixel pitch. Since an improved highly precise system is required, a high-definition rear display or lens array is needed for the densification of pixels in AR display. The most important contribution of this study is that it proved the feasibility of the AR system with IV imaging for clinical use with a registration error of < 1 mm. Our registration frame provided a markerless registration and tracking of IV images and patient, thereby simplifying intraoperative tasks, increasing accuracy and reducing potential discomfort and inconvenience to the patient. Therefore, this modified AR technique with stereo vision has a significant potential for use in clinical applications. In a sense, we think that the method adopted here cannot be rigidly classified into either a methodology or validation paper. In this paper it was termed as methodology because so many aspects of the methods were needed to conduct this work. The repeatability of the method may be in question if it is done only on one patient. Therefore, future works need to include clinical trials of this technology in more number of patients to assess a multitude of potential applications and universalization of this technique.

Abbreviations

AR: Augmented reality; OMS: Oral and maxillofacial surgeries; IV: Integral videography; GCP: Good clinical practice; ADCT: Conditions for the area detector CT; RP: Rapid prototyping; PC: Phase correlation; ROI: Regions of interest; CT: Computed tomography; TRE: Target registration error; SD: Standard deviation.

Competing interest

The authors declare that they have no competing interests.

Authors' contributions

HS conceived of the study, and participated in its design and coordination and drafted the manuscript. HHT and HL contributed to the design and analysis of the study data, and revised the manuscript. KM, TD, KH, and TT provided clinical insight that pervades the manuscript. All authors read and approved the final manuscript.

Acknowledgments

This work was supported by a Grant-in-Aid for Scientific Research (23792318) of the Japan Society for the Promotion of Science (JSPS) in Japan.

Author details

[1]Department of Oral-Maxillofacial Surgery, Dentistry and Orthodontics, The University of Tokyo Hospital, 7-3-1 Hongo, Bunkyo ku, Tokyo 113 8656, Japan. [2]Department of Mechano-Informatics, Graduate School of Information Science and Technology, The University of Tokyo, Tokyo, Japan. [3]Department of Bioengineering, Graduate School of Engineering, The University of Tokyo, Tokyo, Japan. [4]Department of Biomedical Engineering, School of Medicine, Tsinghua University, Beijing, China. [5]Faculty of Advanced Technology and Surgery, Institute of Advanced Biomedical Engineering and Science, Tokyo Women's Medical University, Tokyo, Japan. [6]Department of Mechanical Engineering, School of Engineering, Tokyo Denki University, Tokyo, Japan.

References

1. Lovo EE, Quintana JC, Puebla MC, Torrealba G, Santos JL, Lira IH, et al. A novel, inexpensive method of image coregistration for applications in image-guided surgery using augmented reality. Neurosurgery. 2007;60:366–71.
2. Sielhorst T, Bichlmeier C, Heining SM, Navab N. Depth perception–a major issue in medical AR: evaluation study by twenty surgeons. Med Image Comput Comput Assist Interv. 2006;9:364–72.
3. Kang X, Azizian M, Wilson E, Wu K, Martin AD, Kane TD. Stereoscopic augmented reality for laparoscopic surgery. Surg Endosc. 2014;28:2227–35.
4. Volonte F, Pugin F, Bucher P, Sugimoto M, Ratib O, Morel P. Augmented reality and image overlay navigation with OsiriX in laparoscopic and robotic surgery: not only a matter of fashion. J Hepatobiliary Pancreat Sci. 2011;18:506–9.
5. Fritz J, Thainual P, Ungi T, Flammang AJ, Cho NB, Fichtinger G, et al. Augmented reality visualization with image overlay for MRI-guided intervention: accuracy for lumbar spinal procedures with a 1.5-T MRI system. AJR Am J Roentgenol. 2012;198:W266–73.
6. Mahvash M, Besharati TL. A novel augmented reality system of image projection for image-guided neurosurgery. Acta Neurochir. 2013;155:943–7.
7. Puerto-Souza G, Cadeddu J, Mariottini GL. Toward Long-term and Accurate Augmented-Reality for Monocular Endoscopic Videos. IEEE Trans Biomed Eng. 2014;61:2609–20.
8. Kersten-Oertel M, Chen SS, Drouin S, Sinclair DS, Collins DL. Augmented reality visualization for guidance in neurovascular surgery. Stud Health Technol Inform. 2012;173:225–9.
9. Matsumoto T, Kubo S, Muratsu H, Tsumura N, Ishida K, Matsushita T, et al. Differing prosthetic alignment and femoral component sizing between 2 computer-assisted CT-free navigation systems in TKA. Orthopedics. 2011;34:e860–5.
10. Yokoyama Y, Abe N, Fujiwara K, Suzuki M, Nakajima Y, Sugita N, et al. A new navigation system for minimally invasive total knee arthroplasty. Acta Med Okayama. 2013;67:351–8.
11. Suzuki N, Hattori A, Iimura J, Otori N, Onda S, Okamoto T, et al. Development of AR Surgical Navigation Systems for Multiple Surgical Regions. Stud Health Technol Inform. 2014;196:404–8.
12. Badiali G, Ferrari V, Cutolo F, Freschi C, Caramella D, Bianchi A, et al. Augmented reality as an aid in maxillofacial surgery: validation of a wearable system allowing maxillary repositioning. J Craniomaxillofac Surg. 2014;42:1970–6.
13. Nijmeh AD, Goodger NM, Hawkes D, Edwards PJ, McGurk M. Image-guided navigation in oral and maxillofacial surgery. Br J Oral Maxillofac Surg. 2005;43:294–302.
14. Wang J, Suenaga H, Yang L, Liao H, Kobayashi E, Takato T, et al. Real-time marker-free patient registration and image-based navigation using stereo vision for dental surgery. LNCS. 2013;8090:9–18.
15. Wang J, Suenaga H, Hoshi K, Yang L, Kobayashi E, Sakuma I, et al. Augmented reality navigation with automatic marker-free image registration using 3-D image overlay for dental surgery. IEEE Trans Biomed Eng. 2014;61:1295–304.
16. Lin YK, Yau HT, Wang IC, Zheng C, Chung KH. A Novel Dental Implant Guided Surgery Based on Integration of Surgical Template and Augmented Reality. Clin Implant Dent Relat Res. 2013. doi:10.1111/cid.12119.
17. Kang SH, Kim MK, Kim JH, Park HK, Lee SH, Park W. The validity of marker registration for an optimal integration method in mandibular navigation surgery. J Oral Maxillofac Surg. 2013;71:366–75.
18. Sun Y, Luebbers HT, Agbaje JO, Schepers S, Vrielinck L, Lambrichts I, et al. Validation of anatomical landmarks-based registration for image-guided surgery: an in-vitro study. J Craniomaxillofac Surg. 2013;41:522–6.
19. Liao H, Hata N, Nakajima S, Iwahara M, Sakuma I, Dohi T. Surgical navigation by autostereoscopic image overlay of integral videography. IEEE Trans Inf Technol Biomed. 2004;8:114–21.
20. Liao H, Ishihara H, Tran HH, Masamune K, Sakuma I, Dohi T. Precision-guided surgical navigation system using laser guidance and 3D autostereoscopic image overlay. Comput Med Imaging Graph. 2010;34:46–54.
21. Tran HH, Matsumiya K, Masamune K, Sakuma I, Dohi T, Liao H. Interactive 3-D navigation system for image-guided surgery. Int J Virtual Real. 2009;8:9–16.
22. Suenaga H, Hoang Tran H, Liao H, Masamune K, Dohi T, Hoshi K, et al. Real-time *in situ* three-dimensional integral videography and surgical navigation using augmented reality: a pilot study. Int J Oral Sci. 2013;5:98–102.
23. Wang J, Suenaga H, Liao H, Hoshi K, Yang L, Kobayashi E, et al. Real-time computer-generated integral imaging and 3D image calibration for augmented reality surgical navigation. Comput Med Imaging Graph. 2015;40:147–59.
24. Widmann G, Stoffner R, Bale R. Errors and error management in image-guided craniomaxillofacial surgery. Oral Surg Oral Med Oral Pathol Oral Radiol Endod. 2009;107:701–15.

25. Noh H, Nabha W, Cho JH, Hwang HS. Registration accuracy in the integration of laser-scanned dental images into maxillofacial cone-beam computed tomography images. Am J Orthod Dentofacial Orthop. 2011;140:585–91.
26. Fitzpatrick JM, West JB. The Distribution of Target Registration Error in Rigid-Body Point-Based Registration. IEEE Trans Med Imaging. 2001;20:917–27.
27. Casap N, Wexler A, Eliashar R. Computerized navigation for surgery of the lower jaw: comparison of 2 navigation systems. J Oral Maxillofac Surg. 2008;66:1467–75.
28. Eggers G, Kress B, Muhling J. Fully automated registration of intraoperative computed tomography image data for image-guided craniofacial surgery. J Oral Maxillofac Surg. 2008;66:1754–60.
29. Zhu M, Chai G, Zhang Y, Ma X, Gan J. Registration strategy using occlusal splint based on augmented reality for mandibular angle oblique split osteotomy. J Craniofac Surg. 2011;22:1806–9.
30. Kang SH, Kim MK, Kim JH, Park HK, Park W. Marker-free registration for the accurate integration of CT images and the subject's anatomy during navigation surgery of the maxillary sinus. Dentomaxillofac Radiol. 2012;41:679–85.
31. Bouchard C, Magill JC, Nikonovskiy V, Byl M, Murphy BA, Kaban LB, et al. Osteomark: a surgical navigation system for oral and maxillofacial surgery. Int J Oral Maxillofac Surg. 2012;41:265–70.
32. Marmulla R, Luth T, Muhling J, Hassfeld S. Markerless laser registration in image-guided oral and maxillofacial surgery. J Oral Maxillofac Surg. 2004;62:845–51.
33. Shamir RR, Joskowicz L. Geometrical analysis of registration errors in point-based rigid-body registration using invariants. Med Image Anal. 2011;15:85–95.
34. Khadem R, Yeh CC, Sadeghi-Tehrani M, Bax MR, Johnson JA, Welch JN. Comparative tracking error analysis of five different optical tracking systems. Comput Aided Surg. 2000;5:98–107.

12

Illegal intra-corporeal packets: can dual energy CT be used for the evaluation of cocaine concentration?

Alexandra Platon[1], Minerva Becker[1], Christoph D. Becker[1], Eric Lock[2], Hans Wolff[3], Thomas Perneger[4] and Pierre-Alexandre Poletti[1*]

Abstract

Background: The recent implementation of the dual energy technology on CT-scanners has opened new perspectives in tissue and material characterization. This study aims to evaluate whether dual energy CT can be used to assess the concentration of cocaine of intra-intestinal illegal packets.

Methods: The study was approved by the institutional review board of our institution (CER 13_027_R). From November 2010 to May 2013, all consecutive conveyors in whom a low-dose abdominal CT (LDCT) revealed the presence of illegal intra-corporeal drug packets underwent a dual energy CT series (gemstone spectral imaging) targeted on one container. The mean radiological density (HU) of these packets was measured on the LDCT series, and on the monochromatic dual energy series, at 40 and 140 keV. The difference between the HU at 40 and 140 keV was reported as ΔHU. The effective atomic number Z(eff) was also measured on the monochromatic series. A chemical analysis was performed after expulsion to select cocaine containing packets, and to determine their cocaine concentrations. A correlation analysis was performed between HU, ΔHU and Z(eff), with regard to the percentage of cocaine.

Results: Fifty-four cocaine conveyors were included. The mean cocaine content of the packets was 36.8 % (range 11.2–80, SD 15.4), the mean radiologic density 105 HU, the mean Z(eff) 8.7 and the mean ΔHU 163. The cocaine content was correlated with the ΔHU (0.57, $p < 0.001$), with the Z(eff) ($r = 0.56$, $p < 0.001$) but not with radiologic density ($r = 0.25$, $p = 0.064$). ΔHU >200 was 0.9 (9 of 10) sensitive and 0.82 (36 of 44) specific to predict a cocaine concentration higher than 50 %.

Conclusion: Measuring ΔHU or Z(eff) on dual energy monochromatic CT series can be used to detect ingested packets with cocaine concentration >50 %.

Keywords: Computed tomography, Dual energy body packing, Cocaine

* Correspondence: pierre-alexandre.poletti@hcuge.ch
[1]Department of Radiology, University Hospital of Geneva, 4, rue Gabrielle-Perret-Gentil, 1211, Geneva, Switzerland
Full list of author information is available at the end of the article

Background

Body packing refers to the act of concealing large drug containers (usually >2 cm) within the gastro-intestinal tract. Cocaine and heroin are the most frequent illicit substances smuggled through customs in this way. Standard radiography is often used as a screening test for the detection of intracorporeal body packets, but it is limited by a relatively high rate of false negative interpretations when compared to low-dose CT (LDCT) imaging [1–5]. Therefore, LDCT is now progressively replacing standard radiography in the screening of the persons suspected of conveying body packets. Furthermore, once body packets have been identified, a follow-up LDCT gives also useful information for the detection of potential complications up to the complete evacuation of the packets, such as the absence of progression of a packet through the gastro-intestinal tract, thus increasing the risk of packet rupture [6]. However, it has never been established whether LDCT might bring information about the packets content, which could be clinically relevant in case of impending rupture. The recent implementation of the dual energy technology on CT-scanners has opened new perspectives in tissue and material characterization [7]. Recent in vitro series have suggested that dual energy CT technology (DECT) may be used to differentiate heroin from cocaine in illegal intra-corporeal packets, swallowed by drug smugglers [8, 9], but no studies were performed while packets were still in the gastro-intestinal tract. In our institution, almost all illegal packets contain cocaine, which is due to the specificities of the international drug trafficking pathways. In this setting, knowing the concentration of cocaine contained in the packets may be of great interest for the clinician in charge of the drug conveyer to adapt the therapeutic management in case of impeding rupture.

The aim of the current study is to evaluate whether dual energy CT can be used to assess the concentration of cocaine of intra-intestinal illegal packets.

Methods

The research project was approved by the Institutional Review Board of our institution (Ethics Committee on research involving humans of the University Hospital of Geneva, CER 13_027_R), in compliance with the Helsinki Declaration. Since a better characterization of the packets by a targeted DECT series was considered useful to improve the clinical management of the conveyors, and therefore their safety, the Ethics committee waived the need for consent.

All consecutive adult persons suspected of having ingested drug packets within the Geneva State territory ($n = 720$) during a 30 months period of time (November 2010 to May 2013) were brought to our emergency department for a LDCT examination. LDCT images were immediately interpreted for the presence of drug containers by the radiology resident and the attending physician on call, while the suspect was still on the CT table.

Whenever LDCT was reported positive for body-packets ($n = 120$, 16.5 %), a 3-cm thick CT series was performed, targeted on a drug container, using a dual-energy protocol (Gemstone imaging, GSI).

When the presence of body-packets was reported at LDCT, the conveyors were hospitalized until all packets were collected. For each patient, four of these packets were analyzed by a dedicated laboratory, which evaluated their size and weight, the percentage of cocaine and also performed a qualitative analysis of the cutting agents. These data were retained by the scientific police up to the end of the study.

Exclusion criteria

Cases were excluded from the study when laboratory data could not be obtained or when dual energy series could not be performed. When the cocaine concentrations measured in various packets from the same conveyor were dissimilar (variation of more than 20 % between the highest and the lowest drug concentration), the case was also excluded.

Reference standard

The mean percentage of cocaine obtained from the 4 measures from samples of homogenous drug packets was considered reference standard.

Technical imaging parameters

LDCT were performed with a 64-rows GE 750 HD CT (Discovery 750 HD CT, GE Healthcare, Milwaukee, USA), from lung bases to pelvis, without intra-venous, oral or rectal contrast material, using the following parameters: 64 ×1.25 mm collimation, pitch 1.375, gantry rotation period 0.7 s, tube potential 120 kV, tube charge per gantry rotation 25.2 mAs, reconstruction slice thickness 2.5 mm, using 40 % ASIR (adaptive statistical iterative reconstruction).

GSI series were performed on the same CT scanner as LDCT, on a 3 cm thick area, using the following parameters: 64 ×1.25 mm, pitch 1.375, 140 kV, gantry rotation period 0.6 s, variable potential output of 80 kV and 140 kV, tube charge per gantry rotation 180 mAs.

Effective dose of LDCT and of GSI series

The dose of radiation delivered by low-dose CT and the dual energy series were estimated from the mean normalized values of effective dose per dose-length product (DLP) for the abdomen, as described by Shrimpton et al. [10]. The effective dose for LDCT was 1.4 mSv (DLP = 94.15 [mGy.cm]) for men, and 1.2 mSv for women (DLP 83.54 [mGy.cm]). For the dual energy series, the effective doses were 1.27 mSv and 0.9 mSv for men and women respectively.

CT images analysis

LDCT images and dual CT data were transferred and analyzed on a dedicated GE Advantage workstation (ADW, GE Healthcare, version 4.6), using a GSI viewer 2.0-2L.

LDCT and dual-energy CT images were prospectively analyzed by one of the two board certified attending radiologist of the emergency radiology unit, with 15 and 17 years of experience respectively in reading abdominal CTs. Both radiologists were blinded to the results of the chemical analysis of the packets. The radiologist measured the mean density (HU) in a packet on the LDCT series, using a relatively small (60 mm^2) circular region of interest (ROI), to reduce the risk of partial volume averaging (Fig. 1). The same packet was selected within the 3 cm thick GSI series; the mean effective atomic number Z(eff) (Fig. 2), as well as the mean density (HU) at 40 and 140 keV, were measured in a 60 mm^2 circular ROI. The difference between the attenuations at 40 and 140 keV was calculated and referred to as ΔHU.

Statistical analysis

We obtained mean values and standard deviations of all continuous variables. Then we examined associations between cocaine content (expressed in percent) and various measures of radiologic density using scatterplots and summarized them through Pearson correlation coefficients.

Since the median packet weight in our study population is 10 g, a cocaine content of 35 % or higher is close to the reported lethal threshold (about 3 to 4 g) in case of packet rupture. Therefore, we dichotomized cocaine content as below or above 35 %. We also dichotomized cocaine content as below or above 50 %, to focus on packets with major lethal risk in case of rupture. Then we examined associations between the cocaine concentration at these thresholds with measures of radiologic density by means of receiver operating characteristic curves (ROC) and corresponding areas under the curve (AUC). An AUC of 0.5 means no association while an AUC of 1 reflects perfect discrimination between low-content and high-content containers.

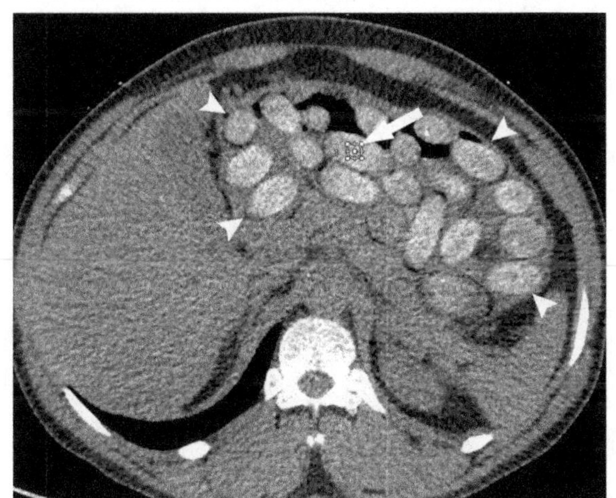

Fig. 1 Thirty-years-old man, positive for conveying drug packets. Axial low-dose CT scan shows numerous drug containers inside the stomach (*arrowheads*); measurement of attenuation is performed within one drug container (*arrow*)

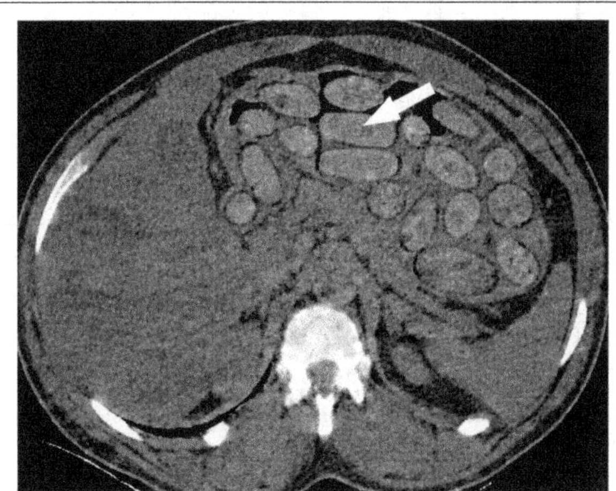

Fig. 2 Thirty-years-old man, positive for conveying drug packets. Dual-energy CT scan shows measurement of the Z(eff) within the same drug container (*arrow*)

For the most promising predictor, we looked at cutoff values that achieved a good compromise of sensitivity and specificity, and reported statistics of test performance.

Analyses were performed using SPSS version 18 (PASW Statistics 18, SPSS Inc, Chicago, USA).

Results

Dual energy CT-scans were not available for 22 of the 120 conveyors in whom drug packets were detected at LDCT; these cases were removed from the study. Forty-four of the 98 remaining cases had to be further excluded, because the laboratory analysis could not be obtained ($n = 26$) or because packets were dissimilar ($n = 18$).

Thus, our study population consisted in 54 conveyors (45 men, 9 women), with a mean age of 34.5 years (range 20–54). The mean amount of packets per conveyor was 34 (range 4–70). The cocaine content ranged from 11 to 80 %, with a mean of 36.8 % (Table 1). The cocaine content was ≤35 in 30 conveyors, >35 % in 24 conveyors, and >50 % in 10. The weight of the packets ranged from 9.6 to 11.8 g (mean 10.04 g).

Table 1 Radiological analyses of packets cocaine content. Means, standard deviations (SD), and correlations between cocaine content, measures of radiologic density (HU) and effective atomic number Z(eff), in 54 drug containers

Variable	Mean (standard deviation)	Pearson r	*P* value
Cocaine content (%)	36.8 (15.4)	–	–
HU low dose CT	105.4 (94.9)	0.25	0.064
Z(eff)	8.71 (0.82)	0.56	<0.001
HU 40 keV	236.7 (174.3)	0.42	0.001
HU 140 keV	73.3 (82.5)	−0.01	0.95
ΔHU[a]	163.4 (130.8)	0.57	<0.001

[a]ΔHU = difference between attenuation at 40 keV and the corresponding 140 keV value

The most frequent cutting substances detected included phenacetin (49 containers, 90.7 %), levamisole (47, 87.0 %), sugars (38, 70.4 %), lidocaine (34, 63.0 %), caffeine (34, 63.0 %), and mannitol (33, 61.1 %).

Associations with radiologic density measures

Cocaine content was moderately associated with Hounsfield units (HU) at 40 keV, but not with HU at 140 keV. However, the difference between these values (ΔHU) showed a very strong correlation with the cocaine content. The results were similar for the Z(eff). Measures of the densities based on the low dose CT scan were only weakly associated with cocaine content (Table 1).

We also confirmed that the ΔHU and the Z(eff) contained practically identical information; the Pearson correlation between these 2 variables was 0.98. Because the method for computing the Z(eff) is proprietary, and therefore only available on a GE system, we displayed our results in ΔHU values only. To obtain the corresponding Z(eff) value from ΔHU, we established a correspondence curve (Fig. 3). The equation of this curve is: $Z(eff) = 7.521 + \Delta HU \times 0.009275 - 0.000008 \times \Delta HU^2$.

The association between ΔHU and cocaine content was continuous, with no evidence of a threshold (Fig. 4). The same pattern of associations was seen when cocaine content was dichotomized at 35 and 50 %. The areas under the ROC curves were 0.83 (95 % CI 0.71 to 0.94) for cocaine content dichotomized at 35 % (Fig. 5), and 0.84 (95 % CI 0.62 to 1.00) for cocaine content dichotomized at 50 % (Fig. 6). ΔHU achieved better sensitivities and specificities for detecting packets with very high cocaine content (>50 %) than for detecting packets with high cocaine content (>35 %), (Table 2).

Discussion

The data from the current studies suggest that DECT can be used to estimate the concentration of cocaine contained in an intracorporeal packet, before its expulsion. DECT achieved a good sensitivity (79 %) and specificity (77 %) for detecting packets with >35 % cocaine concentration, and an even better sensitivity (90 %) and

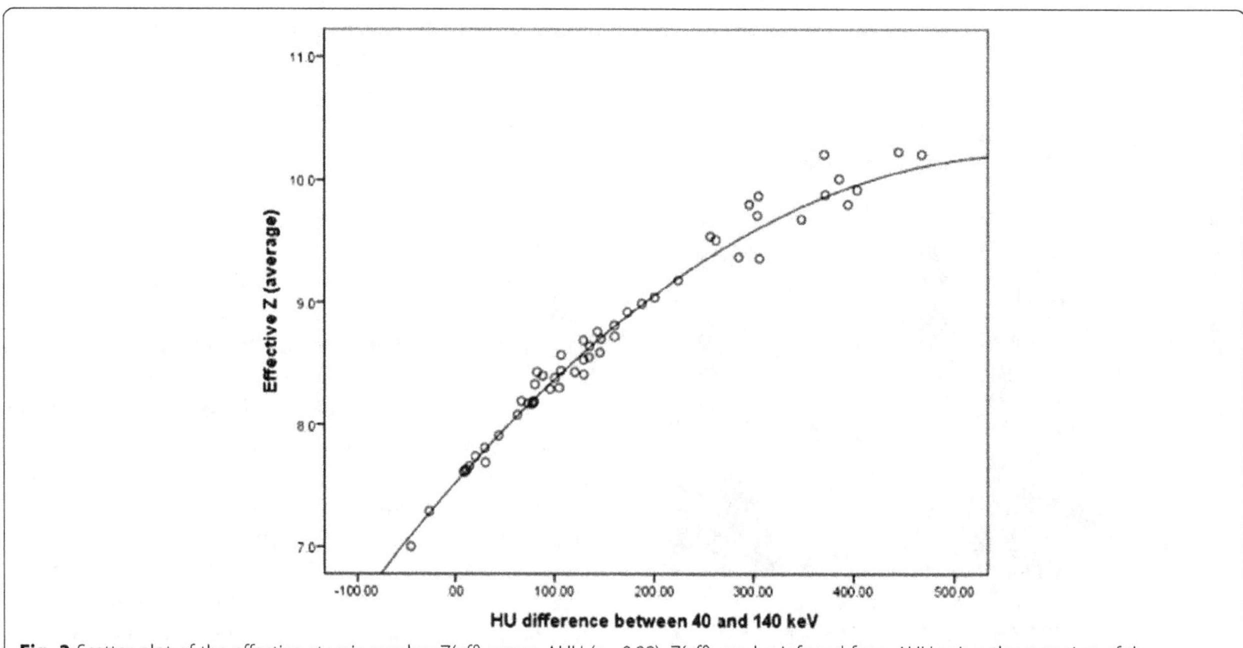

Fig. 3 Scatter-plot of the effective atomic number Z(eff) versus ΔHU (r = 0.98). Z(eff) can be inferred from ΔHU using the equation of the curve: $Z(eff) = 7.521 + \Delta HU \times 0.009275 - 0.000008 \times \Delta HU^2$

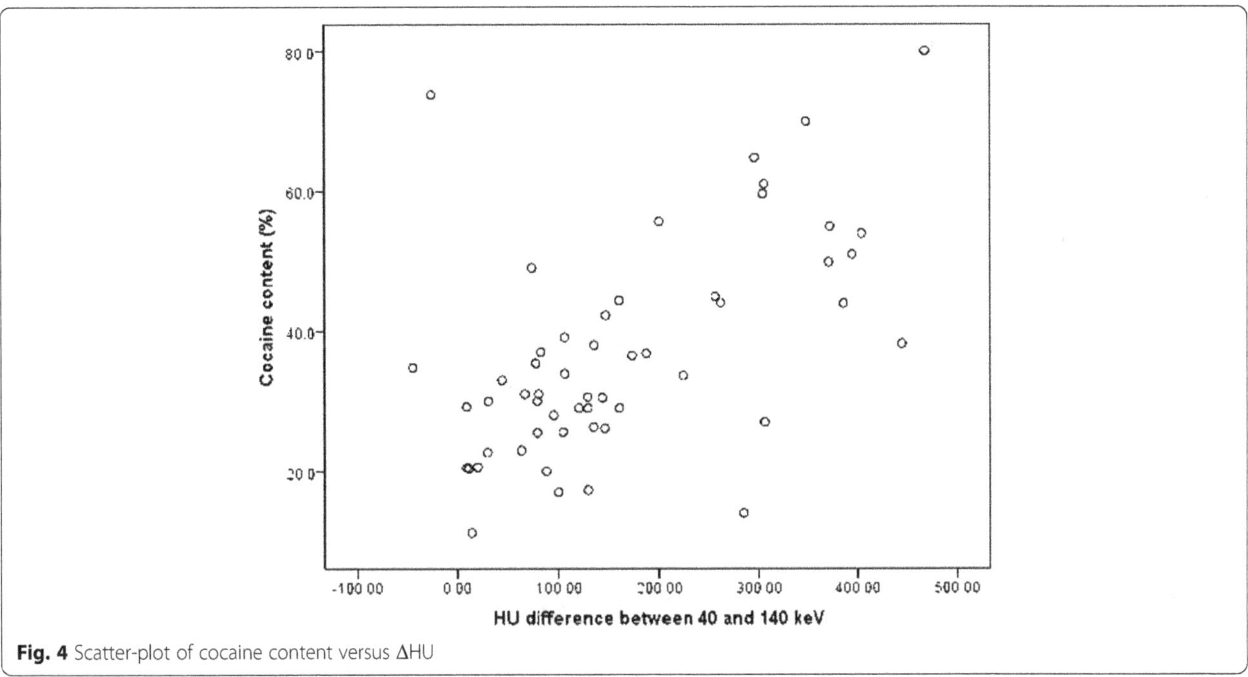

Fig. 4 Scatter-plot of cocaine content versus ΔHU

specificity (82 %) to identify packets with very high cocaine content (>50 %). This improvement in sensitivity could be explained by the fact that the packet content is more homogenous when the percentage of cocaine is higher and, thus, the percentage of cutting agents smaller. Indeed, laboratory analyses of the current study revealed that cocaine was almost always mixed with multiple cutting agents, varying in quality and quantity from one conveyor to the other. Besides, the number of these cutting agents has probably been underestimated, since it is impossible for a laboratory to perform an exhaustive evaluation of all potential substances that may be contained in a packet. Therefore, the influence of the cutting agents on DECT imaging is unpredictable,

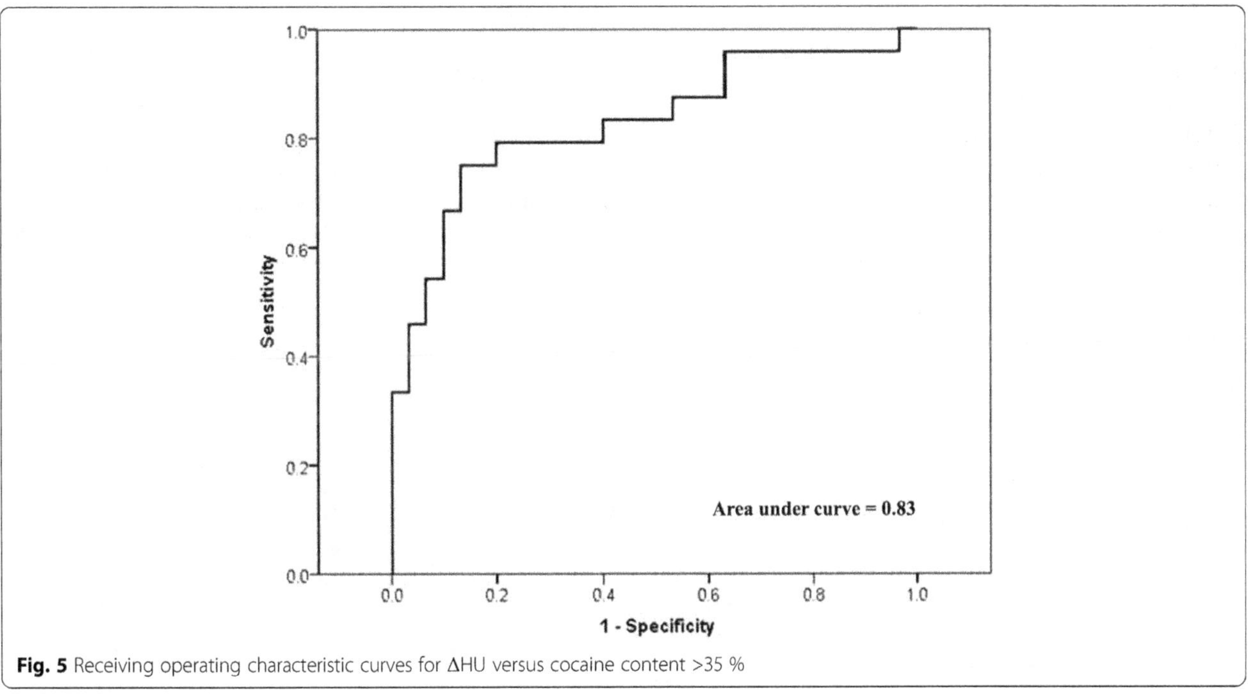

Fig. 5 Receiving operating characteristic curves for ΔHU versus cocaine content >35 %

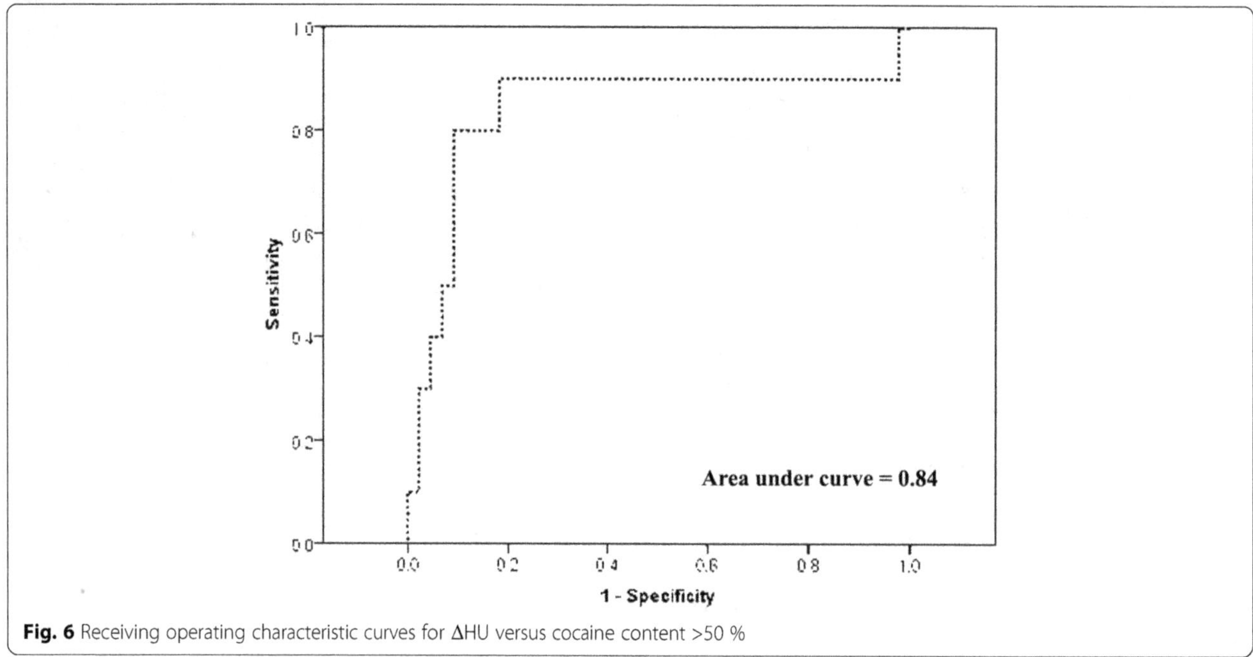

Fig. 6 Receiving operating characteristic curves for ΔHU versus cocaine content >50 %

especially when the percentage of cocaine is low, which certainly constitutes a limitation of the methodology.

Another relevant observation is the linear relationship between ΔHU and Z(eff), and the fact that ΔHU is equivalent to the Z(eff) measures to predict the packet's cocaine concentration. Unlike ΔHU, the algorithm used to measure Z(eff) is proprietary and, therefore, not communicated by the manufacturer. ΔHU, however, can be easily obtained on any dual-energy CT equipment. We therefore recommend using this parameter when reporting results in the scientific literature.

The third observation of the current study is the fact that the cocaine concentration of a packet cannot be assessed by measuring the HU on the standard LDCT images. This can be explained by the fact that the density of the packets varies with the degree of drug compression, as suggested by prior series [1, 8], while the difference in attenuation by DECT, however, would remain unaffected by the compression [8, 9, 11].

Two prior in-vitro series suggested that DECT may be useful to differentiate heroin from cocaine [8, 9]. Since our conveyors population mainly consisted in cocaine smugglers, it was not possible to compare these prior in-vitro qualitative reports with our in-vivo quantitative observations. In a population of cocaine smugglers, the assessment of the percentage of the drug in the packets before expulsion could certainly play a role in the choice of the most appropriate treatment, in case of rupture or impending rupture.

Conclusion

In conclusion, our study showed that DECT may be used for assessing the concentration of cocaine in intracorporeal containers, while the packets are still in the gastrointestinal tract of drug conveyors. Further in vitro

Table 2 Diagnostic performance of ΔHU for 2 levels of cocaine content

Variable	Sensitivity	Specificity	Positive predictive value	Negative predictive value	Odds ratio (95 % confidence interval)
Cocaine content >35 %					
ΔHU >130	0.79 (19/24)	0.77 (23/30)	0.73 (19/26)	0.82 (23/28)	12.5 (3.4–45.7)
ΔHU >140	0.75 (18/24)	0.80 (24/30)	0.75 (18/24)	0.80 (24/30)	12.0 (3.3–43.4)
ΔHU >150	0.71 (17/24)	0.87 (26/30)	0.81 (17/21)	0.79 (26/33)	15.8 (4.0–62.3)
Cocaine content >50 %					
Δ HU >200	0.90 (9/10)	0.82 (36/44)	0.53 (9/17)	0.97 (36/37)	40.5 (4.5–366.8)
Δ HU >250	0.80 (8/10)	0.84 (37/44)	0.53 (8/15)	0.95 (37/39)	21.1 (3.7–121.4)
ΔHU >300	0.70 (7/10)	0.91 (40/44)	0.64 (7/11)	0.93 (40/43)	23.3 (4.3–127.6)

ΔHU: difference between attenuation at 40 keV and the corresponding 140 keV value

series are mandated to increase the precision of the measures by a better understanding of the influence of the cutting agents on DECT results.

Abbreviations

LDCT: Low-dose CT; DECT: Dual energy CT; GSI: Gemstone imaging; Z(eff): Mean effective atomic number; HU: Hounsfield Unit; ΔHU: Difference between the attenuations at 40 keV and 140 keV; ROC: Receiver operating characteristic curve; AUC: Area under the curve; ROI: Region of interest; DLP: Dose-length product.

Competing interests

The authors have no commercial, financial or other interest to disclose with regard to the current submission.

Authors' contributions

PAP and AP did conceive the study. PAP, AP, MB, CDB, HW did equally contribute to the design of the study. AP, PAP; HW and EL did collect the data. TP performed the statistical analysis of the data. AP, PAP, TP, EL, MB, HW, EL carried the data analysis and interpretation. AP, PAP, MB, CDB, HW, TP, EL did participate to the drafting of the manuscript. PAP and CDB did participate to the coordination of the whole study. All authors read and approved the final manuscript.

Acknowledgements

We acknowledge Adjutant Philippe Perret, head of the border guards' narcotics unit of the State of Geneva, for his contribution to this work. Authors received no funding for this study.

Author details

[1]Department of Radiology, University Hospital of Geneva, 4, rue Gabrielle-Perret-Gentil, 1211, Geneva, Switzerland. [2]Scientific Police, Geneva State Police, Geneva, Switzerland. [3]Division of Correctional Medicine and Psychiatry, University Hospital of Geneva, ch. du Petit-Bel-Air 2, 1225, Chêne-Bourg, Switzerland. [4]Division of Clinical Epidemiology, University Hospital of Geneva, 4, rue Gabrielle-Perret-Gentil, Geneva, Switzerland.

References

1. Poletti PA, Canel L, Becker CD, Wolff H, Elger B, Lock E, et al. Screening of illegal intracorporeal containers ("body packing"): is abdominal radiography sufficiently accurate? A comparative study with low-dose CT. Radiology. 2012;265(3):772–9.
2. Gherardi RK, Baud FJ, Leporc P, Marc B, Dupeyron JP, Diamant-Berger O. Detection of drugs in the urine of body-packers. Lancet. 1988;1:1076–8.
3. Kersschot EA, Beaucourt LE, Degryse HR, De Schepper AM. Roentgenographical detection of cocaine smuggling in the alimentary tract. Röfo. 1985;142(3):295–8.
4. Karhunen PJ, Suoranta H, Penttila A, Pitkaranta P. Pitfalls in the diagnosis of drug smuggler's abdomen. J Forensic Sci. 1991;36(2):397–402.
5. Traub SJ, Hoffman RS, Nelson LS. False-positive abdominal radiography in a body packer resulting from intraabdominal calcifications. Am J Emerg Med. 2003;21(7):607–8.
6. Beauverd Y, Poletti PA, Wolff H, Ris F, Dumonceau JM, Elger BS. A body-packer with a cocaine bag stuck in the stomach. World J Radiol. 2011;3(6):155–8.
7. Coursey CA, Nelson RC, Boll DT, Paulson EK, Ho LM, Neville AM, et al. Dual-energy multidetector CT: how does it work, what can it tell us, and when can we use it in abdominopelvic imaging? Radiographics. 2010;30(4):1037–55.
8. Grimm J, Wudy R, Ziegeler E, Wirth S, Uhl M, Reiser MF, et al. Differentiation of heroin and cocaine using dual-energy CT-an experimental study. Int J Legal Med. 2014;128(3):475–82.
9. Leschka S, Fornaro J, Laberke P, Blum S, Alkadhi H, Niederer I, et al. Differentiation of cocaine from heroine body packs by computed tomography: impact of different tube voltages and the dual-energy index. J Forensic Radiol Imaging. 2013;1(2):46–50.
10. Shrimpton PC, Wall BF, Yoshizumi TT, Hurwitz LM, Goodman PC. Effective dose and dose-length product in CT. Radiology. 2009;250(2):604–5.
11. Hergan K, Kofler K, Oser W. Drug smuggling by body packing: what radiologists should know about it. Eur Radiol. 2004;14(4):736–42.

13

Paraneoplastic limbic encephalitis with associated hypothalamitis mimicking a hyperdense hypothalamic tumor

Vipula R. Bataduwaarachchi[1*] and Nirmali Tissera[2]

Abstract

Background: Paraneoplastic limbic encephalitis is an uncommon association of common malignancies such as small cell lung carcinoma, testicular teratoma, and breast carcinoma. The nonspecific nature of the clinical presentation, lack of freely available diagnostic markers, and requirement for advanced imaging techniques pose a great challenge in the diagnosis of this disease in resource-poor settings.

Care presentation: A 64-year-old previously healthy Sri Lankan man was admitted to the general medical unit with subacute memory impairment regarding recent events that had occurred during the previous 3 weeks. Initial noncontrast computed tomography of the brain revealed a hyperdensity in the hypothalamic region surrounded by hypodensities extending toward the bilateral temporal lobes; these findings were consistent with a possible hypothalamic tumor with perilesional edema. The patient later developed cranial diabetes insipidus, which was further suggestive of hypothalamic disease. Interestingly, gadolinium-enhanced magnetic resonance imaging of the brain showed no such lesions; instead, it showed prominent T2-weighted signals in the inner mesial region, characteristic of encephalitis. The possibility of tuberculosis and viral encephalitis was excluded based on cerebrospinal fluid analysis results. Limbic encephalitis with predominant hypothalamitis was suspected based on the radiological pattern. Subsequent screening for underlying malignancy revealed a mass lesion in the right hilum on chest radiographs. Histological examination of the lesion showed small cell lung cancer of the "oat cell" variety.

Conclusion: We suggest that the initial appearance of a hyperdensity in the hypothalamus region on noncontrast computed tomography is probably due to hyperemia caused by hypothalamitis. If hypothalamitis is predominant in a patient with paraneoplastic limbic encephalitis, magnetic resonance imaging will help to differentiate it from a hypothalamic secondary deposit. Limbic encephalitis should be considered in a patient with computed tomographic evidence of a central hyperdensity surrounded by bitemporal hypodensities. This pattern of identification will be useful for early diagnosis in resource-poor settings.

Keywords: Hypothalamitis, Paraneoplastic limbic encephalitis, Cranial diabetes insipidus, Noncontrast computed tomography

* Correspondence: vipbat7@yahoo.com
[1]Department of Pharmacology and Pharmacy, Faculty of Medicine University of Colombo, PO Box 271Kynsey Road, Colombo 8, Sri Lanka
Full list of author information is available at the end of the article

Background

Paraneoplastic limbic encephalitis (PLE) refers to an inflammatory process localized to structures of the limbic system. PLE manifests as a subacute form of encephalitis in later adult life [1]. The occurrence of this disease has been less frequently reported in Asian than in Western countries, probably because of underdiagnosis and under-reporting. PLE is an uncommon association of common malignancies such as small cell lung carcinoma (SCLC) (50 %), testicular teratoma (20 %), and breast carcinoma (8 %); therefore it is considered as a paraneoplastic syndrome [2]. Different types of antineuronal antibodies have been isolated in the cerebrospinal fluid (CSF) of affected patients, including anti-Hu antibodies in patients with SCLC, and anti-Ta antibodies in patients with testicular teratoma [2, 3]. An autoimmune pathogenesis is suggested to play a role in the development of this rare disorder based on the presence of autoantibodies to various neuronal components in the CSF. Although the presence of these autoantibodies may help in the diagnosis, the lack of freely available diagnostic markers and the high number of patients with yet unidentified antibodies and other various tumor types pose a great diagnostic challenge.

Radiological evidence of limbic system involvement is considered to be an excellent supporting tool in the diagnosis of PLE; it helps to exclude other intracranial pathologies as well [2, 4]. A variety of imaging techniques have been used over the years, and the lack of advanced techniques such as magnetic resonance imaging (MRI) and positron emission tomography (PET) in resource-poor settings make the diagnosis more difficult. The PLE-associated mortality rate is considerably high, and treatment success depends on early detection and prompt treatment of the underlying malignancy. The main role of brain imaging in patients with PLE is differentiation between brain metastases and an associated paraneoplastic syndrome. Both of these conditions require entirely different management regimens; therefore, correct differentiation is vital. Although histological examination of brain tissue is ideal in differentiating these two entities, the highly invasive nature of the procedure has made it less popular among neurologists. Therefore, a firm diagnosis supported by imaging is of utmost importance to ensure the best possible care of the patient. Identification of a characteristic radiological pattern on imaging examination is important for proper early evaluation of these patients. We herein report a rare case of PLE associated with SCLC initially misdiagnosed as a hypothalamic tumor by noncontrast computed tomography (CT) imaging of the brain. This is the first such case reported in Sri Lanka.

Case presentation

A previously healthy 64-year-old Sri Lankan man was admitted to the general medical unit because of progressive impairment of his memory regarding recent events that had occurred during the previous 3 weeks. The memory impairment was associated with irritability and confusion. He had been a smoker for 15 pack-years. Physical examination revealed no fever, and his Glasgow coma scale score was 12/15 with alternating irritability and drowsiness. His pupils were equal in size and reactive to light, and no significant neck stiffness was noted. Focal neurological signs were absent. The patient was not cooperative enough to conduct a proper mini-mental examination. His presentation was suggestive of delirium. Basic hematological investigations and renal and liver profiles were not suggestive of an extracranial cause.

Before performing lumbar puncture, we carried out noncontrast CT of the brain to exclude any pathology causing increased intracranial pressure. CT revealed a hyperdensity in the hypothalamic region surrounded by hypodensities extending toward the temporal lobes bilaterally; these findings were consistent with a possible hypothalamic tumor with perilesional edema (Fig. 1a and b).

Electroencephalography showed generalized slowing that was maximal in the bitemporal regions. On the second day of admission, his serum biochemistry parameters became abnormal with a rising serum sodium level (>160 mEq/L) and normal serum potassium level. We noticed a significant increase in his urine output (average of 5.5 L/day) and lowering of his urine osmolality (190 mOsm/kg). Based on the hypovolemic hypernatremia and low urine osmolality associated with the radiological abnormalities in the hypothalamus, we suspected underlying cranial diabetes insipidus in this patient. He was treated with rehydration and intranasal desmopressin, to which he showed only a partial response. The patient was then transferred to the intensive care unit for close monitoring. Once the patient was stable, gadolinium-enhanced MRI of the brain and brain stem was carried out. The transverse section of the brain showed increased T2-weighted signals in the deep temporal lobes, suggesting the involvement of the limbic system (Fig. 2a). The coronal section of the brain showed increased T2-weighted signals in inner mesial regions (Fig. 2b). Interestingly, the mass lesion had disappeared during the previous 3 days. Therefore, viral or autoimmune encephalitis was considered as a more probable diagnosis than a mass lesion. Lumbar puncture was performed at this point, and samples were sent for screening of viral markers (herpes simplex virus, cytomegalovirus, and Japanese encephalitis virus) and tuberculosis polymerase chain reaction; all results were negative. Cytology of the CSF was negative for any malignant cells; however, lymphocytosis was present, suggesting an underlying inflammatory process. Based on the clinical and radiological picture, PLE with associated predominant hypothalamitis was suspected in this patient. Unfortunately, autoimmune markers were

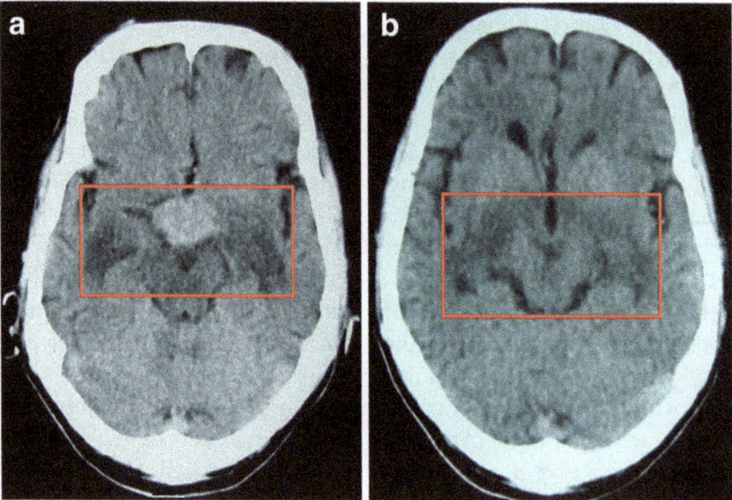

Fig. 1 **a** Non contrast CT images. Transverse section of the brain at the thalamic level. This image showed a high density mass-like lesion in the hypothalamus region with the surrounding hypodense area in the brain. This lesion was initially reported as a mass lesion/ hemorrhage with surrounding edema. **b** Non contrast CT images. Transverse section of the brain at upper brain stem level

not available, and the patient had financial limitations that prevented further investigation. His condition deteriorated with the development of acute kidney injury caused by severe intravascular hypovolemia due to resistant diuresis. Considering the possibility of an associated malignancy, a chest radiograph was obtained and showed a mass lesion in the right hilum. The patient was not fit enough to undergo contrast-enhanced axial CT of the thorax because of his rising serum creatinine level. However, bronchoscopy was performed, and histological examination of the hilar mass showed a SCLC of the "oat cell" variety. Unfortunately, the patient died before the oncology referral while being treated in the intensive care unit.

Conclusions

PLE is a rare neurological syndrome characterized by personality changes, irritability, depression, seizures, memory loss, and sometimes dementia. Common solid tumors such as SCLC, testicular teratoma, and breast cancer are well known to be associated with PLE. Although the exact pathophysiological link is not obvious, the presence of antineuronal antibodies has been documented in some cases. However, the lack of specificity and availability of these markers make testing for these antibodies less helpful for diagnosis. Where these markers are unavailable, brain imaging can be used to support the diagnosis in cases of progressive neurological deterioration.

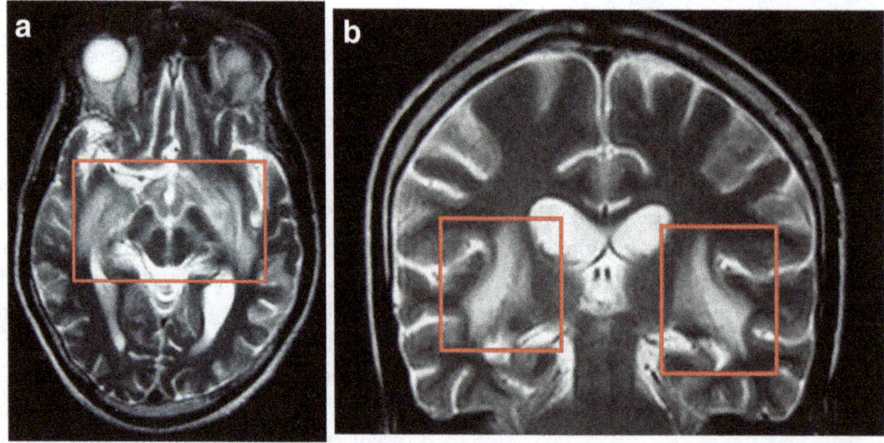

Fig. 2 **a** Magnetic resonance (MR) images on T2 weighted images. Transverse section of the brain. Bilateral hippocampal area and mammillary bodies showed symmetrical high intensity. **b** Magnetic resonance (MR) images on T2 weighted images. Coronal section of the brain. Island and external capsule area showed symmetrical high intensity

Our patient was initially suspected to have a tumor of the hypothalamus with associated cranial diabetes insipidus. We suggest that the initial appearance of a hyperdensity in the hypothalamus could be due to hyperemia secondary to hypothalamitis. This is supported by previous evidence on CT perfusion images that showed a focal increase in the cerebral blood flow and shortening of the mean transit time in the bilateral hippocampi and amygdalae in a patient with encephalitis [5]. Bitemporal hypodensities on a noncontrast CT scan should always raise suspicion for encephalitis, and it is important to arrange an early MRI scan for further evaluation of such lesions. MRI can show unequivocal involvement of temporolimbic structures and helps to exclude other diagnoses [6]. Although MRI is more sensitive than CT for the detection of inflammatory brain lesions because of the higher contrast resolution, CT is still valuable when used with other supporting clinical evidence in settings where other sophisticated scan techniques are not freely available [7]. There are few reported cases of normal CT scans in patients with PLE, and precise epidemiological data are not available [8, 9]. CT evidence of a central hyperdensity surrounded by a bitemporal hyperdensity is a valuable tool with which to identify possible PLE in resource-poor settings. The role of 2-deoxy-2-[F-18] fluoro-D-glucose-positron emission tomography imaging in the clinical management of paraneoplastic neurological syndrome is evolving and thus far has shown much better results than MRI [10]. These investigations are less popular in resource-poor settings because of the lack of availability and higher cost. Hypothalamitis is a less established pathological entity. However, histological diagnosis is not practical because of the highly invasive nature of biopsy and the deep location of the hypothalamus. Several reported cases of diagnostic stereotactic biopsy have revealed inflammatory infiltrates mainly constituting lymphocytic inflammation [11–13]. Based on these findings of a common histological pattern, we suggest that highly invasive biopsy has lower priority than imaging. Other than acute paraneoplastic hypothalamitis, another variety of hypothalamitis is relapsing autoimmune hypothalamitis [14]. However, based on the present case and those described in the literature, we suggest that screening for a hidden malignancy should be an essential step in the initial evaluation of the patient. Another pathological entity that presents with cranial diabetes insipidus is infundibuloneurohypophysitis [15, 16]. Radiological differentiation of pure hypothalamitis from infundibuloneurohypophysitis is rather difficult. Importantly, this demarcation is not essential for appropriate patient management.

In summary, this case report provides useful insights regarding the radiological pattern of limbic encephalitis in noncontrast CT, which may guide physicians in the early diagnosis and prompt management of PLE.

Consent

Written informed consent was obtained from the son on behalf of this patient for publication of this case report and any accompanying images. A copy of the written consent is available for review by the Editor-in-Chief of this journal.

Abbreviations

CT: Computed tomography; CSF: Cerebrospinal fluid; MRI: Magnatic resonance imaging; GCS: Glasgow coma scale; HSV: Herpes simplex virus; CMV: Cytomegalovirus; JE: Japanese encephalitis; PCR: Polymerase chain reaction; EEG: Electroencephalogram.

Competing interests

The author(s) declare that they have no competing interests.

Authors' contributions

VRB participated in the management of this patient and drafted the manuscript. NT involved in the overall supervision and management of this patient. Both authors read and approved the final manuscript.

Authors' information

VRB: MBBS, Pursuing MD in Medicine: Lecturer, Department of Pharmacology and Pharmacy, Faculty of Medicine University of Colombo.
NT: MBBS, MRCP, FCCP: Senior Consultant Physician, Department of Medicine, National Hospital, Ward Place, Colombo, Sri Lanka

Acknowledgements

We thank consultant neurologist Dr (Mrs) Gunaratna P who provided important inputs for clinical decision making in this patient and Dr A Pallewatta who helped in reporting CT/MRI images.

Author details

[1]Department of Pharmacology and Pharmacy, Faculty of Medicine University of Colombo, PO Box 271Kynsey Road, Colombo 8, Sri Lanka. [2]Department of Medicine, National Hospital, Ward Place, Colombo, Sri Lanka.

References

1. Brierley JB, Corsellis JAN, Hierons R, Nevin S. Subacute encephalitis of later adult life. mainly affecting the limbic areas. Brain. 1960;83:357–68.[Article]
2. Gultekin SH, Rosenfeld MR, Voltz R, Eichen J , Posner JB, Dalmau J. Paraneoplastic limbic encephalitis: neurological symptoms, immunological findings and tumour association in 50 patients. Brain. 2000;123;1481–94.
3. Corsellis JA, Goldberg GJ, Norton AR. "Limbic encephalitis" and its association with carcinoma. Brain. 1968;91:481–96.
4. Graus F, Saiz A. Limbic encephalitis: a probably under-recognized syndrome. Neurologia. 2005;20:24–30.
5. Nonaka M, Ariyoshi N, Shonai T, Kashiwagi M, Imai T, Chiba S, et al. CT perfusion abnormalities in a case of non-herpetic acute limbic encephalitis. Rinsho Shinkeigaku. 2004;44(8):537–40.
6. Lawn ND, Westmoreland BF, Kiely MJ, Lennon VA, Vernino S. Clinical, magnetic resonance imaging, and electroencephalographic findings in paraneoplastic limbic encephalitis. Mayo Clin Proc. 2003;78(11):1363.
7. Weber W, Henkes H, Felber S, Jänisch W, Schaper J, Kühne D. Diagnostic imaging in viral encephalitis. Radiologe. 2000;40(11):998–1010.
8. Rimmelin A, Sellal F, Morand G, Quoix E, Clouet PL, Dietemann JL. Imaging of limbic paraneoplastic encephalitis. J Radiol. 1997;78(1):73–76.
9. Lacomis D, Khoshbin S, Schick RM. MR imaging of paraneoplastic limbic encephalitis. J Comput Assist Tomogr. 1990;14(1):115–17.
10. Basu S, Alavi A. Role of FDG-PET in the clinical management of paraneoplastic neurological syndrome: detection of the underlying malignancy and the brain PET-MRI correlates. Mol Imaging Biol. 2008;10(3):131–7.
11. Lecube A, Francisco G, Rodríguez D, Ortega A, Codina A, Hernández C, et al. Lymphocytic hypophysitis successfully treated with azathioprine: first case report. J Neurol Neurosurg Psychiatry. 2003;74(11):1581–3.

12. Yang GQ, Lu ZH, Gu WJ, Du J, Guo QH, Wang XL, et al. Recurrent autoimmune hypophysitis successfully treated with glucocorticoids plus azathioprine: a report of three cases. Endocr J. 2011;58(8):675–83.
13. Zhang S, Ye H, Zhang Z, Lu B, Yang Y, He M, et al. Successful diagnosis of hypothalamitis using stereotactic biopsy and treatment: a case report. Medicine (Baltimore). 2015;94(5), e447.
14. Wang XL, Lu JM, Yang LJ, Lü ZH, Dou JT, Mu YM, et al. A case of relapsed autoimmune hypothalamitis successfully treated with methylprednisolone and azathioprine. Neuro Endocrinol Lett. 2008;29(6):874–6.
15. Takahashi M, Otsuka F, Miyoshi T, Ogura T, Makino H. An elderly patient with transient diabetes insipidus associated with lymphocytic infundibulo-neurohypothysitis. Endocr J. 1999;46(5):741–6.
16. Iwai Y, Yamanaka K, Yoshioka K, Okamoto Y, Sato T. Report of four cases of lymphocytic infundibulo-neurohypothysitis. No Shinkei Geka. 1998;26(9):831–5.

14

Radiomics-based differentiation of lung disease models generated by polluted air based on X-ray computed tomography data

Krisztián Szigeti[1*], Tibor Szabó[2^], Csaba Korom[3], Ilona Czibak[2], Ildikó Horváth[1], Dániel S. Veres[1], Zoltán Gyöngyi[4], Kinga Karlinger[3], Ralf Bergmann[5], Márta Pócsik[2], Ferenc Budán[4,6] and Domokos Máthé[1,2]

Abstract

Background: Lung diseases (resulting from air pollution) require a widely accessible method for risk estimation and early diagnosis to ensure proper and responsive treatment. Radiomics-based fractal dimension analysis of X-ray computed tomography attenuation patterns in chest voxels of mice exposed to different air polluting agents was performed to model early stages of disease and establish differential diagnosis.

Methods: To model different types of air pollution, BALBc/ByJ mouse groups were exposed to cigarette smoke combined with ozone, sulphur dioxide gas and a control group was established. Two weeks after exposure, the frequency distributions of image voxel attenuation data were evaluated. Specific cut-off ranges were defined to group voxels by attenuation. Cut-off ranges were binarized and their spatial pattern was associated with calculated fractal dimension, then abstracted by the fractal dimension – cut-off range mathematical function. Nonparametric Kruskal-Wallis (KW) and Mann–Whitney post hoc (MWph) tests were used.

Results: Each cut-off range versus fractal dimension function plot was found to contain two distinctive Gaussian curves. The ratios of the Gaussian curve parameters are considerably significant and are statistically distinguishable within the three exposure groups.

Conclusions: A new radiomics evaluation method was established based on analysis of the fractal dimension of chest X-ray computed tomography data segments. The specific attenuation patterns calculated utilizing our method may diagnose and monitor certain lung diseases, such as chronic obstructive pulmonary disease (COPD), asthma, tuberculosis or lung carcinomas.

Keywords: Fractal dimension, Radiomics, In vivo micro-CT, Air pollution, Lung disease

Background

"Radiomics" is an approach currently recognized in biomedical image analysis as a tool to define a potentially diverse array of meta-data obtained from images using quantitative radiology image analytics. Some well-selected features of these meta-data can be informative of the health status of the imaged organ system and impact therapy decisions. Such therapy decisions are best taken early in the course of disease. Early therapy decisions have tremendous impact on quality of life in pulmonary diseases.

Fractals are often used to characterize non-Euclidean structures in biology [1]. Utilizing the scaling factor of statistically self-similar and non-overlapping subsets, fractal dimension can be computed [2] providing relevant information describing a structure's complexity and homogeneity [3]. Fractal dimension represents, with certain limitations, the "less or more branching nature" of structures [4, 5] including the respiratory organ [6].

* Correspondence: szigeti.krisztian@med.semmelweis-univ.hu
^Deceased
[1]Department of Biophysics and Radiation Biology, Semmelweis University, Tűzoltó utca 37-47, Budapest H-1094, Hungary
Full list of author information is available at the end of the article

We sought to implement a fractal-based radiomics approach to X-ray computed tomography attenuation data without respiratory gating thereby averting the risk of losing relevant information. Analysis of fractal dimensions in specially binned non-gated X-ray computed tomography image patterns has been the method of our choice.

The currently accepted method of analysing pulmonary fractal dimensions of X-ray computed tomography attenuation data usually consists of segmenting parts of the lung such as the alveolar respiratory units, or pulmonary arteries and veins [7–10]. Al-Kadi and Watson [2] distinguished tumours and blood vessels based on their X-ray attenuation differences (using contrast material) to perform fractal dimension analysis on the image segments. The usually applied methods therefore provide the reader with a fractal dimension value for each of the tissue component segments of lung images. A usual outcome measure e.g. is the fractal dimension of lung arterial vasculature.

Our approach to radiomics has been greatly different from simply calculating fractal dimensions of segmented pulmonary tissue components ("dissected" vessels, bronchi etc.). The examination of fractal dimensions of ideally selected attenuation ranges in relative Hounsfield units (HU) may provide the foundation towards discovering additional hidden tissue features in integrative patterns of lung images instead. These fractal dimension calculations may perhaps detect small scale tissue alterations such as those caused by harmful environmental conditions. Our objective was to unveil possible correlations between air pollutant categories and specific features or patterns of damaged lungs. These features of small magnitude might not be evident in either custom visual X-ray computed tomography image analysis or in the calculation of segmented pulmonary tissue fractal dimensions.

We aimed at distinguishing between different air pollutant effects on the lungs via a radiomic approach with a clinically translatable mathematical algorithm. We preferred using non-gated X-ray computed tomography data. Non-gated data acquisition still contains effects of e.g. hindered chest or lung motion. In our analysis we intended to examine data features reflecting disease-related changes also in lung organ movements rather than anatomical relationships. Thus in our analysis method presented here simple non-gated X-ray computed tomography mouse chest scans have been acquired and evaluated by the calculation of fractal dimension of binary images. We binned voxel sets from each mouse chest X-ray computed tomography volume into numerous attenuation ranges in our study [1, 11], instead of pulmonary tissue-based image segmentation. Additionally we also averted the use of any contrast agent.

Generally speaking, (both in the "classic" and in our novel method), the result of fractal dimension calculation is a number corresponding to how often examined structures (dissected arteries and veins in "classical" methods and voxel 3D patterns with specific attenuation values in our approach) branch and/or fill the space within the chest. However, in our novel approach, the fractal dimension calculation method examines and depicts integrative binary images of lung voxels which are selected according to their attenuation values. We then aimed at the application of our algorithm to discriminate among groups of mice treated with different air pollutants in an early phase of their respective disease models.

Methods

Ethics Statement

The animal experiment was reviewed and approved by the local authorities (Committee on the Ethics of Animal Experiments of Semmelweis University, permit number: PMK ÉBÁI-XIV-I-001/29-7/2012) according to Hungarian animal protection laws in accordance with EU guidelines.

Experimental animals

Three groups of BALBc/ByJ female mice (6–8 weeks old, 18–22 g) were used in the context of our current research. Their exposure was performed in a plexiglass inhalator chamber (30 cm × 30 cm × 50 cm). One group ($n = 5$) was treated with inhalation of sulphur dioxide (SO_2) gas 2 % v/v (SDO group). A second group ($n = 5$) was treated with air diluted, fresh mainstream cigarette smoke from '3R4F' Reference Cigarettes (Kentucky Tobacco Research & Development Center, USA) mixed with ozone-air gas mixture (50 mg/h, 3.7 l/min dilution with air; SAO group). Cigarettes with a shortened filter only (approx. 2 mm) were smoked according to our protocol (1 puff/9 s of 3 s duration and 40 mL volume). The SAO group first received one 20 min long exposure, followed by two 20 min long exposures, and lastly, three 20 min long exposures on the additional remaining days. A control group ($n = 6$) was also used, treated with the inhalation of filtered and humidified (30–40 %), air under identical conditions (CON group). Treatment duration was 14 days, and then imaging was carried out within all groups. An untreated BALB/CyJ female mouse (Janvier, France) was imaged too, in serving the purpose of representation of the attenuation profile of the chest (Fig. 1).

In vivo imaging

X-ray computed tomography information was collected using a NanoX-CT (Mediso Ltd, Hungary) cone-beam in vivo micro-CT imaging system (8 W power of X-ray source, 55 kV source voltage, 3.6x zoom) without using contrast material. It is important to emphasize the

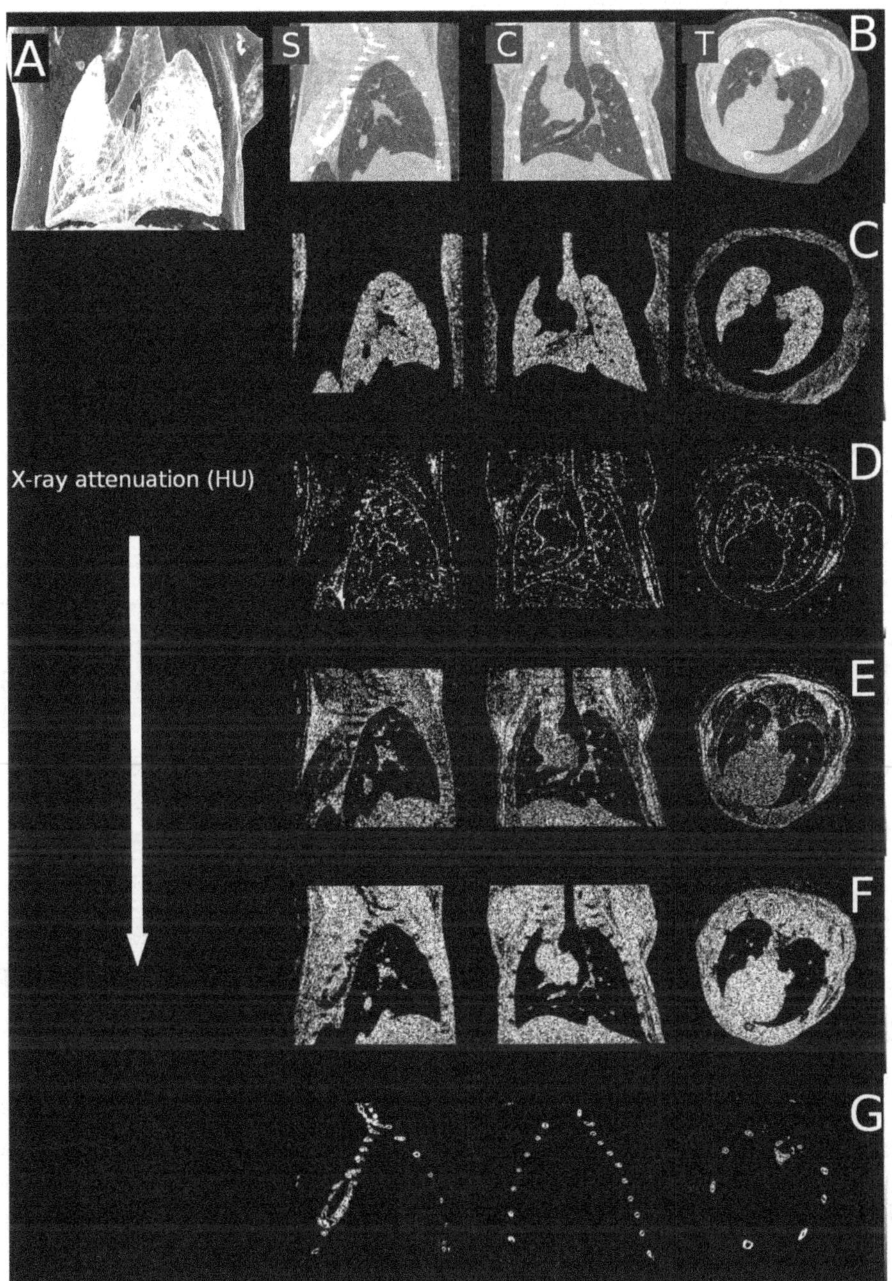

Fig. 1 The reconstruction of the lungs of an untreated mouse shown with the sole intent of representing the attenuation profile of the chest. Sagittal (left **b**), coronal (center **b**), transaxial (right **b**) planes and minimum intensity projection (**a**). Certain attenuation ranges were abstracted from these slices in sagittal, coronal and transaxial planes. **c** −700 – -400 relative HU (lung parenchyma), (**d**): −100 – +200 relative HU (pleura, endothoracic fascia, epipleural fat and interlobar fissures), (**e**): +200 – +500 relative HU (respiratory- and heart muscles, diaphragm), (**f**): +500 – +800 relative HU (blood inside the vessels, aorta and heart, lymphatic fluid and interlobar fissures), and (**g**): +1400 – +3800 relative HU (bones)

physics of cone-beam X-ray computed tomography acquisitions which represents specific technical considerations beyond the scope of our current paper and may distort the direct comparison of attenuation values of the same organs measured with other detection techniques, such as those applied in clinical slice-based X-ray computed tomography systems. Therefore, attenuation values are presented in relative Hounsfield units.

Reconstruction algorithm (Mediso Ltd.) utilizing the Feldkamp-filtered back projection was run on a 64 bit graphics processing unit (GPU). The reconstructed voxel sizes were 54 × 54 × 54 μm in one 370 × 370 × 370 voxel matrix, as region of interest (ROI) following our image acquisition. During data acquisition animals were constantly anaesthetized using a mixture of 2.5 % isoflurane and medical air, and their body temperature was maintained at 38 C. One image acquisition took 4.5 min. Non-respiration-gated data sets were acquired and further analysed.

Fan-beam technology, used earlier and extensively within clinical practice, has today largely been replaced by multislice detector technology. As a result, the difference between pre-clinical and clinical instruments is quickly disappearing and clinical systems are gradually becoming similar to cone-beam computer tomography instruments.

Sensitivity in small animal imaging may be worse when compared to the human counterpart. Voxel size is one tenth or twentieth of the human voxel size, and so the signal-to-noise ratio could be worse (as this ratio is inversely proportional to the third power of voxel volume), however, the measurement time is much longer. In summary, signal-to-noise ratio is better in human measurements, meaning our method will have an increased sensitivity when applied to human cases.

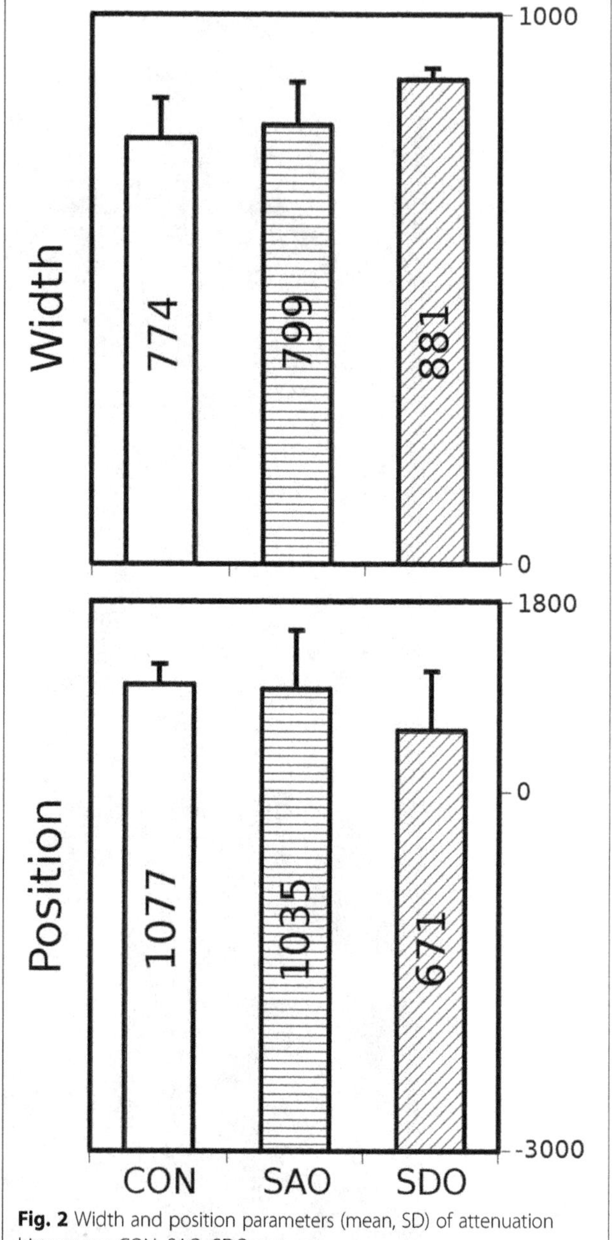

Fig. 2 Width and position parameters (mean, SD) of attenuation histograms. CON, SAO, SDO groups

Evaluation of X-ray attenuation histograms

In the first step, our algorithm segmented the acquired 3D X-ray computed tomography volume reconstructions to contain only the whole lung volumes and to automatically distinguish between the lung tissue, chest bones and other tissues. The attenuation values of lung voxels were represented in a frequency distribution function, commonly referred to as a histogram [12] (data not shown). In the next step of evaluation, Gaussian curves were fitted by a minimum square algorithm (Gnuplot 4.4), featuring height, width and position. We calculated the means and standard deviations of positions and widths of the Gaussian curves of all examined groups (Fig. 2). The height is not presented on Fig. 2 as this parameter is dependent on width and area under histogram by definition.

Characterization by fractal dimension analysis of voxels of various attenuation ranges

Final data analysis was performed in five steps (Fig. 3). The entire attenuation range of the reconstructed chest area of animals was divided into 100 distinct cut-off ranges. Once the attenuation value of a given voxel was within a certain cut-off range, the voxel was represented by “1”, or otherwise, “0”. This generated a binary image. Each such derived binary pattern was then associated with a calculated fractal dimension via box-counting algorithm [13]. The lung morphology was quantified by plotting the fractal dimension of all cut-off ranges in each given X-ray computed tomography 3D attenuation map. This plot is defined as the fractal dimension - cut-off range function.

Here we present the exact details of the mentioned five steps of data analysis with the purpose of demonstrating how the cut-off range associated fractal dimension data were achieved (Fig. 3).

Step 1. The whole attenuation range in the experiments was between −3,000 and +10,000 relative HU. The 100 distinct ranges of attenuation values were chosen by the Freedman-Diaconis rule [14]. A chosen range is defined mathematically as the

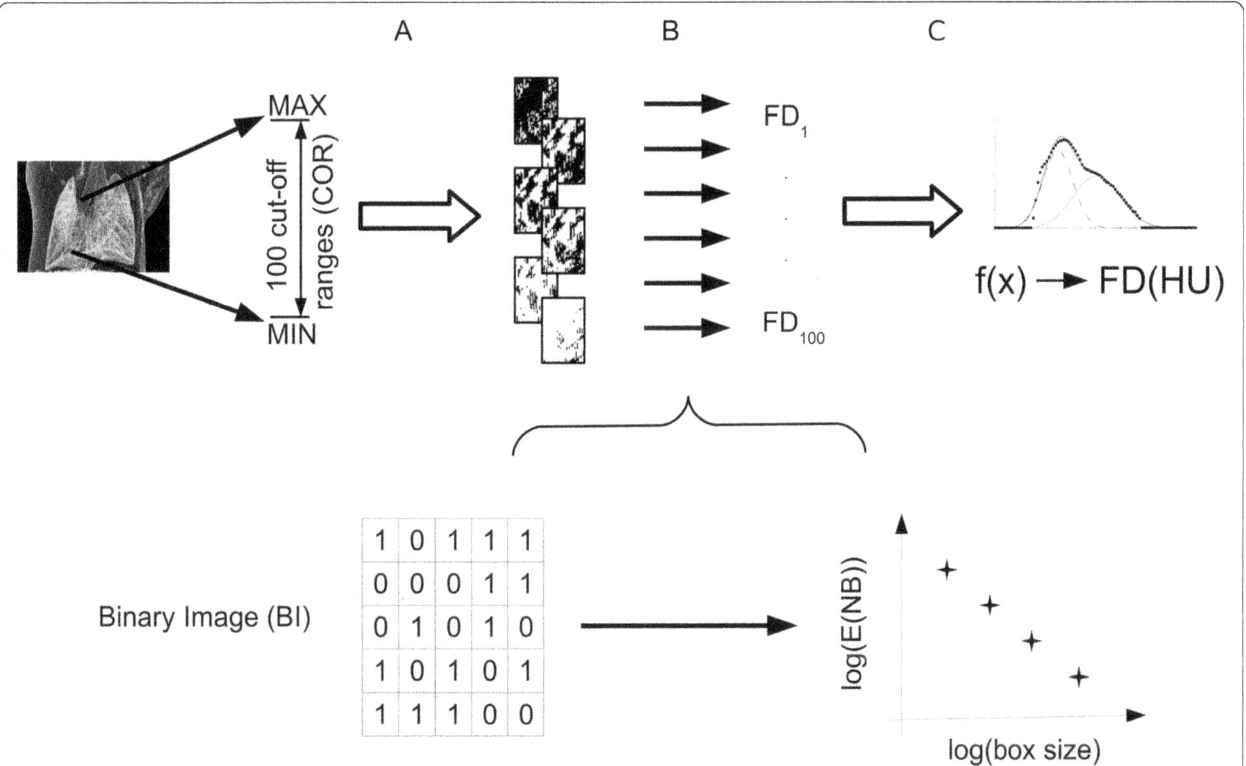

Fig. 3 Representation of the five steps of data analysis. **a**: The entire attenuation range of the reconstructed chest area of animals was divided into 100 distinct cut-off ranges (Step 1). **b**: Binary images are generated (Step 2 and 3) and each such derived binary pattern was next associated with a calculated fractal dimension via box-counting algorithms (Step 4). **c**: The fractal dimension – cut-off range function plot (Step 5)

standard cut-off range. Certain attenuation values ranging between the chosen higher and lower value were ranked into one cut-off range. The 100 cut-off ranges involved the whole scale of the voxel attenuations of all scans and one cut-off range contained 130 relative HU.

Step 2. The X-ray computed tomography images were partitioned into cubic voxels (size: 54 μm in a 370 × 370 × 370 voxel matrix). When the attenuation value of a given voxel was inside a certain cut-off range, then that voxel was associated with "1", or otherwise with "0" in the representation of the cut-off range.

Step 3. This association step was repeated which resulted in a pattern of voxels with "1" and "0" for every cut-off range. These patterns as binary images were used in the next steps. The 100 binary images were derived from 100 previously defined cut-off ranges.

Step 4. The box counting algorithm [13] was used to calculate the fractal dimension number associated with each binary image. See additional details below in the sub-steps labelled a through d.

Sub-step a) In this box-counting algorithm, the length of cubic boxes varied from 1 to 100 voxels. A given box was shifted from one position to another without overlapping in a certain binary image. The number of boxes containing at least one voxel with value "1" was summarized. Thereby, a number was calculated defined as the number of boxes of a given side length (NB).

Sub-step b) The previous sub-step a) was repeated including the difference that the boxes are overlapped. Thus, NB results were produced derived from the shifted overlapped positions. A certain box size in a certain binary image produced two different NB results (from overlapping and non-overlapping boxes). From these two NBs, an average (E(NB)) was calculated and that value was used in further evaluation.

Sub-step c) For each box size, both the a and b sub-steps were repeated. E(NB) was represented as the function of the box size in a certain binary image.

Sub-step d) To determine fractal dimension, the function from sub-step c) was fitted by a power function. The exponent of the power law is the fractal dimension. To each binary image, a fractal dimension number was ordered and calculated utilizing this method.

Step 5. In this step, the cut-off ranges were associated with the calculated fractal dimension. At both the very high and very low cut-off range values, the fractal dimension number is zero, while near the middle values of cut-off ranges the associated fractal dimension number becomes nearly maximal.

The resulting fractal dimension - cut-off range function was fitted by two Gaussian curves (Gaussian curve "A" and "B") using the so-called "least box square" algorithm. The outputs of our algorithm, the height, width and position parameters of these fitted "A" and "B" Gaussian curves, were calculated for all animals (Table 1). Lists these numerical features of the Gaussian curves for every group based on Additional file 1 (supporting data). The lungs of all three groups, SDO, SAO and CON, were characterized by these parameters (Fig. 4).

Lastly, to further attempt significant discrimination of the groups, ratios of all three mean parameters derived from both "A" and "B" Gaussian curves were calculated. The C insets represent the ratios of "A" parameters divided by "B" parameters (where a certain "C" parameter is calculated by dividing the "A" parameter of a given group by the "B" parameter of the same group) (Fig. 5).

These steps were repeated to evaluate the images of each animal.

Statistical analysis

Statistical analysis was performed using the nonparametric Kruskal-Wallis (KW) test for fitted parameters of groups (STATISTICA 7.0, Statsoft Inc., USA). Differences between all groups were evaluated by the Mann–Whitney post hoc (MWph) test (Figs. 2 and 5).

A chi-square test was used to test the reliability ($p < 0.05$) of fit of the histogram and the fractal dimension, or the cut-off range function (either fitted with one single or two independent Gaussian curves).

Table 1 Contains averages and standard deviations of all fitted parameters for all groups of animals

Average	SDO	SAO	CON
Height A	2,161	2,231	2,291
Height B	1,725	1,376	1,276
Position A	181	628	735
Position B	3951	3473	3776
Width A	1133	1036	1086
Width B	2496	1630	1562
STD			
Height A	0,049	0,104	0,042
Height B	0,080	0,063	0,090
Position A	386	540	217
Position B	110	647	277
Width A	61	165	169
Width B	161	169	135

Results

The mean values of width and position of the voxel density histograms demonstrate no significant differences between the three groups (Fig. 2).

The fractal dimension - cut-off range functions were evaluated by fitting them with Gaussian curves "A" and "B" (Fig. 4). These functions can be characterized by height, maximum position and width of the peak. The means of height, width and position of the "A" curve of the CON group do not differ significantly when compared to the SDO or the SAO group. The means of height, width and position are unchanged between the SDO and SAO groups, too (Fig. 5a).

The mean of height of "B" curve of the SDO group increased significantly when compared to the CON group (KW $p = 0.002$, MWph $p = 0.036$) and to the SAO group (KW $p = 0.002$, MWph $p = 0.024$), but not significantly when the CON group was compared to the SAO group (Fig. 5b top). The mean of widths of "B" curves of the SDO group increased significantly (KW $p = 0.016$, MWph $p = 0.036$) compared to the CON group, and also significantly when compared to the SAO group (KW $p = 0.016$, MWph $p = 0.024$), but not significantly when the CON group was compared to the SAO group (KW $p = 0.016$, MWph $p = 0.429$) (Fig. 5b middle). The means of maximum positions are not significantly altered between the SDO, SAO and CON groups (Fig. 5b bottom).

The difference between the ratios of height is significant if the SDO group is compared to the CON group (KW $p = 0.005$, MWph $p = 0.0357$), if the SDO group is compared to the SAO group (KW $p = 0.005$, MWph $p = 0.024$) and if the SAO group is compared to the CON group (KW $p = 0.005$, MWph $p = 0.042$) (Fig. 5c top).

The ratios of width of the SDO and CON groups (KW $p = 0.021$, MWph $p = 0.036$) and the SDO and SAO groups (KW $p = 0.021$, MWph $p = 0.024$) demonstrate a slight but significant difference (Fig. 5c middle), however, the difference between the SAO and CON groups is not significant.

Discussion

Differences between parameters based on the relative HU–frequency histograms of the animals in the three groups, i.e. the differences between mean maximum positions and widths (Fig. 2) could be neither the basis of detection of an altered lung structure nor the categorization

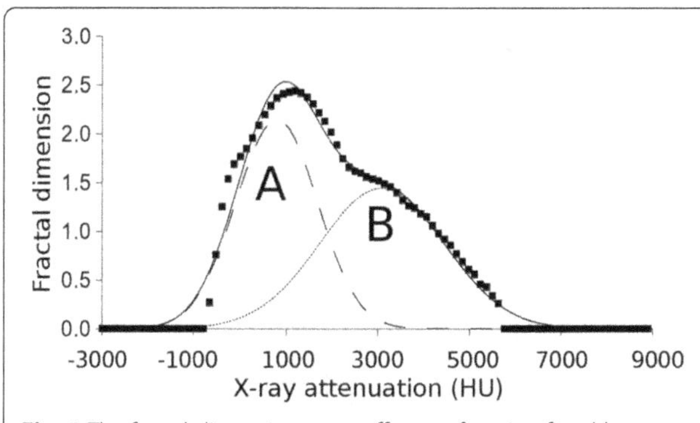

Fig. 4 The fractal dimension – cut-off range function fitted by Gaussian curves "**a**" and "**b**"

of air pollution exposure. Either the absence of gating or the reduced period of mouse model symptom production was likely the reason. Indeed, Sasaki et al. (2015) too could not distinguish the effect of cigarette smoke on lung tissue attenuation in comparison to the control using X-ray computed tomography with gating [15]. However, interestingly enough, a number of differences could be shown using our novel radiomics analysis method.

In our opinion, there are distinctly altered tissue features with respectively changed attenuation patterns in the different mouse models of air pollution related disease. However, the readout of these changes necessitates subtle differentiation and radiomics analysis methods in early phases of lung harm when symptoms are yet considerably subtle.

Severe lung diseases alter the inhalatory and exhalatory movements and these changes can be detected even in mild cases or after relatively short exposure to air pollutants (e.g., the slower exhalation in COPD is evident) [16, 17]. This may be paradoxically advantageous in our approach and likely will help in discerning exposure sources. The hindered motion in the smoke/air and sulphur dioxide groups presumably decreases or even negates spatial and temporal overlapping of different tissues in the same voxel caused by respiratory movement and finally contributes to the mentioned increase of width parameter in the exposed groups. This change in motion dynamics (probably due to inflammation, mucus build-up and entrapped air bubbles) may be an important part of the diagnosis and it is ignored when using respiratory gating. Notably, this finding suggests the fractal dimension- cut-off range function derived radiomic data might unveil some pathologic changes in lung diseases [3, 18]. Possibly the onset of disease as a result of exposure to air pollution could also be observed with our data analysis method.

The Gaussian curves of Fig. 5 display a different pattern of respiratory pulmonary motion in the exposed animals, possibly due to an increase in lung stiffness caused by pollutants.

The height of Gauss curve B is significantly increased in the SDO group compared to the other two groups (Fig. 5b top). We infer this change is attributable to the hindered motion of inflamed tissue.

Sulphurous gases are irritants and induce inflammation, bronchoconstriction and bronchitis resulting in an increase of mucus [3, 19]. Overproduction of mucus can form plugs which entrap air or temporally and partly obstruct the upper airways [20]. Airway clearance of mucus depends on the interactions between physical properties of the mucous gel, serous fluid content, and ciliary function, in addition to airflow [19]. Wagner et al. (2006) discovered in a Sprague–Dawley rat model that 80 ppm concentration of SO_2 (besides overproduction of mucus) caused epithelial cells to lose their ciliae [21]. Nano-sized solid particles originating from fumes tend to accumulate in deeper airways and alveoli [22], as inflammatory agents increase water permeability and dilate cell volume thus thickening airway walls and resulting in the narrowing of the airways (in addition to minor mucus production which cannot be excluded). In our interpretation, this narrowing of the airways causes the different motion dynamics of this group.

The width parameter of the SDO group is significantly increased compared to the other two groups (Fig. 5b center). We believe this change is attributable to the hindered motion of inflamed tissue.

The number of voxels representing thickening airway walls is increased, caused by SO_2 exposure often penetrating into deeper airways and inducing inflammation in the alveoli, leading to the appearance of fluid, derived from necrotic cells [19, 23]. Mucus plugs trap air inside the alveoli and lead to the formation of micro-sized bubbles [24, 25] inside the lung parenchyma. Indeed mucus production is an early response to increased amounts of air pollution [19]. In our interpretation, the increased number of voxels representing thickening airway walls causes the different shape of the fractal dimension - cut-off range function of this group.

Only a slight difference was observed between the means of height of Gaussian curve "B" of SAO and CON groups (Fig. 5b top). In addition to mean values of maximum positions (Fig. 5b bottom), the width parameter of the SAO group was compared to the control group (Fig. 5 middle), however it did not significantly change.

Theoretically speaking, emphysema-diseased areas within the lungs could occur caused by destroyed walls of airways and alveoli [11, 12, 18], however, it appears only in long term experiments [26].

In using the corresponding ratios of parameters of Gaussian curves "A" and "B" (Fig. 5c) and the heights and widths of "B" Gaussian curves (Fig. 5b), all three groups could be distinguished. We believe the difference

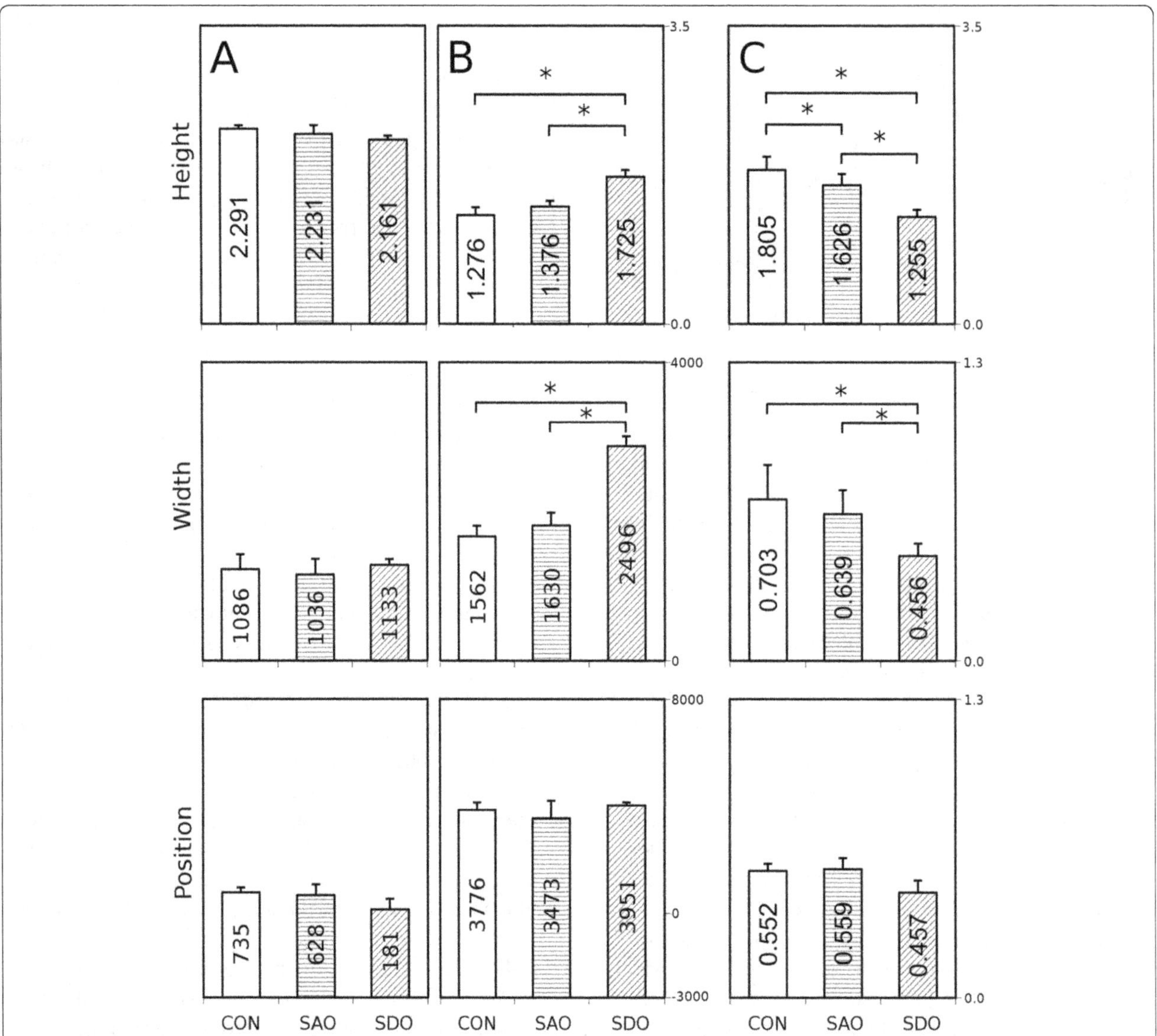

Fig. 5 Calculated height, width and position parameters of the fractal dimension - cut-off range functions. **a**: Height, width and position parameters of Gaussian curve „A" (CON, SDO, SAO groups). **b**: Height, width and position parameters of Gaussian curve „B" (CON, SDO, SAO groups). **c**: The ratios of the relevant parameters of Gaussian curves „A" and „B" (CON, SDO, SAO groups). * $p < 0.05$, Kruskal-Wallis (KW) test with Mann–Whitney post hoc (MWph) test

between the ratios of parameters refers to the different proportion of various kinds of tissue damage caused by different air pollution agents.

The proportion of tissue alterations has a specific pattern in lung diseases of different origin. Altered tissue (e.g., increased mucus production in one model or increased presence of tissue microbubbles in another) was explored.

The mechanism of these changes affecting the respiratory movement remains unclear and warrants further research.

Data acquired in our study (Fig. 5b, c) proved a worthy basis for differentiating specific air pollution caused lung changes in the early stage by direct fractal dimension - cut-off range function pattern analysis. It could be hypothesized that molecular features and presence of mucus in smaller airways [19] and inflammation profile of lung tissues [27] contribute to our fractal dimension analysis-based results. In reference to published literature [19, 28], we postulate that the fractal dimension - cut-off range function calculated with our method may be used as an imaging biomarker. It could be effectively converted to both preclinical applications and clinical use in humans, ideally providing patients the benefit of early warning towards avoiding environmental risks. Additional benefits are expected in the proper treatment at the onset of symptoms of disease, and lastly, to prevent aggravation of disease and exacerbation of COPD and/or asthma bronchiale symptoms. Here, we highlight the importance of length of smoke exposure and genetic susceptibility [28] to emphysema [26], which may later develop and will be reflected in the reported imaging biomarker parameters [3, 18].

The radiomic analysis of the fractal dimension - cut-off range function may be useful in early diagnosis of both exposure to air pollution and lung diseases (such as COPD or asthma), containing information about both the molecular features and patterns of mucus in smaller airways [19] and the inflammation profiles of lung tissues [27]. We propose an increase in the number of structurally quantitative imaging biomarker research studies, towards early detection and follow-up of therapy of other pulmonary diseases, for example, cystic fibrosis, lung carcinomas [3] or tuberculosis [29].

In translational research, our most important goal is to develop methods in animal models which later may be used in clinical practice. In the case of our paper, the translatability of the method is dependent upon three aspects of it. The first is the usability of the algorithm in clinical practice, the second is the relation between anatomy sizes and reconstruction voxels, and the third is the applicability of the algorithm in clinical protocols.

The algorithm does not use specific data, as it only requires a 3D reconstruction, that is attenuation distribution. These data are also available in the clinical setting, so our algorithm proposed here can also be applied for clinical lung computed tomography volumes.

The human body is about 15–20 times longer than the body of the mouse and there is nearly the same difference between spatial resolution (voxel size in preclinical CT is 50 μm and in clinical CT is 500–750 μm). Generally speaking, anatomy size and voxel size change proportionally. Because of the partial-volume effect, though, true resolution does not reach voxel size calculated from reconstruction. It is important to note that the size of alveoli is invariable between species and is around 200 μm. Consequently, neither the pre-clinical nor the clinical instrument can visualize individual alveoli with suitable resolution, but in the case of the pre-clinical instrument, we see one alveolus in the adjacent voxels, whereas in case of the clinical instrument, we see more than one alveoli in one voxel.

Practically speaking, the proposed algorithm can be applied in the clinics and it is not necessary to change protocols, since the usual examinations and unchanged data acquisition chain should be followed by this new "off-line" analysis.

In summary, the use of the algorithm will be self-evident in clinical practice. Naturally, its diagnostic effectiveness needs to be assessed meticulously throughout different diseases.

Conclusions

We discovered a novel diagnostic and disease characterization method providing results within a remarkably short disease model production time compared to the former 8–24 weeks needed to produce detectable lung tissue changes as described in published literature [30]. Additionally, as our method does not apply gating, it may contribute to the simplified and more cost-effective (through higher throughput) data analysis utilizing simple X-ray computed tomography scans in mouse experimental models. The implementation of our data analysis is straightforward and applicable in clinical image data sets and does not require additional hardware. As the early diagnostic potential of COPD-related lung and airway changes was shown here in data containing approximately clinical levels of noise, we remain convinced the translation and validation of our algorithm and data analysis in human clinical trials is warranted [3].

Competing interests

The authors hereby declare they have no competing interests. Tibor Szabó, Ilona Czibak, Márta Pócsik, and Domokos Máthé are employees of CROmed Translational Research Centers. CROmed Translational Research Centers does not have any financial or non-financial interest in the subject matter or materials discussed in this manuscript. Ferenc Budán is an employee/stakeholder of MedProDevelop Kft that has no financial or non-financial interest in the subject matter or materials discussed in this manuscript.

Authors' contributions

DM and TS designed the study; TS, IC, DM and IH did the preclinical imaging work; CK, DSV and FB analyzed the data; KS takes responsibility for the integrity of the data and the accuracy of the data analysis; DM, KS, FB, ZG and MP wrote the paper; KK and RB contributed expert advice and valuable insight. All authors read and approved the final manuscript.

Acknowledgements

Miklós Kellermayer and Jon Marquette are gratefully acknowledged for providing support. The technical help from Mediso's Evaluation Software Team especially László Papp is gratefully acknowledged.

Author details

[1]Department of Biophysics and Radiation Biology, Semmelweis University, Tűzoltó utca 37-47, Budapest H-1094, Hungary. [2]CROmed Translational Research Centers Ltd., Baross utca 91-95, Budapest H-1047, Hungary. [3]Department of Radiology and Oncotherapy, Semmelweis University, Üllői út 78/A, Budapest H-1082, Hungary. [4]Department of Public Health Medicine, University of Pécs, Szigeti út 12, Pécs H-7624, Hungary. [5]Institute of Radiopharmaceutical Cancer Research, Helmholtz-Zentrum Dresden-Rossendorf, Dresden D-01314, Germany. [6]MedProDevelop Kft, Irgalmasok utcája 16, Pécs H-7621, Hungary.

References

1. Mandelbrot BB, Blumen A. Fractal Geometry: What is it, and What Does it do? Proc R Soc A. 1989;423:3–16.

2. Al-Kadi OS, Watson D. Texture analysis of aggressive and nonaggressive lung tumor CE CT images. IEEE Trans Biomed Eng. 2008;55(7):1822–30.
3. van Rikxoort EM, van Ginneken B. Automated segmentation of pulmonary structures in thoracic computed tomography scans: a review. Phys Med Biol. 2013;58:R187–220.
4. Smith TG, Lange GD, Marks WB. Fractal methods and results in cellular morphology - Dimensions, lacunarity and multifractals. J Neurosci Methods. 1996;69(2):123–36.
5. Helmberger M, Pienn M, Urschler M, Kullnig P, Stollberger R, Kovacs G, et al. Quantification of tortuosity and fractal dimension of the lung vessels in pulmonary hypertension patients. PLoS One. 2014;9(1):e87515.
6. Shlesinger MF, West BJ. Complex fractal dimension of the bronchial tree. Phys Rev Lett. 1991;67(15):2106–8.
7. Keller BM, Reeves AP, Henschke CI, Yankelevitz DF. Multivariate Compensation of Quantitative Pulmonary Emphysema Metric Variation from Low-Dose. Whole-Lung CT Scans Am J Roentgenol. 2011;197(3):495–502.
8. Huo Y, Choy JS, Wischgoll T, Luo T, Teague SD, Bhatt DL, et al. Computed tomography-based diagnosis of diffuse compensatory enlargement of coronary arteries using scaling power laws. J R Soc Interface. 2013;10(81):20121015.
9. Gould DJ, Vadakkan TJ, Poche RA, Dickinson ME. Multifractal and Lacunarity Analysis of Microvascular Morphology and Remodeling. Microcirculation. 2011;18(2):136–51.
10. Glenny RW. Emergence of matched airway and vascular trees from fractal rules. J Appl Physiol. 2011;110(4):1119–29.
11. Wright JL, Cosio M, Churg A. Animal models of chronic obstructive pulmonary disease. Am J Physiol Lung Cell Mol Physiol. 2008;295(1):1–15.
12. Smith Jr TG, Lange GD, Marks WB. Fractal methods and results in cellular morphology — dimensions, lacunarity and multifractals. J Neurosci Methods. 1996;69:123–36.
13. Freedman D, Diaconis P. On the histogram as a density estimator: L2 theory. Zeitschrift für Wahrscheinlichkeitstheorie und Verwandte Gebiete. 1981;57:453–76.
14. Sasaki M, Chubachi S, Kameyama N, Sato M, Haraguchi M, Miyazaki M, et al. Evaluation of cigarette smoke-induced emphysema in mice using quantitative micro-computed tomography. Am J Physiol Lung Cell Mol Physiol. 2015;308(10):1039–45.
15. Tantisuwat A, Thaveeratitham P. Effects of Smoking on Chest Expansion, Lung Function, and Respiratory Muscle Strength of Youths. J Phys Ther Sci. 2014;26:167–70.
16. Gagnon P, Guenette JA, Daniel L, Louis L, Vincent M, François M, et al. Pathogenesis of hyperinflation in chronic obstructive pulmonary disease. Int J of Crohn Obstruct Pulmon Dist. 2014;9:187–201.
17. Nagao M, Murase K. Measurement of heterogeneous distribution on Technegas SPECT images by three-dimensional fractal analysis. Ann Nucl Med. 2002;16(6):369–76.
18. Williams OW, Sharafkhaneh A, Kim V, Dickey BF, Evans CM. Airway mucus: From production to secretion. Am J Respir Cell Mol Biol. 2006;34(5):527–36.
19. Kim WD. Lung mucus: A clinician's view. Eur Respir J. 1997;10(8):1914–7.
20. Wagner U, Staats P, Fehmann H-C, Fischer A, Welte T, Groneberg DA. Analysis of airway secretions in a model of sulfur dioxide induced chronic obstructive pulmonary disease (COPD). J Occup Med Toxicol. 2006;1:12.
21. van Dijk WD, Gopal S, Scheepers PT. Nanoparticles in cigarette smoke; real-time undiluted measurements by a scanning mobility particle sizer. Anal Bioanal Chem. 2001;399:3573–8.
22. Castañer E, Gallardo X, Pallardó Y, Branera J, Cabezuelo MA, Mata JM. Diseases affecting the peribronchovascular interstitium: CT findings and pathologic correlation. Curr Probl Diagn Radiol. 2005;34(2):63–75.
23. Bossé Y, Riesenfeld EP, Paré PD, Irvin CG. It's not all smooth muscle: non-smooth-muscle elements in control of resistance to airflow. Annu Rev Physiol. 2010;72:437–62.
24. Moldoveanu B, Otmishi P, Jani P, Walker J, Sarmiento X, Guardiola J, et al. Inflammatory mechanisms in the lung. J Inflamm Res. 2009;2:1–11.
25. Maeno T, Houghton AM, Quintero PA, Grumelli S, Owen CA, Shapiro SD. CD8+ T Cells are required for inflammation and destruction in cigarette smoke-induced emphysema in mice. J Immunol. 2007;178(12):8090–6.
26. Jeffery PK. Structural and inflammatory changes in COPD: a comparison with asthma. Thorax. 1998;53(2):129–36.
27. Churg A, Cosio M, Wright JL. Mechanisms of cigarette smoke-induced COPD: insights from animal models. Am J Physiol Lung Cell Mol Physiol. 2008;294(4):612–31.
28. Chen RY, Dodd LE, Lee M, Paripati P, Hammoud DA, Mountz JM, et al. PET/CT imaging correlates with treatment outcome in patients with multidrug-resistant tuberculosis. Sci Transl Med. 2014;6(265):166.
29. Jobse BN, Rhem RG, Wang IQ, Counter WB, Stämpfli MR, Labiris NR. Detection of lung dysfunction using ventilation and perfusion SPECT in a mouse model of chronic cigarette smoke exposure. J Nucl Med. 2013;54(4):616–23.
30. Beckett EL, Stevens RL, Jarnicki AG, Kim RY, Hanish I, Hansbro NG, et al. A new short-term mouse model of chronic obstructive pulmonary disease identifies a role for mast cell tryptase in pathogenesis. J Allergy Clin Immunol. 2013;131(3):752–62.

Systemic air embolism after percutaneous computed tomography-guided lung biopsy due to a kink in the coaxial biopsy system

Hsu-Chao Chang[1] and Mei-Chen Yang[2,3*]

Abstract

Background: Systemic air embolism is a rare but potentially life-threatening complication of percutaneous computed tomography (CT)-guided lung biopsy. The incidence might be underestimated because of failure to diagnose this adverse event in asymptomatic patients; early recognition is difficult.

Case presentation: We report the case of a 73-year-old man with systemic air embolism, a complication of percutaneous CT-guided lung biopsy, due to a kink in the coaxial biopsy system. Serial post-procedure CT scans demonstrated the causal relationship.

Conclusions: Sequential post-biopsy CT scans demonstrated a causal relationship between this systemic air embolism and percutaneous biopsy, and allowed the radiologist to track the course of the emboli and their resolution. Awareness of air entry via the introducer needle and an early post-biopsy CT scan are crucial for early detection of systemic air embolism. If air embolism occurs in an asymptomatic patient, we recommend performing a delayed chest CT scan to follow the air's course.

Keywords: Complication, Lung mass, Chest imaging

Background

Systemic air embolism after percutaneous computed tomography (CT)-guided lung biopsy is very rare. The estimated incidence is 0.061–0.21% [1, 2], but could be underestimated because of failure to diagnose this adverse event in asymptomatic patients [3]. For example, in a study published in 2012, Freund et al. found that the incidence of radiologically proven systemic air embolism was 3.8%, whereas the incidence of clinically apparent systemic air embolism was 0.49% [4]. Thus, the incidence of post-biopsy systemic air embolism might be higher than is estimated, and sequential CT scans of the entire thorax instead of only the biopsy area might be worth performing to provide a definitive diagnosis of systemic air embolism [5]. Generally, systemic air embolism is thought to occur via two mechanisms. First, if the tip of the biopsy needle is lodged in a pulmonary vein and the inner stylet is removed, air embolism occurs during rapid inspiration when atmospheric pressure exceeds pulmonary venous pressure. Second, when the needle simultaneously traverses an air-containing space and adjacent pulmonary vein, a fistula can occur, resulting in air entering the pulmonary vein when the alveolar pressure is greater than the pulmonary venous pressure [6]. Air can enter via a fistula tract, connecting an air-containing space to a pulmonary vein when alveolar pressure is high, for example, during coughing. To prevent air embolism, the introducer needle should always be occluded by the inner stylet, saline drops, or the operator's finger. Moreover, the patient should be instructed to avoid breathing deeply or coughing forcefully during the procedure [7, 8]. It is believed that, following lung biopsy and needle withdrawal, a large

* Correspondence: mimimai3461@gmail.com
[2]School of Medicine, Tzu Chi University, Hualien, Taiwan
[3]Division of Pulmonary Medicine, Department of Internal Medicine, Taipei Tzu-Chi Hospital, Buddhist Tzu-Chi Medical Foundation, No. 289, Jianguo Rd, Xindian Dist, New Taipei City 23143, Taiwan
Full list of author information is available at the end of the article

number of alveolar-venous or bronchial-venous fistulas can develop along the needle's trajectory. During vascular injury, the walls of small vessels are usually retracted; spontaneous adhesion occurs, forming a seal. When a patient exhibits any symptoms suggestive of air embolism during the lung biopsy procedure, the needle should immediately be removed [8, 9]. The clinical manifestations of air embolism vary, depending on the exact location of the arterial embolus and the volume of air disseminated into the vessels. Once air enters the systemic circulation, it will enter the respective arterial end beds [1, 8]. Functional end arteries can be occluded by even a small volume of air. Only 2 mL of air injected directly into the cerebral circulation is enough to be fatal, and 0.5–1.0 mL of air injected into a coronary artery can lead to cardiac arrest [10]. Initial management includes immediate administration of 100% oxygen and placing the patient in a slight Trendelenburg position [7]. Early hyperbaric oxygen therapy is recommended for patients with cerebral air embolism [5].

Previously reported cases have only demonstrated imaging findings as existing air emboli in post-procedure CT scans. Imaging findings at different times, and the use of those findings to track the course and resolution of air emboli, have not been described. We report a case of systemic air embolism after CT-guided biopsy due to a kink in the coaxial biopsy system, and show the course followed by the emboli, demonstrated on sequential CT scans.

Case presentation

A 73-year-old man with pneumoconiosis, chronic obstructive pulmonary disease, and hypertension who had previously had a cerebrovascular accident and had undergone surgery for gastric cancer ten years earlier, was brought to our emergency department with a one-day history of acute-onset tremor and leg weakness. The chest radiograph and chest CT scan showed a large mass in the right middle lobe (RML) that was out of keeping with his pneumoconiosis. Lung malignancy was of concern; hence, a CT-guided percutaneous lung biopsy was suggested and was performed after obtaining informed consent.

A coaxial biopsy system with a 19-gauge introducer needle and a 20-gauge core biopsy needle (length, 17 cm; Temno, CareFusion, France) was selected for this procedure. Once the introducer needle had reached the lesion, the internal stylet was removed and the core biopsy needle was inserted to procure a specimen. However, after obtaining the first specimen, we were unable to withdraw the core biopsy needle because of a kink. Several attempts to withdraw it resulted in it being pushed forward and kinked again; finally, it was forcibly removed. The core biopsy needle was found to be angulated proximally. Thereupon, free air sprang up from the introducer needle. Hence, the stylet was reinserted and the introducer needle was immediately removed. After withdrawal of the instrument, the patient coughed forcefully. An immediate post-biopsy CT scan was performed; it demonstrated free air with flow-related motion artifact within the RML mass, the left atrium, and the right pulmonary vein (Fig. 1a and b). A follow-up CT scan of the entire thorax demonstrated air collections in the ascending aorta and the right coronary artery (Fig. 1c and d). Because the patient had no symptoms or signs of acute

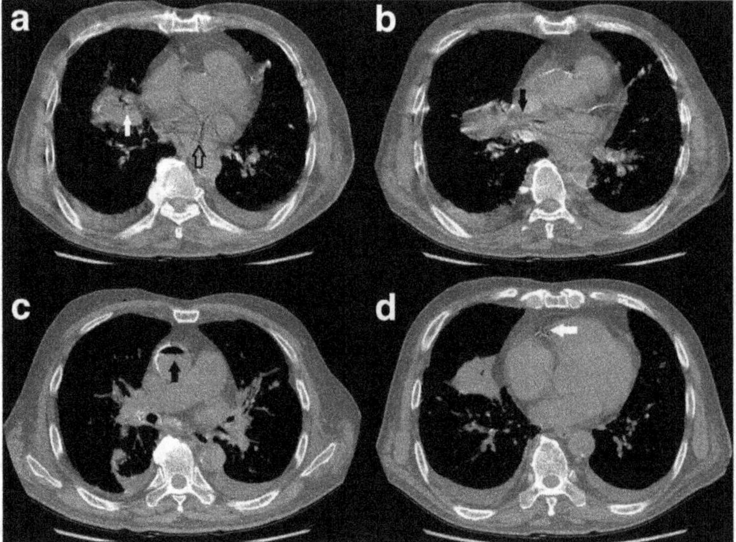

Fig. 1 Series of computed tomography scans demonstrating the movement of the air emboli. Immediate post-procedure computed tomography scans demonstrated free air with flow-related motion artifact in **a** the right middle lobe mass (white arrow), and the left atrium (open arrow), and **b** the right pulmonary vein (black arrow). After 50 s, a follow-up computed tomography scan demonstrated air collections in **c** the ascending aorta (black arrow) and **d** right coronary artery (white arrow)

stroke or myocardial infarction, he was kept in the CT room and oxygen was administered. Ten minutes later, a delayed chest CT scan demonstrated no air collections in the aorta or left heart, and total resolution of the air embolus in the right coronary artery (Fig. 2). The patient's condition was stable and an electrocardiogram showed no ST-segment elevation. He was thus transferred to the intensive care unit for close monitoring.

During his stay in the intensive care unit, neither air embolism nor new neurologic deficits developed, and his troponin I and CK-MB levels were normal. Five days later, brain magnetic resonance imaging was performed; it showed no evidence of acute infarction. The patient was transferred to the ward and was discharged days later in a stable condition. Table 1 shows the timeline of course of events.

Discussion

As demonstrated in this report, post-biopsy sequential CT scans can show the causal relationship between systemic air embolism and percutaneous biopsy, and can track the course and resolution of such emboli. The serial CT scans performed on our patient showed air with flow-related motion artifact in the lung mass, pulmonary vein, left heart, and then in the aorta and coronary artery. Later, the CT scans showed resolution of the air collections in the aorta and left heart, and almost total resolution of the air embolus in the coronary artery. Such evolution occurred quickly. Had the radiologists been unaware of this complication, CT scans would have been delayed and the systemic air emboli would either not have been detected or the diagnosis would have been delayed.

How can one avoid causing an angulation deformity in the core biopsy needle, thereby causing it to kink and get stuck in the introducer needle? Although blood clots can cause the biopsy needle to adhere to the introducer needle, especially when a long instrument is used, such adherence can be managed by flushing the introducer needle. After several experiments, we determined that the core biopsy needle deformity had occurred because the needle had been inappropriately removed from its packaging, resulting in angulation at the fulcrum where pressure was applied (Fig. 3). If the needle is inadvertently kinked, the biopsy set should be instantly discarded to prevent such severe complications as occurred in this case.

In the case presented, the air definitely came from the atmosphere because we witnessed air being drawn into the introducer needle. Moreover, the to-and-fro motion of the kinked core biopsy needle in the introducer needle may have evacuated the mass. Delayed reinsertion of the introducer needle's stylet after forcibly removing the kinked biopsy needle also played an important role. Early awareness of air being drawn into the introducer needle is very important. An immediate series of CT scans to trace the air's course is crucial for early detection of systemic air embolism.

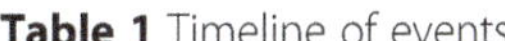

Table 1 Timeline of events

Date	Event
6 Nov	Admission for CT-guided lung biopsy
7 Nov	Systemic air embolism after percutaneous CT-guided lung biopsy due to a kink in the coaxial biopsy system
7 Nov	No ST-segment elevation on electrocardiogram; normal troponin I and CK-MB levels
12 Nov	No acute infarct on brain magnetic resonance imaging
17 Nov	Discharged in a stable condition

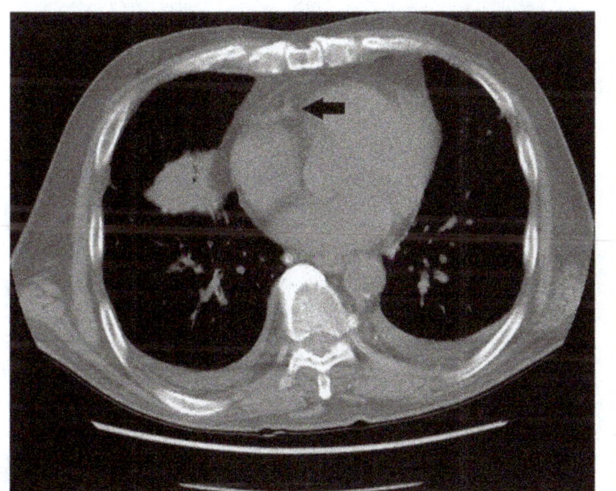

Fig. 2 Delayed chest computed tomography scan, performed after 10 min, demonstrating total resolution of the air embolus in the right coronary artery

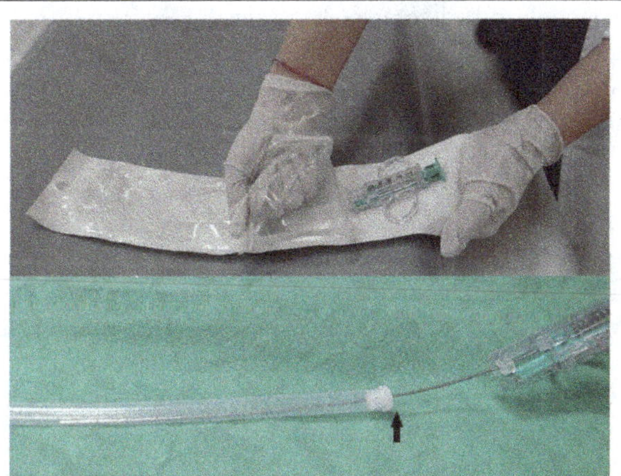

Fig. 3 Inappropriate removal of the core biopsy needle from its packaging. The upper image demonstrates an inappropriate method of removing the core biopsy needle from its packaging, resulting in angulation at the fulcrum where pressure was applied (lower image, black arrow)

Initial management includes immediate administration of 100% oxygen, and placing the patient in a slight Trendelenburg position [7]. Early hyperbaric oxygen therapy is recommended for patients with cerebral air embolism [5]. However, there is no standard protocol for managing asymptomatic patients; we recommend performing delayed post-procedure CT scans to evaluate the air's course.

Two major events need to be considered: Embolic stroke and myocardial infarction. Clinical features that support the diagnosis of cardioembolic stroke include the sudden onset of neurological deficits, an interval from onset to maximal deficit of < 5 min, and rapid regression of symptoms [11]. The symptoms of cerebral arterial air embolism develop suddenly. The clinical presentation is determined by the absolute amount of air and the intracranial vessel territories affected by the embolic event [12]. If delayed post-procedure CT scans show no more air in the left heart or in the thoracic aorta, there is no further concern of cerebral air embolism occurring. However, the symptoms of myocardial infarction may be atypical and silent [13, 14]. The electrocardiogram demonstrates ST-segment elevation rapidly (within 30 s) after manual transient occlusion of a coronary artery [15]. The incidence of acute non-ST elevation myocardial infarction may be higher than acute ST elevation myocardial infarction [16]. In our daily practice, a post-biopsy CT scan is performed routinely in every patient to evaluate complications. If air embolism is detected in a routine post-biopsy CT scan, another delayed CT scan is recommended to follow the air's course in an asymptomatic patient. If this delayed CT scan does not demonstrate air emboli in the coronary artery, left heart, or thoracic aorta, either no air entry occurred or the coronary artery has recanalized. In this patient, we evaluated the coronary arteries in the delayed post-procedure CT scan images to ensure that the air embolism had completely resolved. However, if the air embolism persists or progresses, the patient should be intensively monitored (e.g. symptom and electrocardiogram monitoring, and serial measurement of cardiac enzymes).

Conclusion

Sequential post-biopsy CT scans of this patient demonstrated the causal relationship between systemic air embolism and percutaneous biopsy, and allowed the radiologist to track the course and resolution of the emboli. Awareness of air entry via the introducer needle and an early post-biopsy CT scan are crucial for early detection of systemic air embolism. We recommend that a delayed chest CT scans be performed to follow the air's course when air embolism is detected in an asymptomatic patient.

Abbreviations

CT: Computed tomography; RML: Right middle lobe

Acknowledgements

We would like to thank Editage (www.editage.com) for English language editing.

Funding

This case report was supported by a grant from Taipei Tzu-Chi Hospital, Buddhist Tzu-Chi Medical Foundation (TCRD-TPE-106-RT-1). The funders played no role in the design of the study and collection, analysis, and interpretation of data and in writing the manuscript.

Authors' contributions

HCC collected the data and references, followed up the patient, performed the literature review, and drafted the manuscript. MCY critically revised the manuscript and assisted in the literature review. Both authors have read and approved the final manuscript.

Consent for publication

Written informed consent for publication of the case report was obtained from the patient's daughter-in-law.

Competing interests

The authors declare that they have no competing interests.

Author details

[1]Department of Radiology, Taipei Tzu-Chi Hospital, Buddhist Tzu-Chi Medical Foundation, No. 289, Jianguo Rd, Xindian Dist, New Taipei City 23143, Taiwan. [2]School of Medicine, Tzu Chi University, Hualien, Taiwan. [3]Division of Pulmonary Medicine, Department of Internal Medicine, Taipei Tzu-Chi Hospital, Buddhist Tzu-Chi Medical Foundation, No. 289, Jianguo Rd, Xindian Dist, New Taipei City 23143, Taiwan.

References

1. Tomiyama N, Yasuhara Y, Nakajima Y, Adachi S, Arai Y, Kusumoto M, et al. CT-guided needle biopsy of lung lesions: a survey of severe complication based on 9783 biopsies in Japan. Eur J Radiol. 2006;2006(59):60–4.
2. Ibukuro K, Tanaka R, Takeguchi T, Fukuda H, Abe S, Tobe K. Air embolism and needle track implantation complicating CT-guided percutaneous thoracic biopsy: single-institution experience. AJR Am J Roentgenol. 2009; 2009(193):W430–6.
3. Ghafoori M, Varedi P. Systemic air embolism after percutaneous transthorasic needle biopsy of the lung. Emerg Radiol. 2008;15:353–6.
4. Freund MC, Petersen J, Goder KC, Bunse T, Wiedermann F, Glodny B. Systemic air embolism during percutaneous core needle biopsy of the lung: frequency and risk factors. BMC Pulm Med. 2012;12:2.
5. Blanc P, Boussuges A, Henriette K, Sainty JM, Deleflie M. Iatrogenic cerebral air embolism: importance of an early hyperbaric oxygenation. Intensive Care Med. 2002;28:559–63.
6. Wu CC, Maher MM, Shepard JA. Complications of CT-guided percutaneous needle biopsy of the chest: prevention and management. AJR Am J Roentgenol. 2011;196:W678–82.
7. Bou-Assaly W, Pernicano P, Hoeffner E. Systemic air embolism after transthoracic lung biopsy: a case report and review of literature. World J Radiol. 2010;2:193–6.
8. Hiraki T, Fujiwara H, Sakurai J, Iguchi T, Gobara H, Tajiri N, et al. Nonfatal systemic air embolism complicating percutaneous CT-guided transthoracic needle biopsy: four cases from a single institution. Chest. 2007;132:684–90.
9. Kau T, Rabitsch E, Celedin S, Habernig SM, Weber JR, Hausegger KA. When coughing can cause stroke–a case-based update on cerebral air embolism complicating biopsy of the lung. Cardiovasc Intervent Radiol. 2008;31:848–53.
10. Ho AM, Ling E. Systemic air embolism after lung trauma. Anesthesiology. 1999;90:564–75.

11. Arboix A, Alio J. Cardioembolic stroke: clinical features, specific cardiac disorders and prognosis. Curr Cardiol Rev. 2010;6:150–61.
12. Muth CM, Shank ES. Gas embolism. N Engl J Med. 2000;342:476–82.
13. Valensi P, Lorgis L, Cottin Y. Prevalence, incidence, predictive factors and prognosis of silent myocardial infarction: a review of the literature. Arch Cardiovasc Dis. 2011;104:178–88.
14. Fujino M, Ishihara M, Ogawa H, Nakao K, Yasuda S, Noguchi T, et al. Impact of symptom presentation on in-hospital outcomes in patients with acute myocardial infarction. J Cardiol. 2017;70:29–34.
15. Zalewski A, Goldberg S, Dervan JP, Slysh S, Maroko PR. Myocardial protection during transient coronary artery occlusion in man: beneficial effects of regional beta-adrenergic blockade. Circulation. 1986;73:734–9.
16. McManus DD, Gore J, Yarzebski J, Spencer F, Lessard D, Goldberg RJ. Recent trends in the incidence, treatment, and outcomes of patients with STEMI and NSTEMI. Am J Med. 2011;124:40–7.

Investigations of organ and effective doses of abdominal cone-beam computed tomography during transarterial chemoembolization using Monte Carlo simulation

Yi-Shuan Hwang[1,2], Hui-Yu Tsai[3], Yu-Ying Lin[2] and Kar-Wai Lui[1,2*]

Abstract

Background: To investigate the organ dose, effective dose (ED), conversion factor, and the C-arm rotation angle effects on dose variations of abdominal C-arm cone-beam computed tomography (CBCT) during transarterial chemoembolization (TACE).

Methods: The organ doses and EDs for abdominal C-arm CBCT were retrospectively calculated according to a Monte Carlo technique for 80 patients. Dose variations from projections, ED to dose–area product (DAP) ratios, and effects of body mass index (BMI) on the ED and ED to DAP ratios were also analyzed.

Results: The kidney received the highest dose (14.6 ± 1.2 mSv). Organ dose deviations among C-arm rotation angles was highest for stomach (CV = 0.71). The mean ED of the the CBCT run during TACE was 3.5 ± 0.5 mSv, and decreased with increased BMI ($R^2 = 0.45$, $p < 0.001$). The mean ED to DAP ratio was 0.27 ± 0.04 mSv·Gy^{-1}·cm^{-2} and tended to decrease with increased BMI ($R^2 = 0.55$, $p < 0.001$). The mean ED to DAP ratios were 0.29 ± 0.02, 0.26 ± 0.02, and 0.23 ± 0.03 mSv·Gy^{-1}·cm^{-2} for patients with BMI < 25 kg/m^2, 25–30 kg/m^2, and ≥30 kg/m^2, respectively.

Conclusions: Suitable conversion factors for C-arm CBCT facilitate the use of DAPs for estimating the ED. The patient dose can be varied by adjusting the CBCT rotation angle setting, and dose reduction strategies can be further manipulated.

Keywords: Cone-beam computed tomography, Effective dose, Organ dose, Conversion factor, Dose–area product

Background

C-arm cone-beam computed tomography (CBCT), performed using an angiographic system that rotates a C-arm-mounted, flat-panel detector around the patient, is an imaging technique capable of yielding three-dimensional (3D) volumetric images. Although CBCT is useful for providing additional information on anatomical relationships, detecting tumors, determining the feeding arteries of tumors, and identifying the distribution of the contrast agent injected through the catheter [1], the additional radiation dose resulting from extra 3D imaging acquisitions during interventional procedures is difficult to evaluate in a patient [2].

The effective dose (ED) is considered the most appropriate quantity for estimating the stochastic risk of exposure to ionizing radiation. However, the complexity of dose calculations for C-arm CBCT complicates performing total ED estimations for patients who have undergone interventions, including fluoroscopic procedures and C-arm CBCT runs. Some studies have investigated the patient dose for abdominal CBCT procedures based on Monte Carlo simulations or Thermoluminescent

* Correspondence: kwlui@adm.cgmh.org.tw
[1]Department of Medical Imaging and Intervention, Chang Gung Memorial Hospital at Linkou, 5 Fushing Street, Kweishan, Taoyuan 333, Taiwan, Republic of China
[2]Department of Medical Imaging and Radiological Sciences, College of Medicine, Chang Gung University, Taoyuan, Taiwan
Full list of author information is available at the end of the article

Dosimeter (TLD) measurements [2–6]. To more rapidly estimate the ED, suitable conversion factors should be applied to the dose–area product (DAP) values [7]. Suzuki et al. surveyed three types of angiographic systems from three manufacturers and used three sizes of human-shaped phantoms with Monte Carlo simulations and TLD measurements to assess the doses and effects of the phantom size on the EDs for abdominal C-arm CBCT procedures [2, 5]. Their benchmark studies provided an important reference for abdominal CBCT dose investigations, and demonstrated that conversion factors are protocol specific and may differ among angiographic systems [2, 5].

This study estimated the organ dose, ED, and conversion factors for abdominal C-arm CBCT during transarterial chemoembolization (TACE) by using Monte Carlo simulations for the angiographic systems not included in previous studies. The C-arm rotation angle effects on the organ dose based on the simulations were also investigated. Additionally, the relationship between the ED and patient body mass index (BMI) was investigated, and conversion factors that convert the DAP to ED based on the BMI categories for C-arm CBCT acquisitions in TACE were proposed for more detailed ED estimations.

Methods

Patients

This retrospective study was conducted with approval from institutional review board, and patient informed consent was waived. Eighty patients with hepatocellular carcinoma (HCC; 56 men and 24 women; average age, 65 years) scheduled for TACE between June 2015 and January 2016 were included. None of these patients were optimal candidates for surgery or local treatments, such as radiofrequency ablation.

Patient BMI was calculated from the height and weight listed in the medical records. To further investigate the effects of patient BMI on the dose, the BMI was divided into three categories according to the World Health Organization and National Institutes of Health classification schemes [8]: < 25 kg/m^2 (normal), 25–30 kg/m^2 (overweight), and ≥ 30 kg/m^2 (obese). The mean patient BMI was 25.3 ± 4.0 kg/m^2, and the patient characteristics are summarized in Table 1.

Angiographic system and C-arm CBCT application

In this study, BRANSIST safireVC17 (Shimadzu Corporation, Japan) equipped with a 17-in. direct-conversion flat-panel detector was used as the angiographic system. The system is available for C-arm CBCT applications without automatic exposure control (AEC) adjustments, and the exposure parameters, such as the tube voltage (kV) and current (mA), are kept constant during the C-arm rotation. All technical parameters of the C-arm CBCT application in patients with HCC during TACE are summarized in Table 2. CBCT images were acquired from right anterior oblique (RAO) 120° to left posterior oblique (LAO) 95°, with a total acquisition range of 215°.The DAP values were recorded by technologists and used as the dose index for the dose calculations for each patient.

Organ dose, ED, and conversion factor analysis

Dose evaluations were performed using PCXMC (PCXMC 2.0; Radiation and Nuclear Safety Authority, Helsinki, Finland) according to a Monte Carlo technique. The anatomical data were determined using the hermaphrodite phantom models, and further modified the simulated phantom sizes based on the adult phantom model by adjusting the weights and heights to mimic those of the patients. According to the adjusted weight and height, the program modified the phantom sizes and shapes by using calculated vertical and horizontal scaling factors [9].

In the simulation, the doses were calculated for 29 organs in 44 projections at 5°-intervals from RAO 120° to LAO 95°. To calculate the organ doses for each projection, the projection data including tube voltage (kVp), target angle, filtration, projection angle, X-ray field entrance position, focus to the patient skin distance (FSD), and the field size, were served as input parameters for the program.

The DAP is the input-dose quantity supplied for dose calculations, and organ dose and ED for each projection could thus be calculated subsequently. Notably, the ED was estimated using the tissue weighting factors defined in the International Commission on Radiological Protection report No. 103 [10]. The reported organ dose and ED for each patient was calculated by summing the doses in all 44 projections.

Table 1 Patient characteristics and mean DAPs, EDs, and ED to DAP ratios

	Patient number (Male / Female)	Age	Height (cm)	Weight (kg)	DAP (Gy·cm^2)	ED (mSv)	ED to DAP ratio (mSv·Gy^{-1}·cm^{-2})
All patients	80 (56/24)	65 ± 12 (36–87)	162 ± 8 (146–183)	67 ± 13 (48–120)	12.9 ± 0.8 (11.8–17.1)	3.5 ± 0.5 (2.1–4.5)	0.27 ± 0.04 (0.17–0.35)
BMI < 25 kg/m^2	45 (30/15)	68 ± 11 (37–87)	161 ± 7 (148–176)	59 ± 6 (48–76)	12.9 ± 0.6 (12.3–15.4)	3.8 ± 0.3 (3.0–4.5)	0.29 ± 0.02 (0.24–0.35)
BMI 25–30 kg/m^2	22 (18/4)	62 ± 12 (40–83)	163 ± 7 (146–173)	72 ± 7 (58–86)	12.8 ± 0.6 (11.8–14.8)	3.3 ± 0.4 (2.7–4.2)	0.26 ± 0.02 (0.22–0.30)
BMI ≥ 30 kg/m^2	13 (8/5)	60 ± 13 (36–83)	163 ± 8 (148–183)	85 ± 13 (68–120)	13.2 ± 1.4 (11.9–17.1)	3.0 ± 0.4 (2.1–3.9)	0.23 ± 0.03 (0.17–0.28)

Data are mean ± SD (range)

Table 2 Clinical settings of abdominal CBCT acquisitions for patients undergoing TACE

	Configuration values and acquisition parameters
Acquisition mode	CB-CTAP
Acquisition rate (fps)	30
Radiation time (sec)	12
Rotation speed	20°/sec
Number of frames	Approximate 315 frames
Acquisition range	215°
Focus-to-image distance (FID) (cm)	120
Field of view size (inch)	17
Focus	Large focus
Total filtration (mm)	11.2-mm aluminum equivalent
kV	100
mA	360
Pulse width (msec)	5.6

To further estimate the the angular dependence of the organ dose, the mean and standard deviation (SD) from the 44 projections for each organ dose as well as the coefficient of variation (CV) defined as the SD normalized to the mean were calculated. The ED to DAP ratio, defined as the ED normalized to the DAP value, was also calculated for the C-arm CBCT procedure performed on each patient [2, 5, 11, 12]. Thus, conversion factors for the CBCT performed during TACE were estimated based on the ED to DAP ratios calculated from patient data. Finally, the effects of patient BMI on the ED and ED to DAP ratios were also investigated.

Statistical analysis

SPSS software (version 18.0; SPSS, Chicago, Illinois) was used for statistical analysis. Correlations between patients' BMI and EDs as well as EDs to DAP ratios of CBCT were performed using linear regression. Two-sided p values < 0.05 were considered significant. The magnitudes of the differences of the mean EDs as well as mean ED to DAP ratios between three BMI categories were analyzed by one-way analysis of variance (ANOVA). The differences were considered significant at p values < 0.05.

Results

Organ dose and ED calculations

The mean DAP of the CBCT run during TACE was 12.9 ± 0.8 Gy·cm^2 (11.8–17.1 Gy·cm^2; Table 1). Additionally, Fig. 1 presents the organ dose distributions. The following organs received the highest organ dose: kidney (14.6 ± 1.2 mSv), spleen (12.7 ± 1.3 mSv), adrenal gland (10.9 ± 1.0 mSv), pancreas (7.2 ± 1.0 mSv), and liver (7.0 ± 1.0 mSv). The mean ED per CBCT acquisition was 3.5 ± 0.5 mSv, and ranged from 2.1 to 4.5 mSv.

Effects of patient BMI on ED

Dependence of the ED on patient BMI during the CBCT acquisitions is demonstrated in Fig. 2a, the ED decreased slightly with increased patient BMI ($R^2 = 0.45$, $p < 0.001$). A significant difference was observed in the ED among the three BMI categories ($p < 0.05$, one-way ANOVA). The mean ED values were 3.8 ± 0.3, 3.3 ± 0.4, and 3.0 ± 0.4 mSv for normal, overweight, and obese patients, respectively (Table 1).

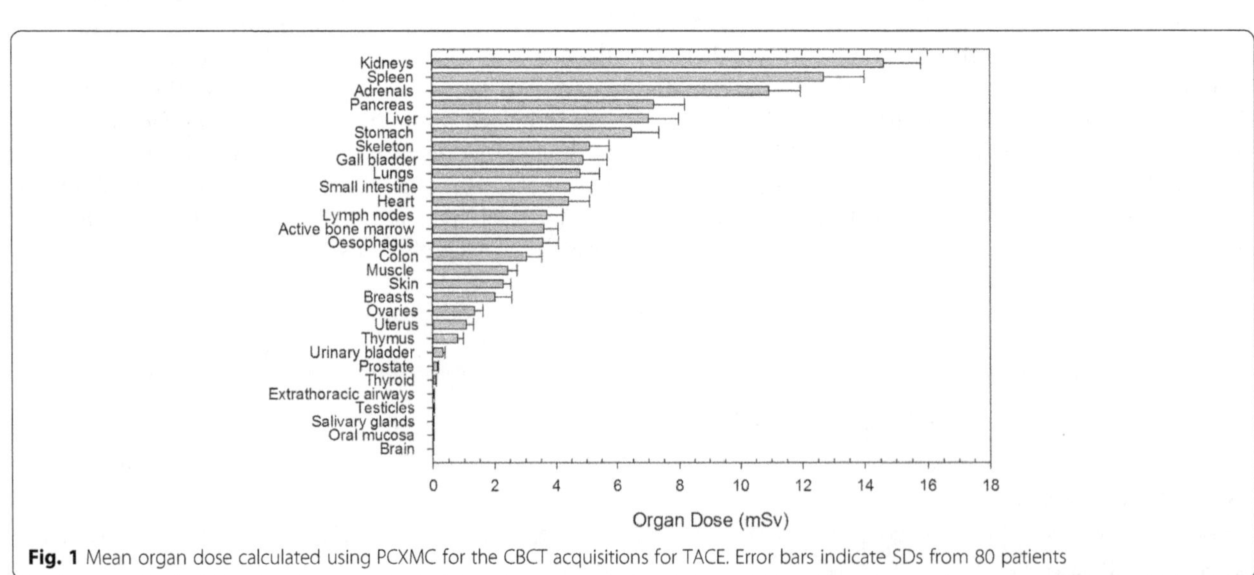

Fig. 1 Mean organ dose calculated using PCXMC for the CBCT acquisitions for TACE. Error bars indicate SDs from 80 patients

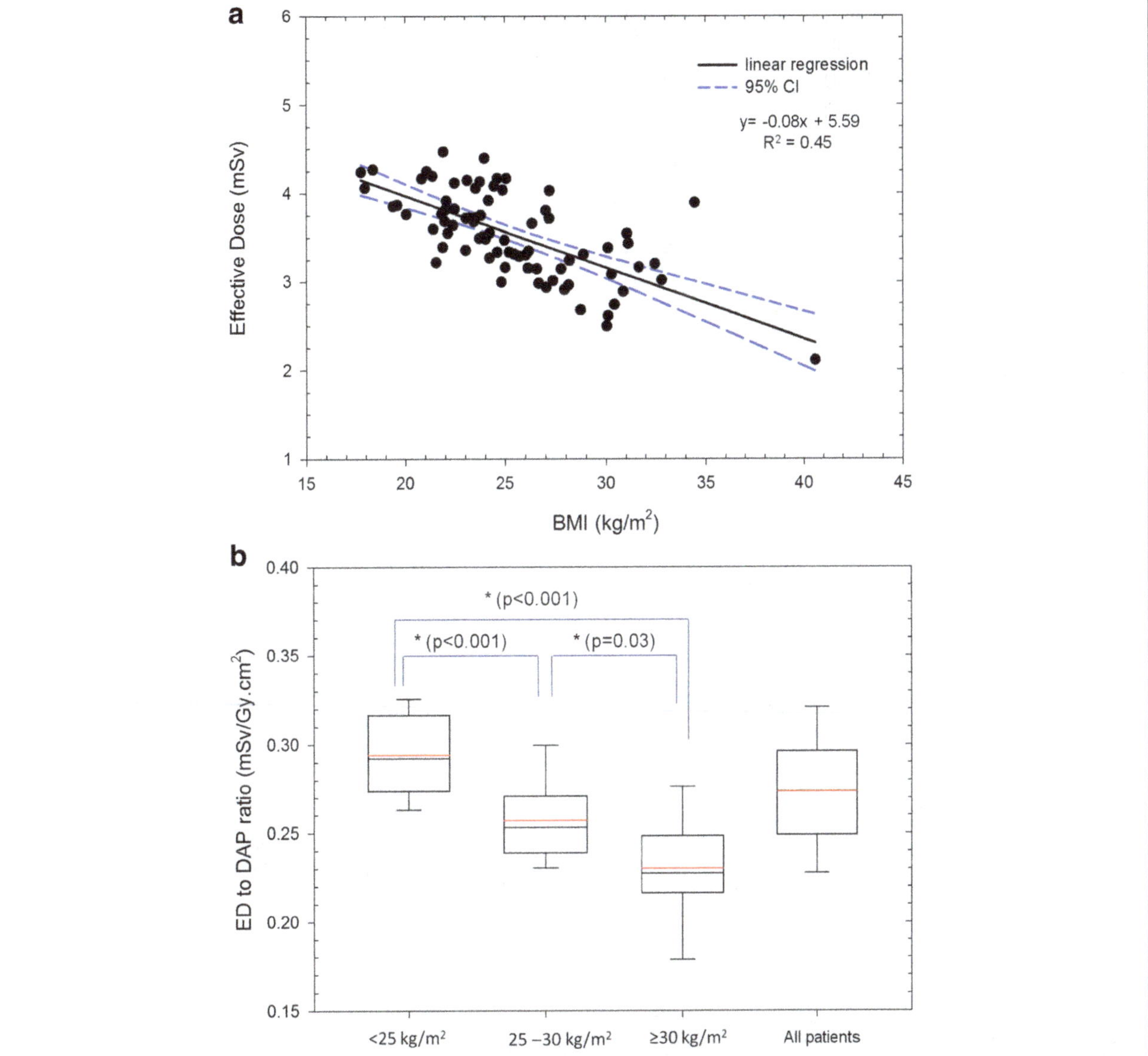

Fig. 2 ED and ED to DAP ratio dependence on patient BMI. **a** An inverse linear relationship between the ED and BMI is demonstrated. Black solid line is the linear regression line between the ED and BMI, and the blue dashed lines display the range of 95% confidence interval (CI). **b** Box plots show the 25%–75% interquartile range of the ED to DAP ratio with patient BMI < 25 kg/m^2, 25–30 kg/m^2, ≥ 30 kg/m^2, and with all the patients. Significant differences were observed in the ED to DAP ratio among the three BMI categories. Red and black lines indicate the mean and median values, respectively

Conversion of DAP values to ED

In the clinical C-arm CBCT acquisitions for TACE investigated, the calculated mean ED to DAP ratio was 0.27 ± 0.04 mSv·Gy^{-1}·cm^{-2} for the entire patient population (0.17–0.35 mSv·Gy^{-1}·cm^{-2}). However, the results also revealed that the ED to DAP ratio was highly dependent on patient BMI and it decreased linearly with increased patient BMI ($R^2 = 0.55$, $p < 0.001$).

Furthermore, significant differences were observed in the ED to DAP ratios among the three BMI categories; specifically, the mean values were 0.29 ± 0.02, 0.26 ± 0.02, and 0.23 ± 0.03 mSv·Gy^{-1}·cm^{-2} for normal, overweight, and obese patients, respectively (Fig. 2b; $p < 0.05$, one-way ANOVA). The mean ED to DAP ratios estimated from the entire patient population and from the BMI categories served as the conversion factors for the Shimadzu angiographic system, and the values are listed in Table 1.

Effects of C-arm rotation angle on organ doses

The CVs of the organ dose calculated from the 44 projections demonstrated deviations among rotation angles are illustrated in Fig. 3a. The results revealed the highest

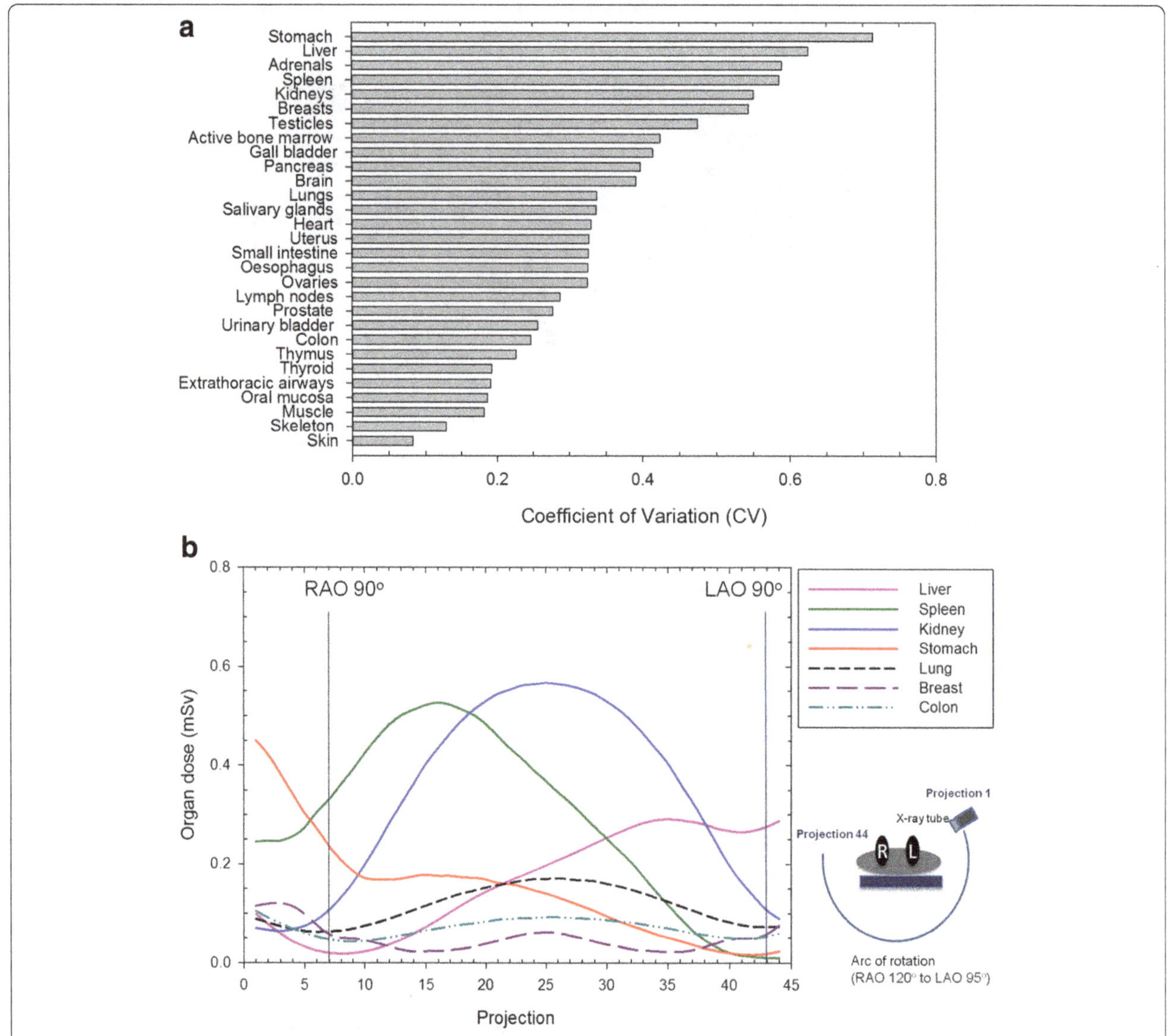

Fig. 3 Dose variations and angular dependence of the organ dose during X-ray tube rotation. **a** Organ dose variations from different X-ray irradiated angle, represent as CVs of the dose from the 44 simulated projections for each organ. **b** The distribution of the demonstrated organ dose per projection for the CBCT procedure

variations for the stomach (CV = 0.71), followed by the liver (CV = 0.62), adrenal gland (CV = 0.59), spleen (CV = 0.59) and kidney (CV =0.55).

To further demonstrate the angular dependence of the dose absorbed by the organs during X-ray tube rotation, Fig. 3b illustrates the organ dose for organs with a higher absorbed dose or higher dose variations from the aforementioned 44 projections (e.g., kidney, spleen, liver, and stomach) and some radiosensitive organs (e.g., lung, breast, and colon) for each projection of the CBCT procedures during the entire tube rotation. An evaluation of the organ locations and projection angles revealed that the dose absorbed by the liver increased from approximately projection 8 to projection 35 (corresponding to RAO 85° to LAO 50°), and the dose distributions for both kidney and spleen demonstrated wide peaks during X-ray tube rotation through the posterior sides of the patients.

Discussion

TACE is an angiographic procedure used to treat patients with hepatic tumors by injecting chemotherapeutic drugs into the selected hepatic artery [13]. To achieve more detailed patient dose investigations during these procedures, the ED obtained through fluoroscopy and CBCT imaging acquisitions should be individually evaluated. Multiple vendors have offered C-arm CBCT applications for angiographic systems, and the dose performance may vary because of the effects of varying designs on the beam quality as well as different protocol settings. To provide additional dose assessment information on abdominal CBCT, in addition to using popular angiographic units used in previous studies [2–6], organ dose and ED for C-arm CBCT acquisitions during hepatic TACE with the angiographic system without AEC capability when performing CBCT acquisitions by using Monte Carlo simulations were investigated.

Studies have investigated the doses for abdominal CBCT, as summarized in Table 3. The mean ED for the CBCT run was determined as 3.5 ± 0.5 mSv in this study. These values were slightly higher than the dose calculated according to the same Monte Carlo technique for the medium phantom with C-arm CBCT acquisitions with a GE INNOVA 4100 (3.1 mSv) but lower than the dose calculated for the large phantom with C-arm CBCT acquisitions using the same GE angiographic system (3.8 mSv) in the study by Suzuki [2].

In this study, BMI scores were used to analyze the relationship between patient size and the ED. The results revealed that the ED during C-arm CBCT acquisitions decreased with increased patient size, which is consistent with the findings of Wielandts et al. [9, 14] but contrasted with those of Ector et al. [8] and Suzuki et al. [2, 5]. Suzuki et al. demonstrated that the DAPs and ED increased with increased phantom size in the abdominal CBCT procedures with all three angiographic systems they investigated [2]. Wielandts et al. calculated CBCT doses for the ablation of arrhythmias and reported that ED is inversely related to patient BMI; this tendency may be because of the very limited increase in the DAP with the BMI despite AEC execution [14]. In this study, because of the technical specifications of the investigated angiographic system, the exposure parameters were preset in the CBCT procedures, regardless of patient size variations, and AEC was not activated in the acquisitions. Thus, DAP values deviated only slightly among the patients in different BMI groups. When the same exposure is used for patients with a higher BMI, the X-ray beam is attenuated more before being absorbed by the organ; thus, the organ doses and EDs would be lower for patients with a higher BMI than for those with a lower BMI. The effects of patient size on the ED for CBCT in systems with fixed-exposure techniques would be similar to those in systems with limited AEC modulations.

The establishment of conversion factors provide an approach for ED estimations when the DAP is available during angiography; however, the conversion factors differ among the angiographic systems and are specific to the used imaging protocols. Suzuki et al. estimated the ED to DAP ratios for three phantom sizes by using three types of angiographic systems for 3D abdominal imaging procedures [2]. Notably, in their survey, patient height and weight affected the ED to DAP ratios slightly, whereas the ED to DAP ratios were 0.37–0.45, 0.26–0.32, and 0.13–0.15 $mSv{\cdot}Gy^{-1}{\cdot}cm^{-2}$ on the Philips Allura Xper FD20/10, GE INNOVA 4100, and Siemens AXIOM Artis dTA systems, respectively, and the conversion factors were estimated to be approximately 0.4, 0.3, and 0.15 $mSv{\cdot}Gy^{-1}{\cdot}cm^{-2}$ on these three systems. Thus, Suzuki et al. concluded that the ED for each patient can be easily estimated using a suitable conversion factor set for each angiographic system [2].

To more conveniently evaluate the EDs for patients, our methodology was based on Monte Carlo simulations, and

Table 3 Previously reported EDs and ED to DAP ratios for abdominal CBCT procedures

Authors	Procedure	Scanner model	Rotation	Dose estimation method	Effective dose (ED) (mSv)	ED to DAP ratio ($mSv{\cdot}Gy^{-1}{\cdot}cm^{-2}$)
This study	Abdominal CBCT imaging: CB CTAP	Shimadzu BRANSIST safireVC17	215°	Using PCXMC based on individual patient data	3.5 ± 0.5 (2.1–4.5)	0.17–0.35
Suzuki et al. [2]	Abdominal 3D imaging	Philips Allura Xper FD20/10	207 °	(1) Placing TLD in the human-shaped phantom (S) (2) Using PCXMC for three human-shaped phantom	(1) TLD: 1.6 (2) PCXMC: 1.9 (S), 2.5 (M), 3.1 (L)	0.37–0.45
		GE INNOVA 4100	194°		(1) TLD: 2.0 (2) PCXMC: 2.2 (S), 3.1 (M), 3.8 (L)	0.26–0.32
		Siemens AXIOM Artis dTA	200°		(1) TLD: 2.6 (2) PCXMC: 2.1 (S), 2.4 (M), 2.6 (L)	0.13–0.15
Braak et al. [3]	CBCT guidance (upper abdomen)	Philips XperCT Allura FD20	240°	Using PCXMC based on individual patient data	4.2 (95% CI 3.8–4.6)	N/A
Kwok et al. [4]	Abdominal CBCT imaging: DynaCT 8-s DR	Siemens Artis zeego	200°	Placing TLD in the human-shaped phantom	15	N/A
	Abdominal CBCT imaging: LCI CTHA Low 10 s	Toshiba Infinix VC-i	200°		25.4	N/A
Sailer et al. [6]	CT abdomen LD roll	Philips XperCT Allura FD20	180°	Using PCXMC based on individual patient data	4.3 (95% CI 3.9–4.8)	N/A

TLD Thermoluminescent Dosimeter, *N/A* not available, *S* small phantom size, *M* medium phantom size, *L* large phantom size

patient data were collected as input for dose calculations. In this study, the mean ED to DAP ratio was 0.27 ± 0.04 mSv·Gy^{-1}·cm^{-2} on a Shimadzu BRANSIST safireVC17 for all patients, and the ratios decreased with increased BMI. The trend was similar with the results of Suzuki et al., and studies have reported that the body volume percentage in the exposure field decreases with increasing phantom size, thus contributing to the effects [2, 5]. The mean ED to DAP ratio estimated from all patients can serve as a conversion factor for easier ED estimations when the DAP is available. However, because of the strong effects of patient BMI on the ED to DAP ratios, using conversion factors without considering patient size may result in the overestimation of ED for obese patients. Using conversion factors adapted to patient size in addition to the DAP can serve as a feedback mechanism for providing clinicians with more details on ED estimations when performing C-arm CBCT.

The variation in the relative position of the organs to the X-ray tube during the C-arm rotation explains the fluctuations in the projection-by-projection radiation dose. The dose was higher when the organ was irradiated by the incident beam. During the C-arm rotation, dorsal organs, such as kidneys, received a higher dose during the major portions of the projections because the C-arm rotated from the left to the right side of the patient and went through the posterior side during the acquisitions. Among the 44 projections, dose variation was the highest for the stomach, followed by the liver, possibly because the stomach and liver were irradiated directly in the start and end positions, respectively, of the C-arm rotation. The dose absorbed by the liver increased during the rotation because the liver was more directly irradiated with the incident beam aimed at the anterior right side of the patient. By contrast, the stomach absorbed higher doses in the initial projections because of the direct X-ray irradiation in the beginning of the rotation trajectory, and the dose decreased during the rotation.

When totaling the organ doses from all 44 projections, the simulated results revealed that total doses to the organs in the upper abdomen were higher than those to the other organs. This is because the liver was the target organ during C-arm CBCT acquisitions. Therefore, the radiation window was always positioned in the upper abdomen during the C-arm rotation. In this study, dorsal organs, such as the kidney and adrenal gland, received the highest total dose during C-arm CBCT acquisitions, which likely occurred because the C-arm was rotated through the posterior side of the patients during the acquisitions, and the mentioned organs were localized in the direct-irradiated FOV for major portions of the projections during the exposure procedure. Notably, this phenomenon is in strong concordance with the results of Suzuki et al. [2, 5].

ED is calculated as a weighted sum of organ doses; therefore, its value is mainly determined by the organs that are highly irradiated and those that have more crucial weighting factors [9]. Based on the finding that the organ dose would vary in all radiation projections, ED for patients can be varied by adjusting the C-arm CBCT rotational angle. The stomach is one of the most radiosensitive organs (tissue weight factor, 0.12) [10] in the irradiated FOV; therefore, decreasing stomach dose by adjusting the C-arm CBCT rotational angle may lead to largely decrease total ED. C-arm rotation angle, FOV locations as well as the C-arm rotating around the anterior or posterior sides of the patients markedly affected patient doses, and this indicated that dose reduction strategies can be further manipulated from C-arm rotation angle setting or X-ray irradiated field location.

Our study has some limitations. First, the applicability of the results may be restricted. A system without AEC for C-arm CBCT applications was used in this study, and the results may be applicable to similar system configurations but not to those with AECs. However, the methodology described herein can still be used as a reference for patient dose evaluations of C-arm CBCT acquisitions. To provide more feasible clinical applications, the conversion factors for C-arm CBCT acquisitions should be further evaluated for different protocols and other angiographic systems from diverse manufacturers. Second, the use of the BMI as a patient size indicator has limitations. For example, a muscular patient with a narrow waist and an overweight patient can have a similar BMI, and a patient with ascites may have a low BMI but increased abdominal girth, which would affect the organ dose as well as the ED; this may not be reflected in the simulations.

Conclusions

We calculated the organ dose and ED according to a Monte Carlo technique for C-arm CBCT acquisitions during TACE by using a Shimadzu BRANSIST safireVC17 system. The ED to DAP ratios may differ with the protocols, systems, and patient sizes; however, overall, both ED and ED to DAP ratios decrease with increasing patient size. Suitable conversion factors for C-arm CBCT acquisitions facilitate the use of DAPs for estimating the ED during CBCT procedures and thus provide convenient patient dose estimations. The radiation dose absorbed by patients can be varied by adjusting the C-arm CBCT rotational angle settings, and dose reduction strategies can be further manipulated.

Abbreviations

3D: Three-dimensional; AEC: Automatic exposure control; ANOVA: Analysis of variance; BMI: Body mass index; CBCT: Cone-beam computed tomography; CV: Coefficient of variation; DAP: Dose–area product; ED: Effective dose; FSD: Focus to the patient skin distance; HCC: Hepatocellular carcinoma; kV: Tube voltage; LAO: Left posterior oblique; RAO: Right anterior oblique; SD: Standard deviation; TACE: Transarterial chemoembolization; TLD: Thermoluminescent Dosimeter

Acknowledgements

This study was supported by the grants of Chang Gung Memorial Hospital (CMRPG3F0691and CMRPG3F0692). The authors thank the Dose Assessment Core Laboratory of Institute for Radiological Research for assistance regarding dose assessment. Hui-Yu Tsai is supported by the Ministry of Science and Technology, R.O.C. (MOST 105-2314-B-182-003).

Funding

This study was supported by the grants of Chang Gung Memorial Hospital (CMRPG3F0691and CMRPG3F0692). HYT is supported by the Ministry of Science and Technology, R.O.C. (MOST 105-2314-B-182-003).

Authors' contributions

YSH, HYT, and KWL conceived the study and participated in its design, data collection, statistical analysis and drafting of the manuscript. YYL participated in data collection and data analysis. All authors read and approved the final manuscript for publication.

Consent for publication

Not applicable.

Competing interests

The authors declare that they have no competing interests.

Author details

[1]Department of Medical Imaging and Intervention, Chang Gung Memorial Hospital at Linkou, 5 Fushing Street, Kweishan, Taoyuan 333, Taiwan, Republic of China. [2]Department of Medical Imaging and Radiological Sciences, College of Medicine, Chang Gung University, Taoyuan, Taiwan. [3]Institute of Nuclear Engineering and Science, National Tsing Hua University, Hsinchu 300, Taiwan.

References

1. Orth RC, Wallace MJ, Kuo MD. Technology assessment Committee of the Society of interventional radiology. C-arm cone-beam CT: general principles and technical considerations for use in interventional radiology. J Vasc Interv Radiol. 2008;19:814–20.
2. Suzuki S, Yamaguchi I, Kidouchi T, Yamamoto A, Masumoto T, Ozaki Y. Evaluation of effective dose during abdominal three-dimensional imaging for three flat-panel-detector angiography systems. Cardiovasc Intervent Radiol. 2011;34:376–82.
3. Braak SJ, van Strijen MJL, van Es HW, Nievelstein RAJ, van Heesewijk JPM. Effective dose during needle interventions: cone-beam CT guidance compared with conventional CT guidance. J Vasc Interv Radiol. 2011;22:455–61.
4. Kwok YM, Irani FG, Tay KH, Yang CC, Padre CG, Tan BS. Effective dose estimates for cone beam computed tomography in interventional radiology. Eur Radiol. 2013;23:3197–204.
5. Suzuki S, Furui S, Yamaguchi I, Yamagishi M, Watanabe A, Abe T, et al. Effective dose during abdominal three-dimensional imaging with a flat-panel detector angiography system. Radiology. 2009;250:545–50.
6. Sailer AM, Schurink GWH, Wildberger JE, de Graaf R, van Zwam WH, de Haan MW, et al. Radiation exposure of abdominal cone beam computed tomography. Cardiovasc Intervent Radiol. 2015;38:112–20.
7. Compagnone G, Giampalma E, Domenichelli S, Renzulli M, Golfieri R. Calculation of conversion factors for effective dose for various interventional radiology procedures. Med Phys. 2012;39:2491–8.
8. Ector J, Dragusin O, Adriaenssens B, Huybrechts W, Willems R, Ector H, et al. Obesity is a major determinant of radiation dose in patients undergoing pulmonary vein isolation for atrial fibrillation. J Am Coll Cardiol. 2007;50:234–42.
9. Wielandts J-Y, Smans K, Ector J, De Buck S, Heidbüchel H, Bosmans H. Effective dose analysis of three-dimensional rotational angiography during catheter ablation procedures. Phys Med Biol. 2010;55:563–79.
10. ICRP, 2007. The 2007 Recommendations of the International Commission on Radiological Protection. ICRP Publication 103. Ann. ICRP 37 (2-4). http://www.icrp.org/publication.asp?id=ICRP%20Publication%20103.
11. Wang C, Nguyen G, Toncheva G, Jiang X, Ferrell A, Smith T, et al. Evaluation of patient effective dose of neurovascular imaging protocols for C-arm cone-beam CT. AJR Am J Roentgenol. 2014;202:1072–7.
12. Li JH, Haim M, Movassaghi B, Mendel JB, Chaudhry GM, Haffajee CI, et al. Segmentation and registration of three-dimensional rotational angiogram on live fluoroscopy to guide atrial fibrillation ablation: a new online imaging tool. Heart Rhythm. 2009;6:231–7.
13. Paul J, Jacobi V, Farhang M, Bazrafshan B, Vogl TJ, Mbalisike EC. Radiation dose and image quality of X-ray volume imaging systems: cone-beam computed tomography, digital subtraction angiography and digital fluoroscopy. Eur Radiol. 2013;23:1582–93.
14. Wielandts J-Y, De Buck S, Ector J, LaGerche A, Willems R, Bosmans H, et al. Three-dimensional cardiac rotational angiography: effective radiation dose and image quality implications. Europace. 2010;12:194–201.

The segmentation of bones in pelvic CT images based on extraction of key frames

Hui Yu[1], Haijun Wang[1*], Yao Shi[1], Ke Xu[2], Xuyao Yu[3] and Yuzhen Cao[1]

Abstract

Background: Bone segmentation is important in computed tomography (CT) imaging of the pelvis, which assists physicians in the early diagnosis of pelvic injury, in planning operations, and in evaluating the effects of surgical treatment. This study developed a new algorithm for the accurate, fast, and efficient segmentation of the pelvis.

Methods: The proposed method consists of two main parts: the extraction of key frames and the segmentation of pelvic CT images. Key frames were extracted based on pixel difference, mutual information and normalized correlation coefficient. In the pelvis segmentation phase, skeleton extraction from CT images and a marker-based watershed algorithm were combined to segment the pelvis. To meet the requirements of clinical application, physician's judgment is needed. Therefore the proposed methodology is semi-automated.

Results: In this paper, 5 sets of CT data were used to test the overlapping area, and 15 CT images were used to determine the average deviation distance. The average overlapping area of the 5 sets was greater than 94%, and the minimum average deviation distance was approximately 0.58 pixels. In addition, the key frame extraction efficiency and the running time of the proposed method were evaluated on 20 sets of CT data. For each set, approximately 13% of the images were selected as key frames, and the average processing time was approximately 2 min (the time for manual marking was not included).

Conclusions: The proposed method is able to achieve accurate, fast, and efficient segmentation of pelvic CT image sequences. Segmentation results not only provide an important reference for early diagnosis and decisions regarding surgical procedures, they also offer more accurate data for medical image registration, recognition and 3D reconstruction.

Keywords: CT segmentation, Pelvis, Key frame extraction, Skeleton, Marker-based watershed algorithm

Background

Recently, traffic accidents, falls and other serious high-energy trauma have often led to pelvic fractures. Researches show that the incidence of heavy-vehicle injury has increased over the years [1] and patients with pelvic fractures who present in shock have a mortality of 30–50% [2]. Pelvic fracture is the third most common cause of death in traffic trauma [3]. Rapid and accurate diagnosis and treatment are not only important to reduce the mortality caused by pelvic fractures, but also helpful for the functional reconstruction and correction of deformities of the pelvis. Medical imaging and processing are crucial in the process of diagnosis and treatment. The computed tomography (CT) images and 3D reconstruction by CT are commonly used to display the anatomical structure of pelvis and characteristics of the lesions [4]. Analysis based on CT images is important for the description of pelvic anatomy, the planning of surgical procedures and the evaluation of the post-operative effects [5]. And the most important step of analysis is bone segmentation, which is crucial to quantitatively evaluate the degree of fracture, detect the location of bleeding, and judge the condition of injury [6]. Therefore, the accuracy of segmentation will affect the doctor's judgment of the disease, the selection of the best surgical approach, etc.

At present, the pelvic region is manually marked for surgical procedures in the clinic. This process is time-consuming and error prone [7]. Therefore, it is necessary

* Correspondence: wanghaijun336@163.com
[1]Department of Biomedical Engineering, Tianjin University, Tianjin, China
Full list of author information is available at the end of the article

to propose a fast, accurate, and efficient method for pelvic segmentation.

Image segmentation is a hot topic in medical image processing. Recently, various segmentation methods have been proposed [8], some of which are based on thresholding [9–12]. The central idea of threshold segmentation is to transform the segmentation problem into pixel classification problem. Considering the fact that bone mineral density is heterogeneous, the connection between the femoral head and acetabulum is narrow, and a weak edge can be caused by disease, it is difficult to select a universal threshold. Other methods are based on the region growing technique, in which pixels with similar properties are set up as a region [13–15]. However, this method requires a long time and a large amount of space. In recent years, classification and clustering have also been used for medical image segmentation, and the relevant research focuses on the improvement of robustness [16–18]. Methods based on deformable models [19–25] and active shape models [26–30] have become a hot topic. For example, Calder et al. [20]proposed a segmentation method based on level set. Truc et al. [21] included density distance enhancement in a C-V model, and Martinez et al. [22] applied multi-scale edge detection to adjust a geometric model. Wu et al. [26] combined the active shape model with template matching, and Li et al. [27] combined the active shape model with a clustering model. However, most segmentation algorithms put more attention to the characteristics of a single CT image, so that the characteristics of CT sequences are usually ignored. Although there are many existing algorithms for medical image segmentation, an effective and accurate algorithm for the segmentation of pelvic CT image sequences has not been proposed. To assist doctors in diagnosis and treatment, an accurate segmentation of pelvic structure is essential. However, considering factors such as individual differences among different patients, bone mineral density unevenness, and narrowing of the hip joint space, it is difficult to rely only on gray scale information for accurate segmentation.

This paper proposes a novel segmentation method based on CT images of the pelvis. In the sequence of CT slices, because of the small shooting distance, the morphological characteristics between two adjacent CT images have high similarity. Thus, the key frames can be extracted. And the results of key frames are used to direct the segmentation of the remaining pelvic CT images according to the watershed algorithm based on skeleton markers. The proposed method greatly decreases the diagnostic time, and it's helpful for the early diagnosis of patients, selection of surgical planning, etc.

Methods

In this algorithm, we will select some CT images as key frames by using the method of key frame extraction. Then, experts will manually mark key frames to appoint the bone topological structure of these CT images. The segmentation results of key frames will be applied to describe the bone topology of other images. Next, the bone topology of the CT images will be used as a marker, and the watershed algorithm based on skeleton markers will be used to realize the automatic segmentation of pelvic structure. The algorithm consists of four parts: pre-processing of the CT image, key frame extraction in the CT image sequence, interactive marking and the watershed algorithm based on skeleton markers. The pretreatment process is used to denoise, extract regions of interest, and resize the image, reducing the amount of data in a single CT image. The CT sequence key frame extraction process is divided into two steps, and this process is used to reduce the number of CT images required for manual segmentation. In addition, the aim of interactive marking is to specify the bone topology of key frames. By matching key frames, the bone topology of each CT image can be acquired so that the accuracy of pelvic segmentation can be guaranteed. Finally, based on the interactive marking of key frames, the watershed algorithm based on skeleton markers is used to automatically segment all the CT images. The overall schematic diagram of the algorithm is shown in Fig. 1. In the following sections, the method is explained in detail.

Dataset

The dataset has been obtained from Tianjin Medical University General Hospital and Tianjin Nankai Hospital. Data has been randomly collected from 20 patients with traumatic pelvic injuries. These patients are in the 35- to 60-year age range and both sexes account for half. For each CT image sequence, the size of the planning CT images in the axial plane is 512×512 pixels, with 1 mm image resolution and 2–7 mm slice thickness. Besides, a total of 245 images are collected from each patient.

Pre-processing

Pre-processing removes surrounding artifacts from the original image, such as the CT platform and cables. Moreover, the image size is also adjusted in this process. The pelvis area is segmented from the original image as follows:

1. Only extract the image part of each DICOM file. The image data is 16 bits and there are 65,536 Gy levels. Considering the limited resolution of the human eyes and the limitations of experimental

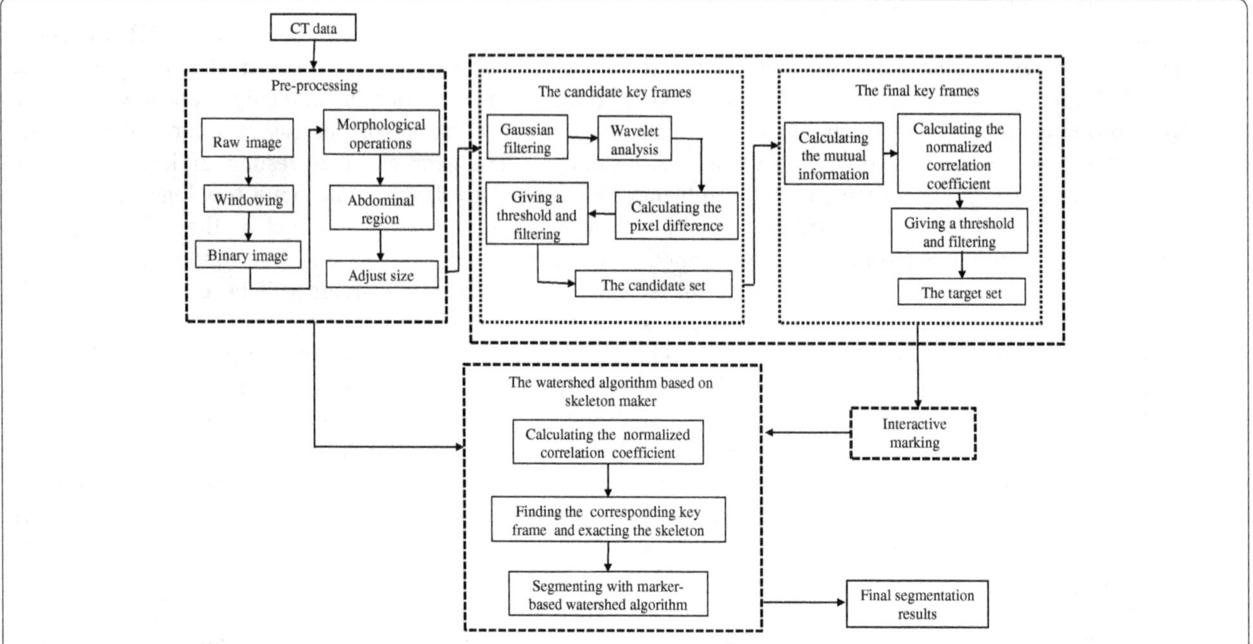

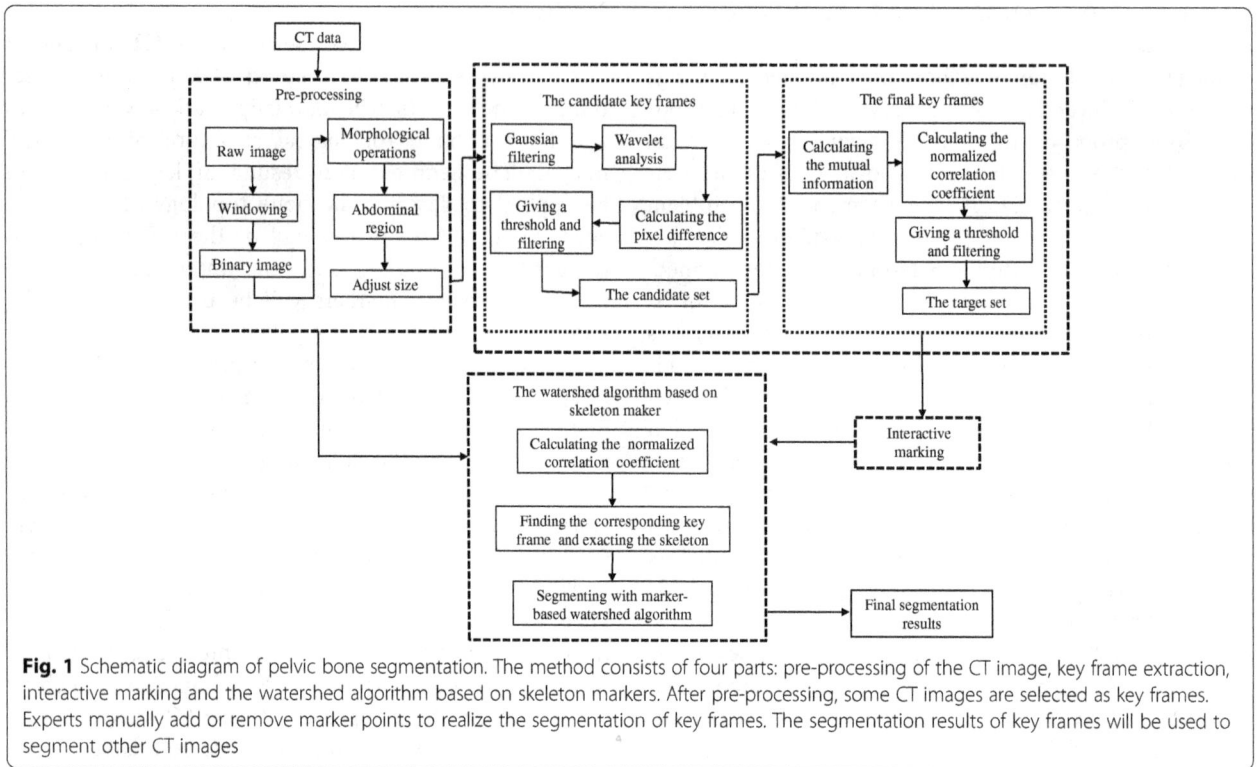

Fig. 1 Schematic diagram of pelvic bone segmentation. The method consists of four parts: pre-processing of the CT image, key frame extraction, interactive marking and the watershed algorithm based on skeleton markers. After pre-processing, some CT images are selected as key frames. Experts manually add or remove marker points to realize the segmentation of key frames. The segmentation results of key frames will be used to segment other CT images

facilities, convert the data in the image using (1) with data compression to 256 Gy levels.

$$f(x)=\begin{cases}0 & x\le c-\frac{w}{2}\\ \left[x-\left(c-\frac{w}{2}\right)\right]\times\frac{255}{w} & c-\frac{w}{2}<x<c+\frac{w}{2}\\ 255 & x\ge c+\frac{w}{2}\end{cases} \quad (1)$$

Here, f is a bitmap gray value, x is image data, w is window width, and c is window level.

2. Create a binary version of the original image according to (2).

$$f(x)=\begin{cases}0 & x=0\\ 1 & else\end{cases} \quad (2)$$

3. Apply morphological operations to the binary image so that the different objects can be separated and that the object which has the largest area is the pelvis. Next, all the pixels in this object will be set to 1, and others become 0. The binary image is called the "mask image".
4. Conduct an image convolution with the mask image and the original image, removing the CT platform, artifacts and other interference. At this time, the image is reserved for only the pelvis region; the remainder has been set to 0.
5. Adjust the size of the image by cutting out the non-pelvis area as much as possible. From now on, the pre-processed image is called the "input image".

The method of key frame extraction

After pre-processing, key frame extraction from the CT image sequence becomes the focus of the method. In this paper, key frames refer to the CT images of a CT sequence that have obvious changes in bone structure. As we can see from Fig. 2, there are four consecutive CT images. The first two CT images have similar bone structures. From the graph, we also find that the bone structure of (c) has obvious topological differences from the previous images. (b) has three bone topologies, while (c) has four obvious bone topologies. Therefore, (c) can be selected as a key frame. The method of key frame extraction consists of two steps. The first step is to obtain the candidate key frames. The last step is to obtain the final key frames.

To obtain candidate key frames, we extract the approximate region of bone as a region of interest so that the computation can be reduced. The pixel difference of the adjacent images is used to determine whether a new candidate key frame is required. The pixel difference of the adjacent images is defined as (3).

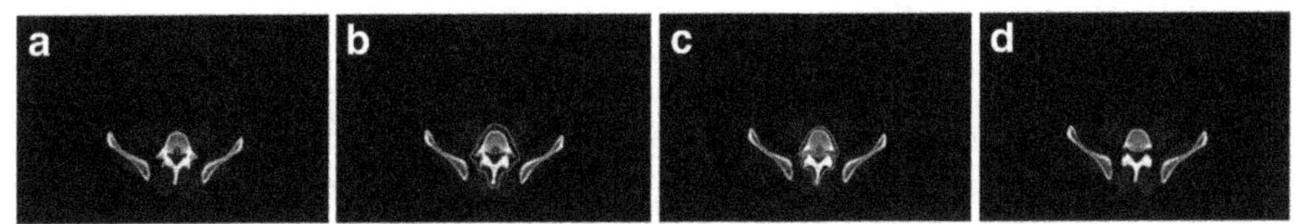

Fig. 2 Four consecutive CT images of Patient 1. (**a**) and (**b**) have similar bone topologies. We believe that each has three bone topologies, while (**c**) and (**d**) have four obvious bone topologies. The differences are shown in red

$$Dif = y_{j+1} - y_j \tag{3}$$

The greater the value is, the lower the degree of similarity is. Therefore, when the pixel difference of the adjacent images is greater than the threshold, it is considered that the difference between the adjacent images is large and that the similarity is not obvious. Thus, a new candidate key frame is added to the candidate set.

To summarize, the extraction of candidate key frames is implemented as follows:

1. Use a Gaussian filter on the input image.
2. Perform wavelet analysis of the filtered image and conduct image reconstruction using the approximation matrix.
3. Calculate T_1 based on (4).
4. Create a binary image based on (5).
5. Convolute the binary image with the filtered image and the resulting image is called the "interesting image".
6. Sort the interesting images in accordance with the spatial order and import CT data$\{y_1, y_2, y_3, \cdots, y_L\}$.
7. For $i = 1$ to $L - 1$
   Calculate the pixel difference of the adjacent images
   If the difference is greater than T_2
      the $i + 1$image is added to the candidate set
   Endif
   Endfor
8. The candidate set of key frames $\{g_1, g_2, g_3, \cdots, g_l\}$ is gained.

During the extraction of the candidate key frames, T_1 is the mean value of the reconstructed image of the non-zero area. It is defined as (4) and used to create a binary image. (4) and (5) are combined to obtain the approximate region of bones. In particular, the key frames in the candidate set are the pre-processed images and not the reconstructed images.

$$T_1 = \sum_{x=0}^{N-1}\sum_{y=0}^{M-1} f(x,y)/[N \times M - Zeros(S)] \tag{4}$$

Where $f(x, y)$ is a bitmap gray value, N is the width of image, and M is the height of image. $S = \{(x, y) | f(x, y) = 0\}$ is the set of background pixels and zero pixels. $Zeros(S)$ is the notation used for the cardinality of set S.

$$Mask(x,y) = \begin{cases} 1 & f(x,y) > T_1 \\ 0 & f(x,y) \le T_1 \end{cases} \tag{5}$$

Where $Mask(x, y)$is the binary image of reconstructed image.

To illustrate the key frame extraction process, we will use data of Patient 1 to explain the process in detail. After generating the interesting images, these images are numbered from 1 to 245 according to the anatomic structure. Figure 3 shows the pixel difference value of the example. To avoid missing key frames, T_2 is defined as (6), and it is described in blue in Fig. 3. After the extraction of the candidate set, there are 196 CT images to be selected out.

$$T_2 = 0.7 \times mean(Dif) \tag{6}$$

To obtain the target key frames, mutual information [31] and the normalized correlation coefficient [32] are utilized. The mutual information is defined as (7), and the normalized correlation coefficient is defined as (8). The mutual information reflects the gray correlation of the image; a greater mutual information value indicates that the gray difference of the two images is smaller. However, there is a lack of spatial location information so that redundant key frames will be extracted only when using mutual information. Thus, the normalized correlation coefficient is proposed to reduce the redundant key frames; a greater normalized correlation coefficient value indicates that the two images have higher similarity. The experimental results show that using the normalized correlation coefficient can effectively reduce the number of redundant key frames.

$$I(x,y) = \sum_{a\in f_1, b\in f_2} P_{f_1 f_2}(a,b) \log\left[P_{f_1 f_2}(a,b)/P_{f_1}(a)P_{f_2}(b)\right] \tag{7}$$

Where $P_{f_1}(a)$ is the probability density of imagef_1, and $P_{f_2}(b)$ is the probability density of image f_2. $P_{f_1 f_2}(a,b)$ is the joint probability density of image f_1 and image f_2.

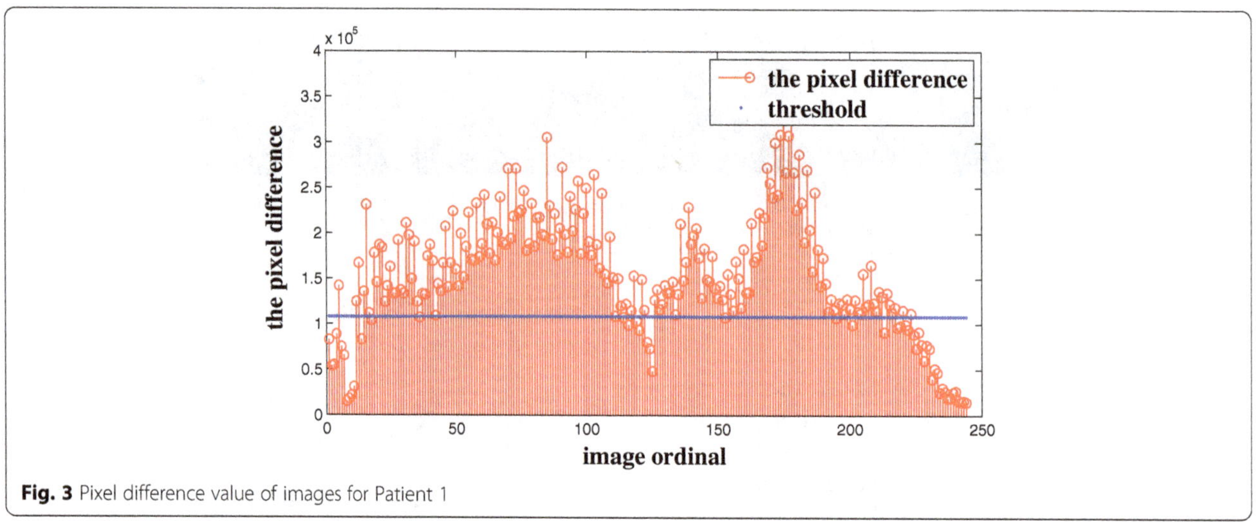

Fig. 3 Pixel difference value of images for Patient 1

$$R(x,y) = \frac{\sum_{i=0}^{M-1}\sum_{j=0}^{N-1}\left[f_1(i,j)-\overline{f_1}\right]\left[f_2(i,j)-\overline{f_2}\right]}{\sqrt{\sum_{i=0}^{M-1}\sum_{j=0}^{N-1}\left[f_1(i,j)-\overline{f_1}\right]^2\sum_{i=0}^{M-1}\sum_{j=0}^{N-1}\left[f_2(i,j)-\overline{f_2}\right]^2}} \tag{8}$$

Here, $f_1(i,j)$ is the pixel value of image f_1, $f_2(i,j)$ is the pixel value of imagef_2, $\overline{f_1}$ is the average gray value of image f_1, and $\overline{f_2}$ is the average gray value of imagef_2 .

The extraction of the target set from the candidate set is illustrated as follows:

1. Import the candidate set$\{g_1, g_2, g_3, \cdots, g_l\}$.
2. For $i = 1$ to l - 1
   Calculate the mutual information
   If ($(I(i+1, i) \leq T_3)$)
   the $i+1$image is added to the intermediate set
   Endif
   Endfor
3. For $j = 1$to k - 1
   Calculate the normalized correlation coefficient
   If ($(R(j+1, j) \leq T_4)$)
   the $j+1$image is added to the target set
   Endif
   Endfor
4. The target set of key frames $\{k_1, k_2, k_3, \cdots, k_t\}$ is gained.

The mutual information value of the candidate set is shown in Fig. 4. In this case, T_3 is the mean mutual information value and is shown in blue. In addition, when the mutual information value of adjacent candidate key frames is less thanT_3, the candidate key frames will be selected out to calculate the normalized correlation coefficient. As we can see from Fig. 5, there is no significant change in the bone topology of these images in the intermediate set, and these images can use the segmentation results of the same key frame as the reference. Therefore, it is necessary to take measures to remove redundant key frames in the intermediate set. Figure 6 shows the normalized correlation coefficient value of images in the intermediate set. T_4 is the mean normalized correlation coefficient and is shown in blue. An image will be chosen as a key frame in the target set when the normalized correlation coefficient is less than T_4. Finally, there are 31 images in the target set.

To describe the distribution of the key frames in the CT image sequence, Fig. 7 shows the interval between key frames. And the interval refers to the difference of each key-frame slice from the previous key-frame slice. At the same time, we equidistantly extract 31 images from the CT image sequence as a reference. It is found that the key frames are not evenly distributed. As a result, we can draw a conclusion that the key frames can effectively reflect the changes in pelvic structure and that it is meaningful to extract key frames.

Based on the above procedure, the target set of key frames $\{k_1, k_2, k_3, \cdots, k_t\}$ can be extracted. After the extraction of key frames, the number of CT images required for manual marking is greatly reduced.

Interactive marking

For each image in the target set, the first step is creating a binary version of the image. Next, marker points are obtained by extracting the skeleton from the binary image. The method of extracting the skeleton is introduced in the next section. Finally, the initial contours can be automatically generated through the watershed algorithm based on skeleton markers, which will also be introduced in next section. However, the results may be inconsistent with the topological structure of the human pelvis so that the segmentation

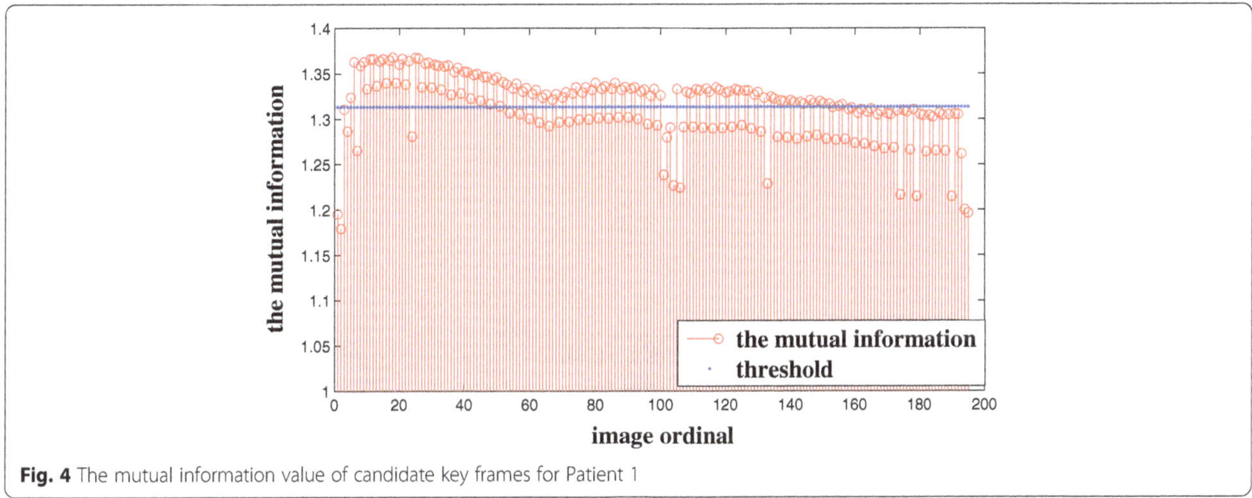

Fig. 4 The mutual information value of candidate key frames for Patient 1

results of this automatic algorithm cannot meet the requirements of clinical guidance. Therefore, the resulting image will be provided to experts, who will manually add or remove marker points to correct the initial contours. The segmentation results of key frames will be used to segment other CT images.

The watershed algorithm based on skeleton marking

The method is divided into two parts: skeleton extraction and the marker-based watershed algorithm. Before segmentation, it is first necessary to search for the key frame matching the CT image. When a CT image is processed, the corresponding key frame image is obtained by calculating the normalized correlation coefficient between the CT image and key frames in the target set. In the corresponding key frame image, the bone region segmentation results will be regarded as foreground, and the remaining region will be regarded as background. Next, the skeleton of foreground and background can be obtained via skeleton extraction. On the other hand, the gradient image of CT image should be gained. Then, using skeleton image mark the gradient image and shield the original minimum pixels in gradient image. Therefore, the new gradient image will be acquired. Finally, the segmentation results are obtained by using watershed transform for the new gradient image.

Skeleton extraction

The skeleton can provide information about the size and shape of targets in an image [33]. In this paper, we use the skeleton to describe location and topology information for pelvic bones. The method of thinning is used for skeleton extraction [34]. Whether or not a boundary point is converted into a background point is

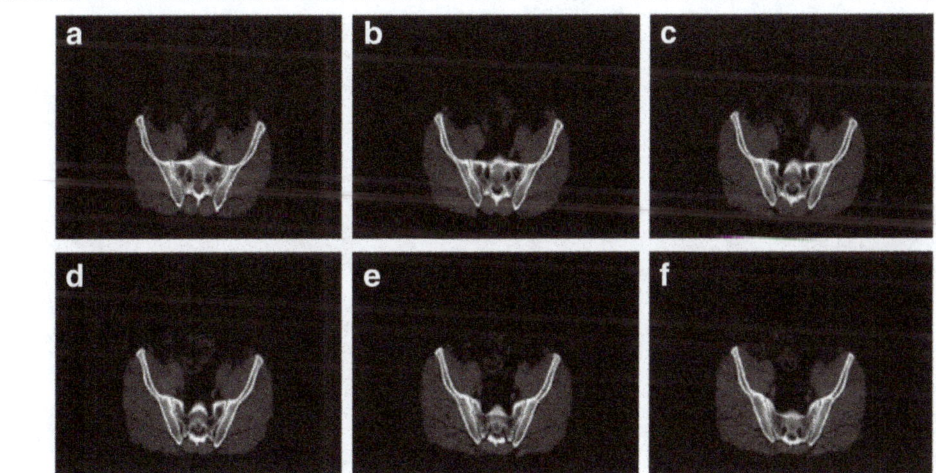

Fig. 5 Example of some consecutive key frames in an intermediate set for Patient 1. After using the mutual information, some obtained key frames still have similar bone topologies. As seen from (**a** - **f**), all frames have three bone topologies

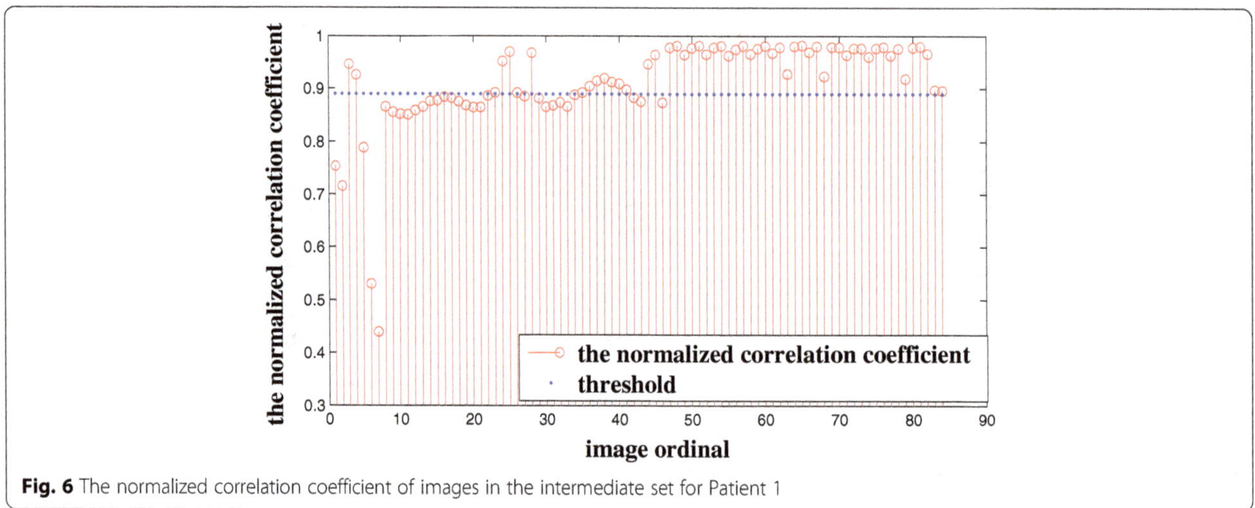

Fig. 6 The normalized correlation coefficient of images in the intermediate set for Patient 1

determined by the neighboring relations, and the iterative process is ended up with a pixel width. Supposing that the foreground pixel value is 1, the background pixel value is 0, $n(p_1)$ is the number of non-zeros in the neighborhood, and $s(p_1)$ is the total number of adjacent pixels from 0 to 1. Figure 8 shows the relationship between a pixel p_1 and eight-neighboring pixels. Whether a point can be removed or not depends on the eight adjacent points. In this paper, we consider mainly the following three cases [35]: υ_1 indicates whether the deletion will cause region splitting or not; υ_2 indicates whether it is the east, south, or northwest border; υ_3 indicates whether it is the north, west, or southeast border. These values can be described as in (9).

$$\begin{aligned}
\upsilon_1 &= \{p_1 | 2 \le n(p_1) \le 6, s(p_1) = 1\} \\
\upsilon_2 &= \{p_1 | p_2 \times p_4 \times p_6 = 0, p_8 \times p_4 \times p_6 = 0\} \\
\upsilon_3 &= \{p_1 | p_2 \times p_4 \times p_8 = 0, p_8 \times p_2 \times p_6 = 0\}
\end{aligned} \tag{9}$$

$$\begin{aligned}
D_1 &= \{p_1 | p_1 = 1, p_1 \in \upsilon_1, p_1 \in \upsilon_2\} \\
D_2 &= \{p_1 | p_1 \in \upsilon_1, p_1 \in \upsilon_3\}
\end{aligned} \tag{10}$$

The skeleton extraction algorithm is divided into two steps. First, the boundary pixels that satisfy the condition D_1 in the whole image are sought. The pixel

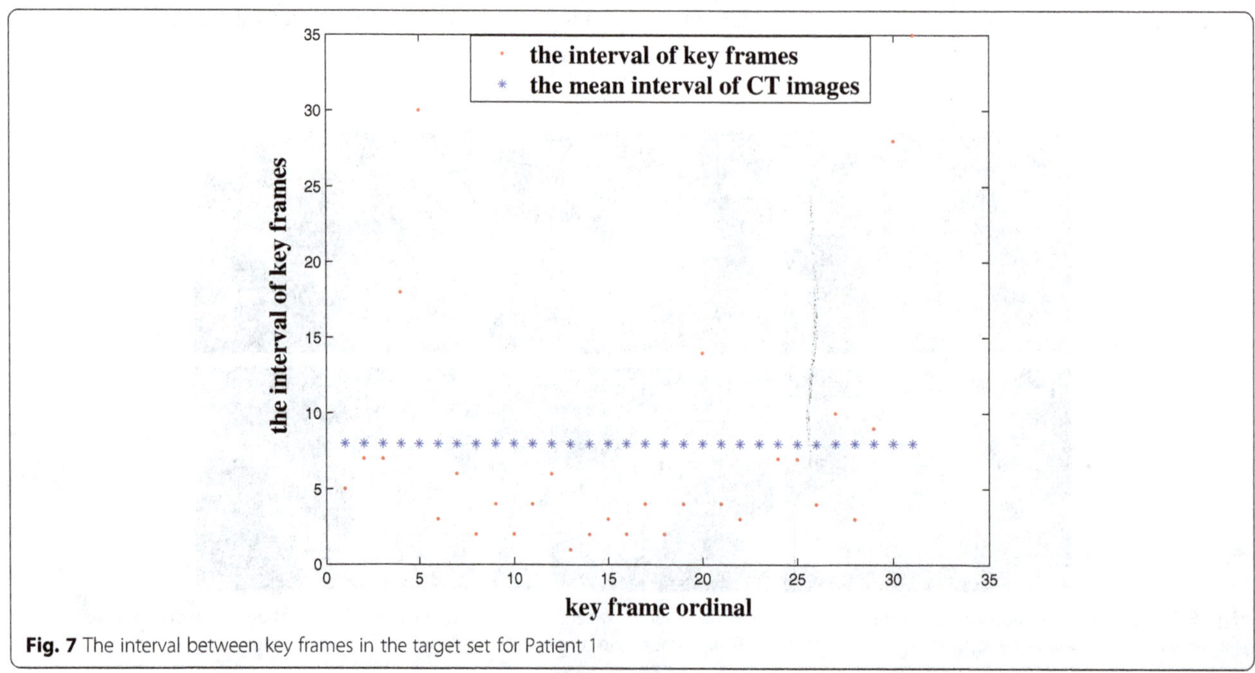

Fig. 7 The interval between key frames in the target set for Patient 1

p_9	p_2	p_3
p_8	p_1	p_4
p_{97}	p_6	p_5

Fig. 8 The relationship between neighboring pixels

points that we find are the ones that can be deleted. The pixels are converted to the background points after traversing the whole image. Then, the boundary pixels that meet condition D_2 in the transformed image are sought. Similarly, the pixels are converted after traversing the whole image. After this process is the next iteration, until there are no points that can be deleted between the two steps. In addition, the two conditions are presented as in (10).

As for key frames, the skeleton of the foreground (I_F) and background (I_B) can be generated by utilizing the skeleton extraction algorithm. The skeleton is shown as $S_H = Skel(I_F, I_B)$ and it will be the marker points for the marker-based watershed algorithm.

The marker-based watershed algorithm

The marker-based watershed algorithm [36] is based on a gradient image. Therefore, creating a gradient image is the first step in this process. In this method, the gradient image is obtained using the Sobel operator. The convolution templates (S_x, S_y) can be described as follows:

$$S_x = \begin{bmatrix} 1 & 2 & 1 \\ 0 & 0 & 0 \\ -1 & -2 & -1 \end{bmatrix} \quad S_y = \begin{bmatrix} 1 & 0 & -1 \\ 2 & 0 & -2 \\ 1 & 0 & -1 \end{bmatrix} \tag{11}$$

The gradient of pixel p_1 can be gained by calculating the convolution of the templates and the eight neighboring pixels in Fig. 8. The solution is as follows:

$$\begin{aligned} G_x &= p_9 + 2 \times p_2 + p_3 - (p_7 + 2 \times p_6 + p_5) \\ G_y &= p_9 + 2 \times p_8 + p_7 - (p_3 + 2 \times p_4 + p_5) \end{aligned} \tag{12}$$

The gradient image can be described as $\nabla f(x, y)$, and $\nabla f(x, y) = [G_X, G_Y]^T$, where G_x is the gradient along the X direction, and G_y is the gradient along the Y direction.

The skeleton S_H is used to mark the gradient image $\nabla f(x, y)$ At the same time, the original minimum pixels in gradient image will be shielded. In other words, in the marked gradient image, the local minimal value corresponds to the pixel region that is the non-zero area in the skeleton image. Finally, segmentation of the pelvic structure is achieved by using the watershed transform for the marked gradient image.

Results

The proposed segmentation method is tested on 20 patients. Each patient has 245 pelvic CT images. Patient 1 is used as an example to display the results from different stages of the method and they are presented in this section as follows.

Figure 9 shows the pre-processing results for the example. The results show that the edges of bone tissue are clearly defined by the window technology. Therefore, adjusting the window is necessary. In addition, the pelvis area can be extracted completely from the CT image after the removal of artifacts, platforms, etc.

Figure 10 shows the results obtained by the watershed algorithm based on skeleton markers. The results show that the distribution of pelvic structure can be well described by the skeleton and that the pelvic structure can be segmented accurately in a single CT image using this method.

Figure 11 shows the segmentation results of four CT images that are consecutive in the anatomic structure by the proposed method. The results show that the distribution of pelvic structure is well described by the marker points that were obtained from the corresponding key frame. Furthermore, the results also indicate that the proposed method can reliably segment the CT image sequence.

Figure 12 shows the segmentation results using the proposed method in fracture areas. (a), (b), (c) and (d)

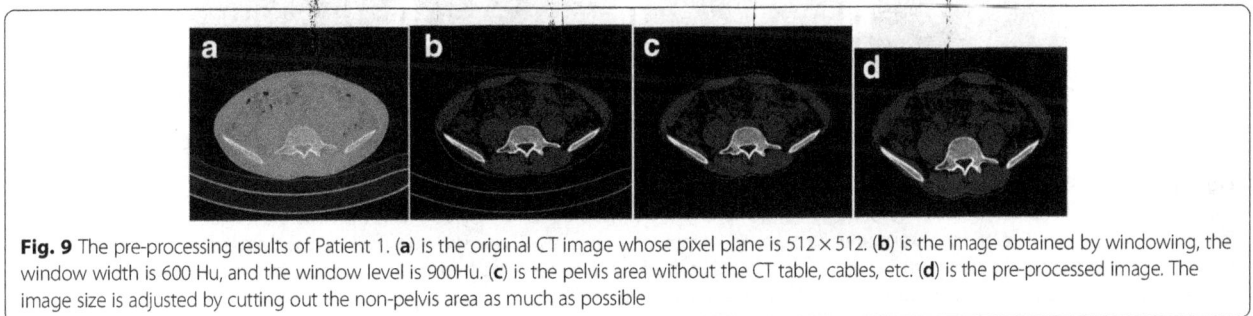

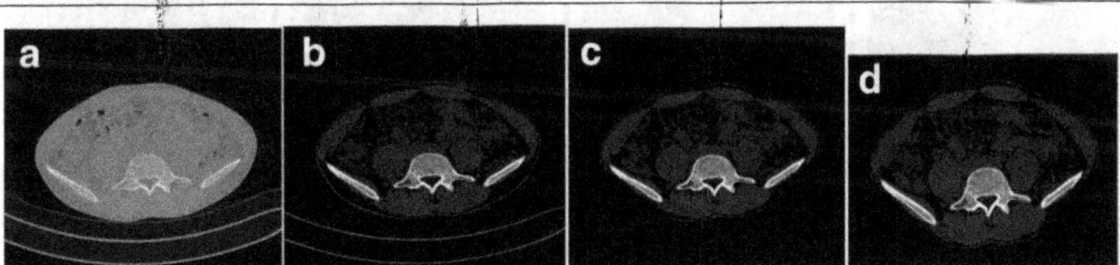

Fig. 9 The pre-processing results of Patient 1. (**a**) is the original CT image whose pixel plane is 512 × 512. (**b**) is the image obtained by windowing, the window width is 600 Hu, and the window level is 900Hu. (**c**) is the pelvis area without the CT table, cables, etc. (**d**) is the pre-processed image. The image size is adjusted by cutting out the non-pelvis area as much as possible

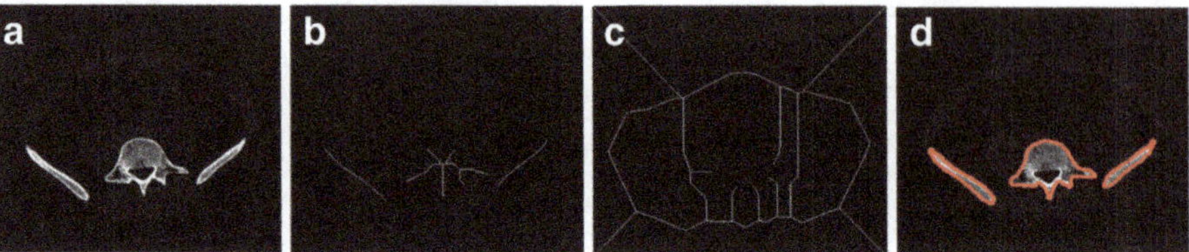

Fig. 10 Example results of Patient 1 obtained by the watershed algorithm based on skeleton markers. (**a**) is the input image as well as the pre-processed image. (**b**) is the skeleton image the for foreground and indicates the location of the pelvic structure. (**c**) is the skeleton image for the background and indicates the location of the other structures. (**d**) is the segmentation result and it is shown in the pre-processed image. The automatically segmented pelvic structure contours are displayed in red

are consecutive and these images are from Patient 3. These images show the segmentation results of CT images with sacrum bone fracture. (e), (f), (g) and (h) are also consecutive and they are from Patient 7. And they display the contours of bones in ischium bone fracture area. As can be seen from Fig. 12, the proposed method can accurately segment the fracture area.

Table 1 shows the number of key frames in each CT sequence. The results show that the ratio between the number of key frames and the total CT sequence number is approximately 13%. Thus, the number of images that need to be manually marked will be greatly reduced by extracting key frames.

Discussion

In this section, some measures are taken to evaluate the performance of the proposed algorithm. A quantitative comparison is performed between the manual segmentation and the computed segmentation. In addition, a three-dimensional display of the segmented bone structure is rendered. Besides, the performance of the watershed algorithm based on skeleton markers and gradient vector flow (GVF) is compared. And the

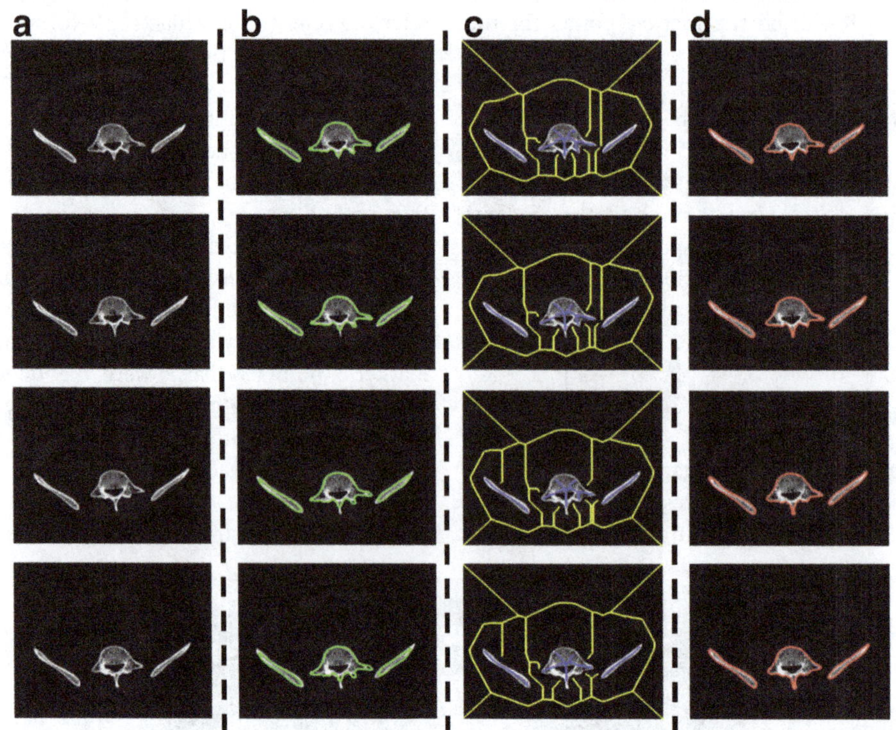

Fig. 11 Example results of Patient 1 obtained by the proposed method. (**a**) is the input image as well as the pre-processed image. (**b**) is the manual segmentation results for the corresponding key frame, and the edges are shown in green. (**c**) is the skeleton images. The skeleton of foreground is shown in blue and the skeleton of background is displayed in yellow. These skeletons will be used as marker points for the marker-based watershed algorithm. (**d**) is the segmentation result of the proposed method and it is shown in the pre-processed image. The automatically segmented pelvic structure contours are displayed in red

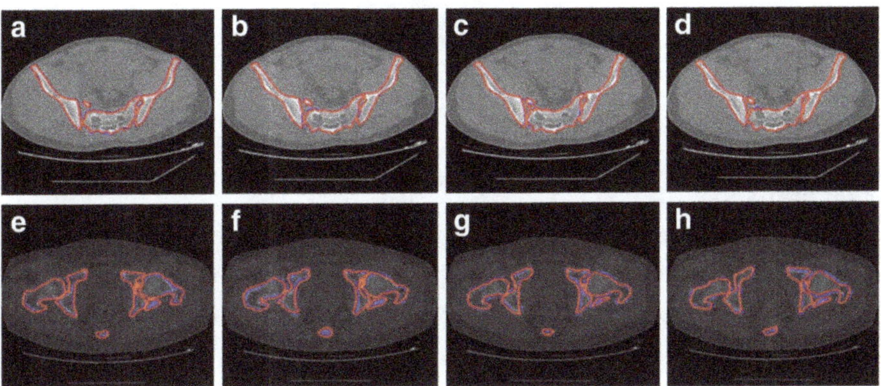

Fig. 12 Example of segmentation results using proposed method in the fracture area. (**a**), (**b**), (**c**) and (**d**) are from Patient 3. (**e**), (**f**), (**g**) and (**h**) are from Patient 7. The segmentation results of the proposed method are shown in the original image. The manual segmentation results by experts are displayed in blue while the automatically segmented pelvic structure contours are displayed in red

running time of the proposed algorithm is also an important index.

Evaluation measures

The overlapping area and the mean deviation distance are used to quantify the accuracy [37]. In this section, 245 CT images will be manually segmented by experts for each patient and the results will be the ground truth.

Table 1 Shows the number of key frames in each CT sequence

Images	Total no. of CT images	Total no. of the candidate set	Total no. of the target set
Patient 1	245	178	28
Patient 2	245	153	32
Patient 3	245	148	30
Patient 4	245	164	33
Patient 5	245	157	33
Patient 6	245	177	31
Patient 7	245	169	32
Patient 8	245	163	27
Patient 9	245	157	31
Patient 10	245	182	35
Patient 11	245	178	31
Patient 12	245	159	27
Patient 13	245	170	30
Patient 14	245	170	33
Patient 15	245	144	29
Patient 16	245	138	27
Patient 17	245	169	31
Patient 18	245	173	33
Patient 19	245	165	29
Patient 20	245	154	30

S_1 represents surface obtained by the proposed method and S_2 represents surfaces obtained by experts manually. Besides, L_1 represents a set of contour points obtained by the proposed method andL_2 represents a set of contour points manually obtained by experts. As for two surfaces, we define A_1 as the area for surface $S_1$and A_2as the area for surface S_2.

The overlapping area O of two surfaces S_1 and S_2 is defined as:

$$O = \frac{A_1 \cap A_2}{A_2} \times 100\% \qquad (13)$$

The mean deviation distance Mad of two contour points sets L_1 and L_2 is defined as:

$$Mad = \frac{1}{K}\sum_{n=1}^{K} d(l_n, L_2) \qquad (14)$$

Where l_n denotes each contour point inL_1,Kdenotes the total number of contour points in L_1. Deviation distance refers to the distance between the contours obtained by the proposed algorithm and the ground truth. The deviation distance between L_1 and $L_2$is defined as:

Table 2 Shows the segmentation results and the overlapping area of CT images from five patients'

Images	The average overlapping area	Accurate	Fair	Unacceptable
Patient 1	96.3%	95.1%(233/245)	3.7%(9/245)	1.2%(3/245)
Patient 2	94.1%	93.5%(229/245)	4.5%(11/245)	2%(5/245)
Patient 3	97.4%	96.7%(237/245)	2.9%(7/245)	0.4%(1/245)
Patient 4	94.8%	94.7%(232/245)	4.1%(10/245)	1.2%(3/245)
Patient 5	95.6%	95.9%(235/245)	3.3%(8/245)	0.8%(2/245)

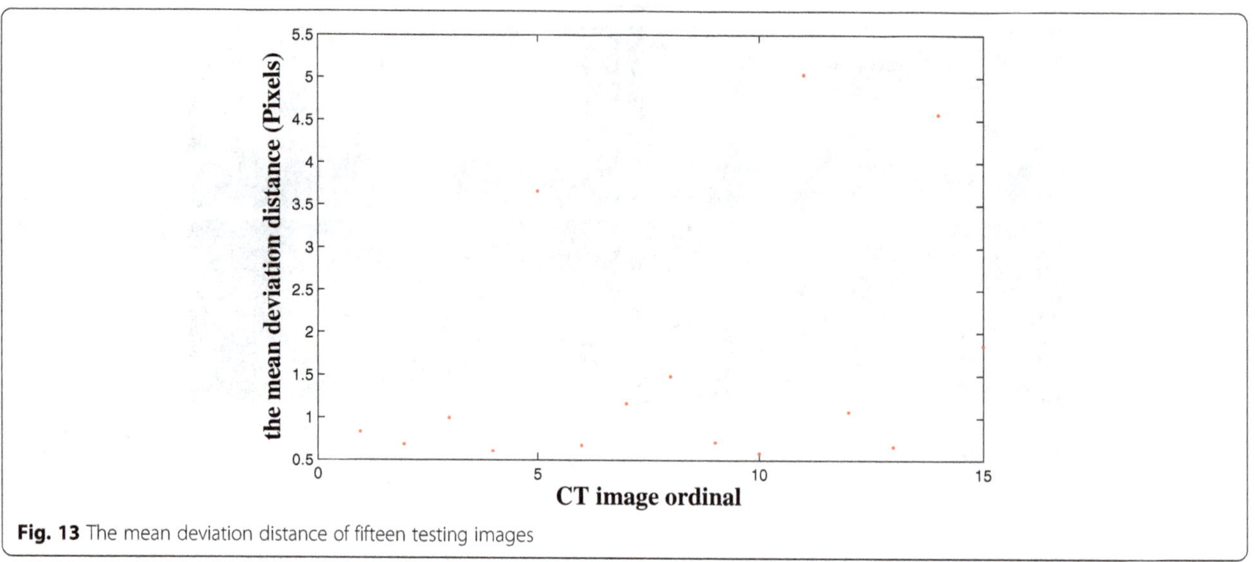

Fig. 13 The mean deviation distance of fifteen testing images

$$d(l_n, L_2) = \min_{l_i \in L_2} \|l_n - l_i\|_2 \quad (15)$$

Five patients of the 20 patients are randomly selected, and their CT images are used to calculate the overlapping area O. The shapes presenting with an overlapping area of more than 90% are classified as "accurate", the shapes presenting with an overlapping area of 90–80% are classified as "fair", and the shapes presenting with an overlapping area of less than 80% are classified as "unacceptable" [37].

Table 2 shows the segmentation results and the overlapping area of CT images from five patients'. The results show that the average overlapping area of all the data is more than 94%. More than 93.5% of the results are classified as "accurate", and less than 2% of the results are classified as "unacceptable". The unacceptable results may be caused by blurred edges of bones, uneven gray value of bones, lack of appropriate key frames, etc.

Figure 13 shows the mean deviation distance of fifteen testing images. These images are randomly selected from Patient 1 to Patient 5.The maximum mean deviation distance is 5.03 pixels, and the minimum mean deviation distance is approximately 0.58 pixels. Without the impact of the method, an unsmooth contour may also lead to a large mean deviation distance. The results show that the proposed method is reliable for accurate pelvic segmentation.

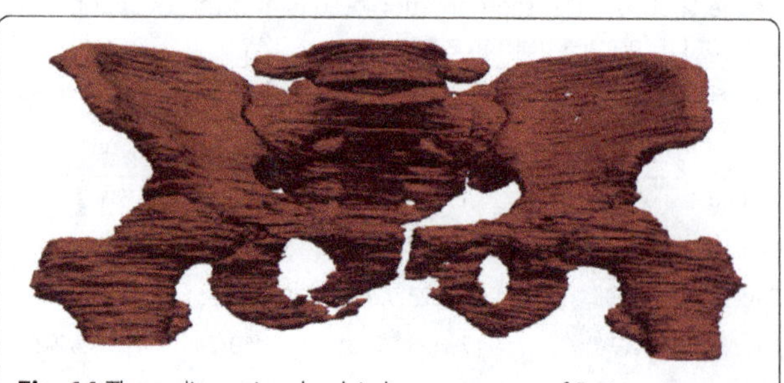
Fig. 14 Three-dimensional pelvic bone structure of Patient 4

After segmented sequences of CT slice images are obtained, a three-dimensional model of pelvic bone structure can be reconstructed utilizing these segmented bone structures. In addition, three-dimensional visualization may be used for further validating the accuracy of the proposed method. The segmentation results are visually inspected as shown in Fig. 14. As can be seen from this figure, the three-dimensional structure of pelvic bone is clearly presented and the detected fracture exits in the pelvic region.

The gradient vector flow (GVF) model

In this section, the segmentation performance using the watershed algorithm based on skeleton markers and the GVF model is compared. The GVF model was introduced by Xu and Prince [38] in 1998. In relation to the traditional snake model, the sensitivity of the initial curve position and the convergence of the concave area are improved. In this paper, the segmentation results of the key frames are taken as the initial curve in the GVF model.

Figure 15 shows the example of segmentation results using the two methods. As can be seen from Fig. 15b, the results of key frames cannot accurately describe the edges of pelvic bones in intervening images. However, the contours of bones in key frames can offer location and topology information of pelvic bones in the intervening images. Location information can be used to indicate the possible areas of bones and the topology information can be used to indicate the possible number of bones. From Fig. 15d, we can find that the information given by key frames cannot make GVF

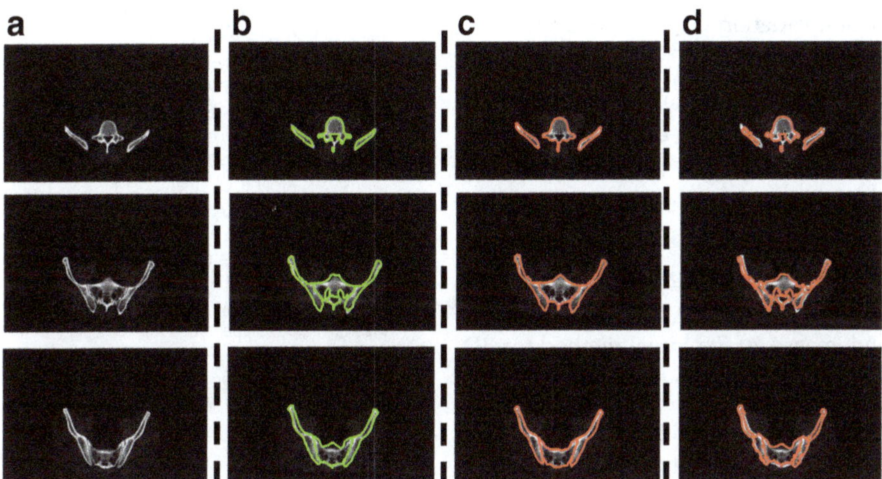

Fig. 15 Example results using the watershed algorithm based on skeleton markers and the GVF model. These testing images are from Patient 1. (**a**) is the input image as well as the pre-processed image. (**b**) is the manual segmentation results of the corresponding key frame, and the edges are shown in green. (**c**) is the automatic segmentation results of the watershed algorithm based on skeleton markers, and the edges are shown in red. (**d**) is the segmentation results of the GVF model, the edges are shown in red and they are shown in the pre-processed image

model obtain good segmentation results. Through this comparison of the segmentation results, it can be found that the watershed algorithm based on skeleton markers has better segmentation effect than the GVF model.

Algorithm running time

In this section, the test environment is as follows: the CPU is Inter-Core i3–2120 3.3 GHZ, the system memory is 4 GB, and the programming environment is MatLabR2014. Table 3 shows the running time of the proposed method except for the time of manual marking. As we can see from the graph, the average running time is approximately 2 min for one patient with 245 CT images.

Interactive marking has an approximate time of 30 s for each key frame image because the experts only need to manually add or remove a small number of marker points. The experimental results show that there are approximately 30 CT images that are selected for manual marking. Therefore, the proposed method takes approximately 15 min for one patient with 245 CT images. Such performance suggests a considerable reduction in processing time compared with manual segmentation.

Table 3 Shows the Running Time of the Proposed Method

Procedure	Average Running Time
Pre-processing	27.657s
Extraction of candidate key frames	36.288s
Extraction of final key frames	45.482s
The watershed algorithm based on skeleton markers	21.834s
Total algorithm	131.261s

In conclusion, the proposed method not only ensures the accuracy of pelvic segmentation but also reduces the time of segmentation.

Conclusions

A novel segmentation method based on CT image sequences of the pelvis is presented in this paper. The key parts of the method are the method of key frame extraction and the watershed algorithm based on skeleton markers. By using the method of key frame extraction, the number of manually marked CT images decreases to approximately 30. Based on the method of skeleton extraction, the distribution of pelvic structure can be well described in key frames. Considering that anatomical structures have characteristics of spatial continuity, the skeleton can be used to describe the location and topological information of pelvic bones in other CT images. Appling the watershed algorithm based on skeleton markers can achieve accurate, fast and efficient segmentation of pelvic structure. And segmentation results not only provide an important reference for early diagnosis and decisions regarding surgical procedures, they also offer more accurate data for medical image registration, recognition and 3D reconstruction.

In this paper, the performance of the proposed method depends on the accuracy of key frame extraction. When a crucial CT image is not selected, the accuracy of segmentation using the method will be affected. In addition, the performance is also affected by blurred edges of bones, variation of bones, etc. since the watershed algorithm is applied.

Future work will focus on the following points: 1) Propose a more efficient method to extract key frames. This method should ensure that the key frames are not redundant and that crucial CT images will not be missing. In addition, the running time of the method should also be considered. 2) Apply this method to segment other organs. 3) Using this method to process MRI and ultrasound images. 4) Explore a method for 3D reconstruction relying only on the key frames.

In conclusion, the proposed method is able to achieve accurate, fast, and efficient segmentation of pelvic CT image sequences.

Abbreviations

CT: Computed tomography; GVF: The gradient vector flow (GVF) model

Acknowledgments

The dataset used for this project was provided by Tianjin Medical University General Hospital and Tianjin Nankai Hospital.

Funding

This work was supported by the National Natural Science Foundation of China (NSFC) under Grant 61475116.

Authors' contributions

HY and HW conceived and designed the experiments; HW performed the experiments; YS and XY analyzed the data; KX and YC provided dataset and medical guidance; HW wrote the manuscript. All authors read and approved the final manuscript.

Competing interests

The authors declare that they have no competing interests.

Author details

[1]Department of Biomedical Engineering, Tianjin University, Tianjin, China. [2]Department of Orthopedic, Tianjin Medical University General Hospital, Tianjin, China. [3]Department of Radiation Oncology, Tianjin Medical University Cancer Institute & Hospital, Tianjin, China.

References

1. Naumann RB, Dellinger AM, Zaloshnja E, Lawrence BA, Miller TR. Incidence and total lifetime costs of motor vehicle-related fatal and non-fatal injury by road user type in the United States. Traffic Inj Prev. 2010;11(4):353.
2. Management of Exsanguinating Pelvis Injuries:An algorithm for the management of exsanguinating pelvic trauma. http://www.trauma.org/index.php/main/article/668/.Accessed 20 May 2008.
3. Fulkerson EW, Egol KA. Timing issues in fracture management: a review of current concepts. Bull Hosp Jt Dis. 2009;67(1):58.
4. Zhao JB, Liu J. Application value of three-dimensional CT reconstruction in diagnosis and treatment of pelvic fracture-dislocation. China J Orthop Traumatol. 2006;19(7):403–4.
5. Foshager MC, Walsh JW. CT anatomy of the female pelvis: a second look. Radiographics A Rev Publ Radiol Soc North America Inc. 1994;14(1):64–6.
6. Najarian K, Vasilache S, Smith R, et al. Accurate pelvic fracture detection for X-ray and CT images: US, US 8538117 B2[P]. 2013. http://www.freepatentsonline.com/8538117.pdf.
7. Dalinka MK, Arger P, Coleman B. CT in pelvic trauma. Orthop Clin N Am. 1985;16(3):471–80.
8. Collier DC, Burnett SS, Amin M, Bilton S, Brooks C, Ryan A, Roniger D, Tran D, Starkschall G. Assessment of consistency in contouring of normal-tissue anatomic structures. J Appl Clin Med Phys. 2003;4(1):17–24.
9. Norouzi A, Rahim MSM, Altameem A, Saba T, Rad AE, Rehman A, Uddin M. Medical image segmentation methods, algorithms, and applications. IETE Tech Rev. 2014;31(3):199–213.
10. Li Y. Bone segmentation in human CT images. J Biomed Eng. 2004;21(2):169.
11. Natsheh AR, Ponnapalli PV, Anani N, Benchebra D. Segmentation of bone structure in sinus CT images using self-organizing maps. In: IEEE international conference on imaging systems and techniques: 2010; 2010. p. 294–9.
12. Aguirreramos H, Avinacervantes JG, Cruzaceves I. Automatic bone segmentation by a Gaussian modeled threshold. In: Medical Physics: Fourteenth Mexican Symposium on Medical Physics: 2016; 2016. p. 883–94.
13. Janc K, Tarasiuk J, Bonnet AS, Lipinski P. Genetic algorithms as a useful tool for trabecular and cortical bone segmentation. Comput Methods Prog Biomed. 2013;111(1):72–83.
14. Mehnert A, Jackway P. An improved seeded region growing algorithm. Pattern Recogn Lett. 1997;18(10):1065–71.
15. Vasilache S, Ward K, Cockrell C, Ha J, Najarian K. Unified wavelet and gaussian filtering for segmentation of CT images; application in segmentation of bone in pelvic CT images. Bmc Med Inform Decis Making. 2009;9(Suppl 1):1–8.
16. Nguyen NT, Branzan-Albu A, Branzan-Albu A. A new segmentation method for MRI images of the shoulder joint. In: Computer and robot vision, 2007 CRV '07 fourth Canadian conference on: 2007; 2007. p. 329–38.
17. Kim E, Li H, Huang X. A hierarchical image clustering cosegmentation framework. In: Computer Vision and Pattern Recognition, vol. 2012; 2012. p. 686–93.
18. Camastra F, Vinciarelli A. Machine learning for audio, image and video analysis: theory and applications. London: Springer; 2008.
19. Mantas J. Methodologies in pattern recognition and image analysis—a brief survey. Pattern Recogn. 1987;20(1):1–6.
20. Calder J, Tahmasebi AM. A variational approach to bone segmentation in CT images. Proc SPIE Int Soc Opt Eng. 2011;7962(3):346–54.
21. Truc PTH, Lee S, Kim TS. A density distance augmented Chan-Vese active contour for CT bone segmentation. In: Conference: international conference of the IEEE engineering in Medicine & Biology Society IEEE engineering in Medicine & Biology Society Conference, vol. 2008; 2008. p. 482–5.
22. Martínez F, Romero E, Dréan G, Simon A, Haigron P, De CR, Acosta O. Segmentation of pelvic structures for planning CT using a geometrical shape model tuned by a multi-scale edge detector. Phys Med Biol. 2014;59(6):1471.
23. Chen L, Chen Y, Wang Z, Zhao W, Chen J. Segmentation of the pelvic bone using a generalized gradient vector convolution field snake model. J Med Imaging Health Inform. 2015;5(7):1482–7.
24. Gao Y, Shao Y, Lian J, Wang AZ, Chen RC, Shen D. Accurate segmentation of CT male pelvic organs via regression-based deformable models and multi-task random forests. IEEE Trans Med Imaging. 2016;35(6):1532–43.
25. Kardell M, Magnusson M, Sandborg M, Carlsson GA, Jeuthe J, Malusek A. Automatic segmentation of pelvis for brachytherapy of prostate. Radiat Prot Dosim. 2016;169(1–4):398.
26. Wu J, Davuluri P, Ward K, Cockrell C, Hobson R, Najarian K. A new hierarchical method for multi-level segmentation of bone in pelvic CT scans. Annual International Conference of the IEEE Engineering in Medicine and Biology Society. 2011; 2011(4):3399–3402.
27. Li D, Zang P, Chai X, Cui Y, Li R, Lei X. Automatic multiorgan segmentation in CT images of the male pelvis using region-specific hierarchical appearance cluster models. Med Phys. 2016;43(10):5426.
28. Zhang W, Liu J, Yao J, Summers RM. Segmenting the thoracic, abdominal and pelvic musculature on CT scans combining atlas-based model and active contour model. Proc SPIE Int Soc Opt Eng. 2013;8670(4):08.
29. Chen X, Bagci U. 3D automatic anatomy segmentation based on iterative graph-cut-ASM. Med Phys. 2011;38(8):4610.

30. Bakir H, Charfi M, Zrida J. Automatic active contour segmentation approach via vector field convolution. Signal Image Video Proc. 2016;10(1):1–10.
31. Steuer R, Kurths J, Daub CO, Weise J, Selbig J. The mutual information: detecting and evaluating dependencies between variables. Bioinformatics. 2002;18(suppl_2):S231–40.
32. Gao GZ, Zhongwu LI, Lifu YU. Application of the normalized cross correlation coefficient in image sequence object detection. Comput Eng Sci. 2005;27(3):38–40.
33. Cornea N D, Silver D, Min P. Curve-skeleton properties, applications, and algorithms. IEEE Transactions on Visualization & Computer Graphics. 2007; 13(3):530.
34. Shu C, Mo Y. Morphological thinning based on image's edges. In: International conference on communication technology proceedings: 1998, vol. 1; 1998. p. 5.
35. Hui YU, Changsheng QU, Jinhang LI. Method for hand profile extraction in complicated conditions. Comput Eng Appl. 2015;51(14):170–4.
36. Wiese T, Yao J, Burns JE, Summers RM. Detection of sclerotic bone metastases in the spine using watershed algorithm and graph cut. Proc SPIE. 2012;8315(6):36.
37. Wu J, Belle A, Hargraves RH, Cockrell C, Tang Y, Najarian K. Bone segmentation and 3D visualization of CT images for traumatic pelvic injuries. Int J Imaging Syst Technol. 2014;24(1):29–38.
38. Xu C, Prince JL. Generalized gradient vector flow external forces for active contours 1. Signal Process. 1998;71(2):131–9.

18

CT features of lung agenesis – a case series (6 cases)

Jamshid Sadiqi* and Hidayatullah Hamidi

Abstract

Back ground: Lung agenesis is a rare congenital anomaly. The main etiology of the disease is unknown whereas genetic, iatrogenic and viral factors as well as vitamin A deficiency during early pregnancy may result in developmental failure of primitive lung bud causing unilateral pulmonary agenesis. Affected patients usually present with variable respiratory symptoms and recurrent chest infection at any age. Plain film demonstrates opaque unilateral lung while chest CT scan can definitely diagnosis the disease. The anomaly has three types. Type I is pulmonary agenesis, type II is called pulmonary aplasia and type III is pulmonary hypoplasia.

Cases' presentation: Six patients with main complaint of dyspnea underwent contrast enhanced chest CT in radiology department of French Medical Institute for Mothers and children, Kabul and were diagnosed lung agenesis. Three patients were categorized as type II pulmonary agenesis (aplasia). Two patients, three months old boy and a seven year- old girl demonstrated right lung aplasia. Another patient boy of eighteen years old presented with left lung aplasia.

Two boys of four and seven months of age were classified as type I pulmonary agenesis (agenesis).

A boy of one year old was diagnosed pulmonary agenesis type III, right lung hypoplasia.

Conclusion: Six patients were diagnosed with pulmonary agenesis by Chest CT scan. The clinicians should consider possibility of congenital pulmonary agenesis in dyspneic patients with opaque unilateral hemithorax in plain film.

Keywords: Pulmonary agenesis- pulmonary aplasia- pulmonary hypoplasia

Background

Pulmonary agenesis is an extremely rare congenital entity which can occur unilateral or bilaterally. Almost all cases are unilateral since bilateral agenesis in not compatible with life [1]. Unilateral pulmonary agenesis for the first time was discovered by Depozze in a female autopsy in 1673 [2]. In 50% of cases, lung agenesia accompanies other congenital anomalies like cardiovascular [3], central nervous system [4] gastrointestinal, genitourinary system, skeletal system, Down syndrome and Klippel Feil syndrome [5]. The clinical features vary from asymptomatic to variable respiratory complaints such as dyspnea and respiratory distress with history of recurrent chest infections. The symptoms may occur as early as in neonatal period or later on during childhood and even adult life [1–5]. Physical examination of patients shows asymmetrical chest wall movements with absent or decrease respiratory sounds in unilateral hemithorax [5]. Chest x-ray demonstrates white-out hemithorax whereas further examinations like chest CT scan, bronchoscopy, bronchography and pulmonary angiography are needed for definitive diagnosis [6]. The treatment is often medical however surgical intervention may be required for some cases especially when other congenital anomalies coexist [7]. Here we present six patients from 1 month old to 18 years of age with different types of pulmonary agenesis.

Case presentation

Six patients whom underwent contrast enhanced chest CT scan in radiology department of French Medical Institute for Mothers and children in Kabul were diagnosed lung agenesis during 2015 to 2018.

According to Boyden classification; two patients had type I pulmonary agenesis (agenesia) which was confirmed by total absent of unilateral lung, main bronchus and its

* Correspondence: jamshidsadiqi79@gmail.com
Department of Radiology, French Medical Institute for Mothers & Children (FMIC), behind Kabul Medical University, Jamal mina, P.O. Box: 472, Kabul, Afghanistan

pulmonary vessels. Two boys of four months and seven months of age with respiratory distress and history of recurrent chest infection showed evidence of right lung agenesis with mediastinal shift and right side position of the heart in both patients (Fig. 1, 1b and Fig. 2).

Three patients had type II pulmonary agenesis (aplasia) which is characterized by complete absence of unilateral lung and its pulmonary vessels with a small rudimentary blind ended main bronchus. A boy of three months of age with respiratory distress demonstrated right side aplasia (Fig. 3 and Fig.3b). Another case of right lung aplasia with mediastinal shift was noted in a seven years old girl whom presented with dyspnea and chest infection (Fig. 4). Third patient was a young boy of eighteen years old with left lung aplasia and left sided heart with mild kyphoscoliotic changes along the thoracic spine (Fig. 5).

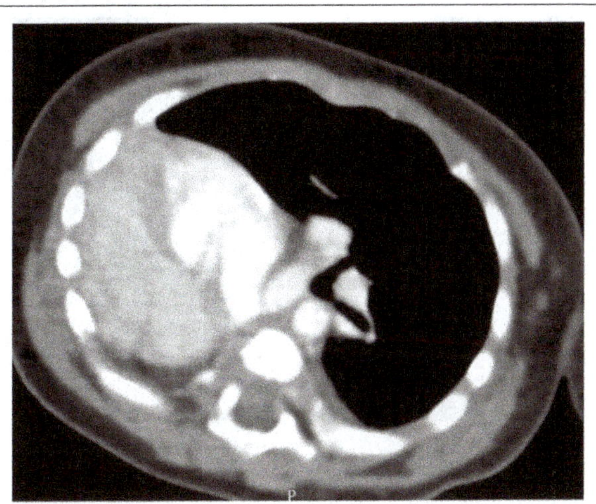

Fig. 2 Mediastinal window CT image in axial section shows complete absent of right lung, bronchus and vessels with malposition of the heart in the right hemithorax. (Seven months' boy)

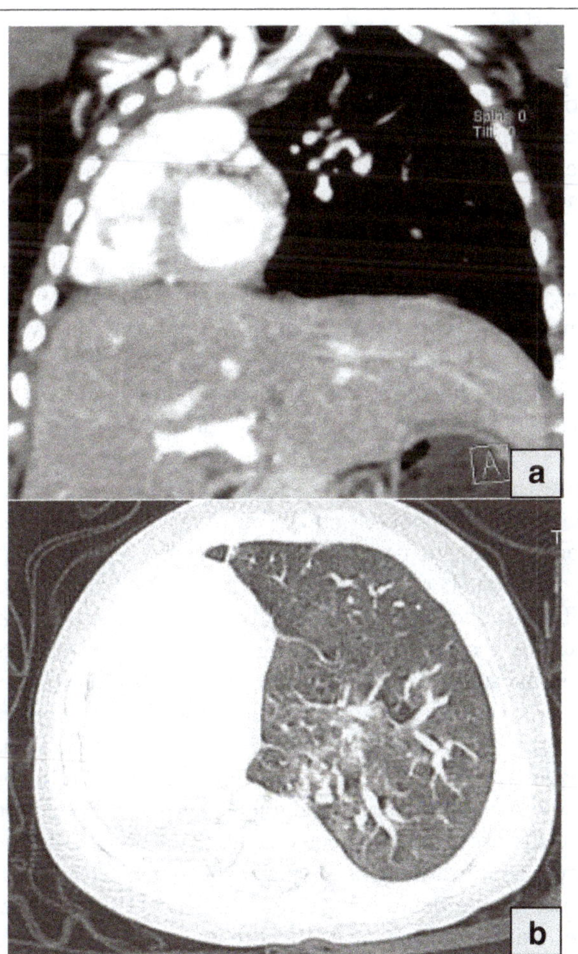

Fig. 1 a Coronal CT image in mediastinal window shows complete absent of right lung, bronchus and vessels with complete heart and mediastinal shift into the right hemithorax. Fig. 1:**b** CT axial image in lung window demonstrates absence of right lung parenchyma with its vasculature and location of heart and great vessels in the right side. (Four months' boy)

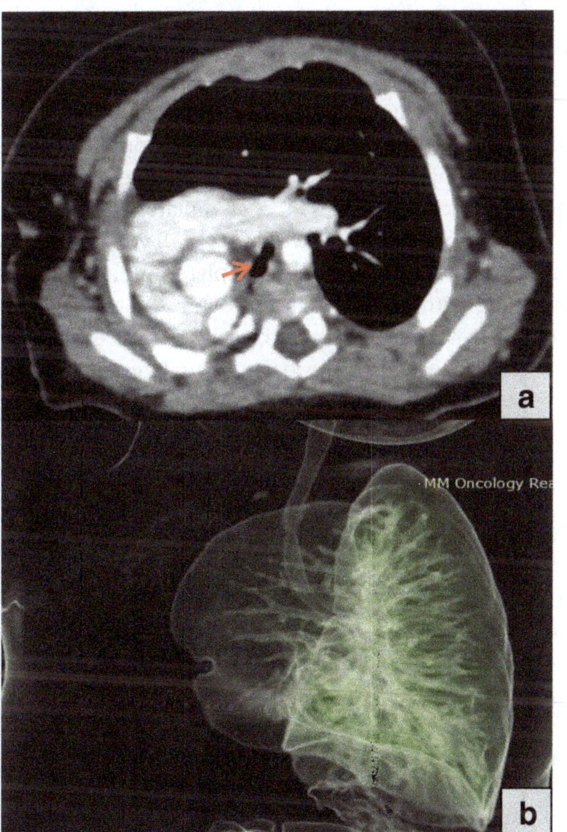

Fig. 3 a Axial CT image of three months old baby in mediastinal window shows absent right lung with rudimentary right main bronchus (red arrow) associated with right cardiac and great vessels position with extension of left lung towards the right side. Fig. 3:**b** Volume rendered image shows unilateral left lung with complete absent right lung and its bronchus in seven months baby

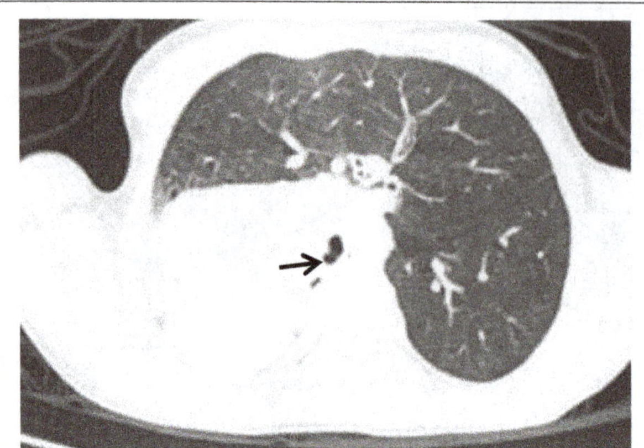

Fig. 4 Axial lung window CT images also demonstrating rudimentary right bronchus (black arrow) with absent right lung and herniation of left lung to the right side

Type III pulmonary agenesis (hypoplasia) was observed in a one year old boy with mild shortness of breath and opacity in the right upper lung zone. The chest CT images demonstrated partial right lung in the lower zone with displacement of heart in the right upper lung (Fig. 6).

Discussion and conclusion

For the first time pulmonary agenesis was classified by Schneider [8] which later on was modified by Boyden [9] into three groups according to development of their primitive lung bud. Type I which is called pulmonary agenesis is complete absence of unilateral lung parenchyma, its bronchus and vasculature. Type II is named pulmonary aplasia which is complete absence of unilateral lung with a rudimentary bronchus. Type III is pulmonary hypoplasia characterized by partial existence of branchial tree with some parts of unilateral pulmonary parenchyma and its vessels [2]. Although the main etiology of the disease is unknown, lack of vitamin A during pregnancy, viral agents, genetic as well as iatrogenic factors [10] have been mentioned as possible causes [2]. The lungs normally develop from foregut during the 4th and 5th weeks of gestation. The failure of bronchial analogue to divide equally between two lungs with possible abnormal blood flow in dorsal aortic arch during this period may result in hypoplasia, aplasia and agenesis of unilateral pulmonary parenchyma. In the meantime the contra lateral lung produces almost twice alveoli in compensation [11]. As during this period of time the migration of heart also occurs, therefore some cases may coexist with congenital heart anomalies [10]. Pulmonary hypoplasia may occur due to secondary reasons as well such as chest wall deformity, diaphragmatic hernia, cystic adenomatoid malformations, and pleural effusion. Bilateral pulmonary hypoplasia can also happen due to thoracic dystrophies and oligohydramnios [6]. For diagnosis of pulmonary agenesis different imaging techniques can be used. Plain chest shows unilateral opaque lung with mediastinal shift whereas for final diagnosis CT scan, MRI [12], bronchography, bronchoscopy and pulmonary angiography are used. Sometimes the disease can be detected in prenatal life by help of prenatal ultrasound showing hyperechoic hemithorax however the definitive diagnosis is hard [13] which can be confirmed by Fetal MRI [12]. According to the literature, left side agenesis is more common comparing to the right side with longer life expectancy. However in our cases just one patient had left lung agenesis while the other five cases had right side agenesis. Right lung agenesis happens with more incidences of cardiovascular abnormalities and patient may have more severe

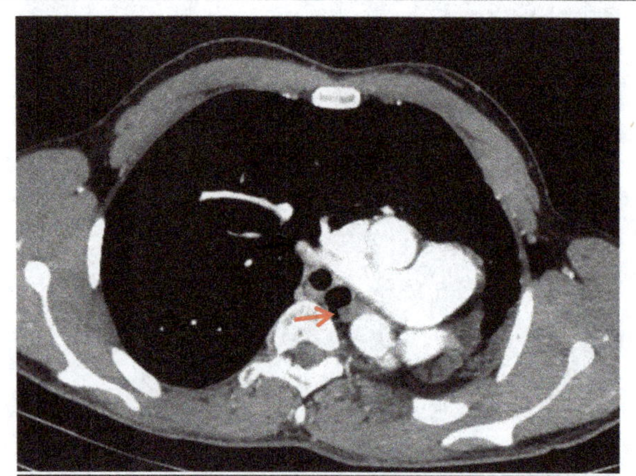

Fig. 5 Axial CT image of eighteen years old boy in mediastinal window shows absent left lung with rudimentary left bronchus (red arrow) with left posterior position of cardiac and great vessels and right lung significant extension towards the left hemithorax

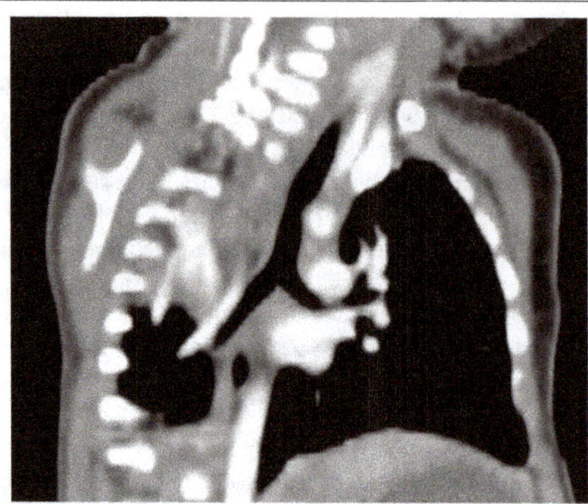

Fig. 6 Coronal CT image of one year old boy in mediastinal window shows partial absent right lung (upper and middle) with existence of right lower lobe with its bronchus. The heart locates in the right upper zone

symptoms due to pronounced carina malformation and cardiac and mediastinal shift [10]. Treatment strategies contain medical management and surgical repair. Medical treatments comprise control of recurrent chest infection, bronchodilators and controlling other complications. Surgery is usually needed in associated congenital anomalies. The prognosis usually depends to functionality of the unilateral existed lung and associated anomalies [2].

As this anomaly can occur at any age, the possibility of lung agenesis should be in differential diagnosis of patients having decrease to absent breath sounds with less or no movement of unilateral chest wall and opaque hemithorax in plain film. For confirmation, diagnostic imaging such as chest CT scan, MRI, bronchoscopy and chest angiography can be done. The early detection of the pulmonary agenesis is essential to reduce the development of fibrosis in patient's unilateral lung which can occur as result of recurrent chest infection. The surgical procedures should also be in consideration in presence of other congenital anomalies or complications.

Abbreviations
CT: Computed tomography; MRI: Magnetic resonance imaging

Acknowledgements
Not applicable.

Funding
No financial support was provided for this study.

Authors' contributions
JS did the literature review, prepared the images, drafted the manuscript and submitted the draft manuscript for the journal according to journal policy as well as being as corresponding author; HH edited the drafted manuscript and provided the images of the cases. Both authors read and approved the final manuscript.

Competing interest
It is stated that both authors have no conflict of interest.

Consent for publication
A written consent was obtained from parents of the patient's for publication of the report and any accompanying images. Since all 6 patients were children.

References

1. Biyyam DR, Chapman T, Ferguson MR, Deutsch G, Dighe MK. Congenital lung abnormalities: embryologic features, prenatal diagnosis, and postnatal radiologic-pathologic correlation. Radiographics. 2010;30(6):1721–38.
2. Kisku KH, Panigrahi MK, Sudhakar R. Agenesis of lung-a report of two cases. Lung India: official organ of Indian chest. Society. 2008;25(1):28.
3. Johnson RJ, Haworth SG. Pulmonary vascular and alveolar development in tetralogy of Fallot: a recommendation for early correction. Thorax. 1982; 37(12):893–901.
4. Cooney TP, Thurlbeck WM, Mathers J. Lung growth and development in anencephaly and hydranencephaly. Am Rev Respir Dis. 1985;132(3):596–601.
5. Cooney TP, Thurlbeck WM. Pulmonary hypoplasia in Down's syndrome. N Engl J Med. 1982;307(19):1170–3.
6. Pathania M, Lali BS, Rathaur VK. Unilateral pulmonary hypoplasia: a rare clinical presentation. BMJ case reports. 2013;2013:bcr2012008098.
7. Katsenos S, Antonogiannaki EM, Tsintiris K. Unilateral primary lung hypoplasia diagnosed in adulthood. Respir Care. 2014;59(4):e47–50.
8. Schneider P, Schawatbe E. E. Die Morphologie der Missbildungen Des Menschen Under Thiere. Jena: Gustav Fischar. 1912;3 Part.2:817–822.
9. Boyden E. Developmental anomalies. Am J Surg, 1955;89:79–88. [PubMed].
10. Agarwal A, Maria A, Yadav D, Bagri N. Pulmonary agenesis with Dextrocardia and hypertrophic cardiomyopathy: first case report. J Neonatal Biol. 2014; 3(141):2167–0897.
11. Yetim TD, Bayaroğullari H, Yalçin HP, Arıca V, Arıca SG. Congenital agenesis of the left lung: a rare case. J clin. imag scie. 2011:1.
12. Kuwashima S, Kaji Y. Fetal MR imaging diagnosis of pulmonary agenesis. Magn Reson Med Sci. 2010;9(3):149–52.
13. Dembinski J, Kroll M, Lewin M, Winkler P. Unilaterale pulmonale Agenesie. Aplasie und Dysplasie Zeitschrift für Geburtshilfe und Neonatologie. 2009; 213(02):56–61.

19

An alternative method for quantifying coronary artery calcification: the multi-ethnic study of atherosclerosis (MESA)

C Jason Liang[1], Matthew J Budoff[2], Joel D Kaufman[3], Richard A Kronmal[1] and Elizabeth R Brown[1,4*]

Abstract

Background: Extent of atherosclerosis measured by amount of coronary artery calcium (CAC) in computed tomography (CT) has been traditionally assessed using thresholded scoring methods, such as the Agatston score (AS). These thresholded scores have value in clinical prediction, but important information might exist below the threshold, which would have important advantages for understanding genetic, environmental, and other risk factors in atherosclerosis. We developed a semi-automated threshold-free scoring method, the spatially weighted calcium score (SWCS) for CAC in the Multi-Ethnic Study of Atherosclerosis (MESA).

Methods: Chest CT scans were obtained from 6814 participants in the Multi-Ethnic Study of Atherosclerosis (MESA). The SWCS and the AS were calculated for each of the scans. Cox proportional hazards models and linear regression models were used to evaluate the associations of the scores with CHD events and CHD risk factors. CHD risk factors were summarized using a linear predictor.

Results: Among all participants and participants with AS > 0, the SWCS and AS both showed similar strongly significant associations with CHD events (hazard ratios, 1.23 and 1.19 per doubling of SWCS and AS; 95% CI, 1.16 to 1.30 and 1.14 to 1.26) and CHD risk factors (slopes, 0.178 and 0.164; 95% CI, 0.162 to 0.195 and 0.149 to 0.179). Even among participants with AS = 0, an increase in the SWCS was still significantly associated with established CHD risk factors (slope, 0.181; 95% CI, 0.138 to 0.224). The SWCS appeared to be predictive of CHD events even in participants with AS = 0, though those events were rare as expected.

Conclusions: The SWCS provides a valid, continuous measure of CAC suitable for quantifying the extent of atherosclerosis without a threshold, which will be useful for examining novel genetic and environmental risk factors for atherosclerosis.

Background

Coronary artery calcium (CAC) as detected by computed tomography (CT) is a known marker of subclinical atherosclerosis [1,2] and is a powerful predictor of the risk of coronary events [3-16]. Most commonly, the Agatston, mass, and volume scores have been used to quantify the amount of CAC [17-20].

The Multi-Ethnic Study of Atherosclerosis (MESA), a prospective study with 6814 participants free of cardiovascular disease (CVD) at baseline, was designed to include CT scanning at 4 time points (with two scans per individual at each time point). The CVD exclusion was for those with known clinical disease, and based on self-reported information. The CT reading protocol used a conservative algorithm for lesion detection with high specificity for detection of lesions at the sacrifice of sensitivity. Any voxels not meeting the lesion definition in the algorithm were not used in calculating CAC scores. As such, participants early in the disease progression stages with small calcifications that showed up on the CT scan as less than four contiguous voxels or 130 Hounsfield units (HU) may have been classified as having an undetectable level of CAC. Roughly 50% of the participants in the MESA cohort received a zero CAC score while almost certainly

* Correspondence: elizab@uw.edu
[1]Department of Biostatistics, University of Washington, Seattle, WA, USA
[4]Vaccine and Infectious Disease and Public Health Sciences Divisions, Fred Hutchinson Cancer Research Center, Seattle, WA, USA
Full list of author information is available at the end of the article

many of these have quantifiable, though less substantial, calcified atherosclerotic lesions. This classification as "zero" has a small impact on our ability to identify individuals at high risk of a coronary event since the high threshold is still adequately sensitive for risk prediction; however, having excess zeros due to misclassification adversely impacts our ability to use CAC measures for modeling and understanding subclinical disease extent and progression.

An ancillary study in MESA focused on ambient air pollution exposures in cohort members is studying the effect of pollutant concentrations on progression of atherosclerosis over 10 years of follow-up [21]. While the relationship between air pollution exposure and CAC is a wholly different question not pursued in this study, it was a motivating factor in developing a valid scoring method to quantify CAC extent throughout the range of detected calcium. More specifically, there are multiple reasons to explore new approaches to quantifying CAC in the MESA. First, current scoring techniques ignore much of the information available in the CT scan that may prove useful in identifying calcified lesions. Second, many of the participants with an Agatston Score (AS) of zero may have had CAC present that did not meet the definition for CAC on the image. Therefore, current CAC measures can fall short as measures of subclinical disease burden while very successfully serving as surrogates for risk of clinical events. Third, the high proportion of zero scores complicates analysis of CAC data. We thus propose an alternative score, the spatially weighted calcium score (SWCS), that uses spatial information in the image combined with voxel-specific weights derived from the phantom, thereby making use of more of the information in the CT scans and also providing a continuous measure of CAC.

Methods

Data collection

The MESA was established to study the prevalence, progression, and risks of subclinical cardiovascular disease. Details of the study design have been previously published [22]. A cohort of 6814 men and women, aged 45–84, without known clinical cardiovascular disease was recruited between July 2000 and September 2002 from six urban communities (Baltimore City and Baltimore County, Maryland; Chicago, Illinois; Forsyth County, North Carolina; Los Angeles County, California; New York, New York; and St. Paul, Minnesota). Each of the six centers recruited a population-based sample while oversampling blacks, Chinese, and Hispanics based on self-reported ethnicity at time of enrollment. Institutional review boards at each site approved the study, and all participants gave written informed consent. Further documentation regarding data collection and protocols can be found at www.mesa-nhlbi.org [23].

Risk factors

Information about risk factors and demographics was obtained at enrollment and during the baseline examination. Participants were given questionnaires to obtain information about tobacco usage, passive smoke exposure, alcohol use, medical conditions, medical care access, family history of CVD, reproductive history, and medication use and history. Physical activity was measured using a questionnaire from the Cross-Cultural Activity Participation Study; diet was measured using a modified version of the Insulin Resistance Atheroslecrosis study instrument; anger and anxiety were measured using questionnaires administered on the Spielberger trait anger and anxiety scales; depression was measured on the Center for Epidemiologic Studies Depression scale. Height, weight, and waist and hip circumferences were measured. Blood pressure was measured three times using an automated oscillometric sphygmomanometer (Dinamap Pro 1000; Critikon, Tampa, Florida). Blood samples were taken after a 12-hour fast, and were analyzed by a central laboratory at the University of Vermont for many different measurements including total cholesterol, lipids and lipoproteins (including HDL and LDL), insulin resistance, plasma glucose, triglycerides, high-sensitivity C-reactive protein, and creatinine measurements. Diabetes was defined as use of insulin or oral hypoglycemic agents, or fasting glucose of 126 mg/dL or greater. Body-mass index was defined as weight in kilograms divided by the square of height in meters. Documentation further detailing the questionnaire and measurement protocols can be found at www.mesa-nhlbi.org [23] and Bild et al. [22].

Cardiovascular events (follow-up)

We followed all participants for cardiovascular events for an average of 6.0 years. Interviewers called each participant at intervals of 9–12 months to obtain information about new CVD conditions, CVD interventions, hospitalizations, treatments, changes in life habits, and death. Detailed descriptions of MESA events definitions and follow-up procedure have been previously published [11,15]. For our analyses, we separately considered any CHD (definite or probable myocardial infarction, definite CHD death, or definite or probable angina) and hard CHD (definite or probable myocardial infarction or definite CHD death) events. We note that probable angina cases were only classified as a CHD event if accompanied with a revascularization procedure.

CT scanning

A detailed report of the CT scanning and reading protocol has been previously reported [24]. At the baseline examination, each participant was given two consecutive unenhanced chest CT scans. The Chicago, Los Angeles, and New York sites used electron-beam CT systems (Imatron C150; GE Medical Systems, Milwaukee, Wisconsin), which scan at a slice thickness of 3.0 mm. The Baltimore, Forsyth County, and St. Paul sites used multi-detector CT systems (Lightspeed QXi, Lightspeed Plus; GE Medical Systems, Milwaukee, Wisconsin; Volume Zoom; Siemens, Erlangen, Germany), which scan at a slice thickness of 2.5 mm. To allow for calibration to compensate for inter-scan variability, radiographic phantoms with known densities of calcium hydroxyapatite (0, 50, 100, and 200 mg/mL) were placed beneath the thorax of each participant for each scan. Participants over 100 kg and at sites using multi-detector CT systems were scanned using slightly different settings.

CT scan reading

Each scan was read by one of two physician readers at the CT reading center (Los Angeles Biomedical Research Institute at Harbor-UCLA, Torrance, California). As each participant received two consecutive scans, the scans were randomized to lessen the possibility of analysts consecutively reading scans from the same participant. Reading was done using an interactive system to identify the phantoms, determine the artery trajectories and classify candidate calcified plaques. For all techniques presented in this paper, the search for calcified lesions was restricted to be within an 8 mm radius of the trajectories defined by the readers. Further details can be found in previously published reports [24].

Calculation of the Agatston score

After arterial trajectories were determined and a phantom-based adjustment was applied, candidate calcified plaques were identified by the software with the criteria that each plaque be composed of at least 4 contiguous voxels with an attenuation level of 130HU or greater. The analysts then reviewed each candidate plaque and accepted or rejected its classification as calcified plaque.

To calculate the AS, each accepted lesion was assigned a score by multiplying the lesion volume by a coefficient based on its maximum HU (coefficient of 1 if maximum = 130–199, 2 if 200–299, 3 if 300–399, 4 if > = 400). The AS is the sum of the scores across all accepted lesions. As each participant received two scans, for purposes of this study the average of the two Agatston scores are used for each participant. Use of the average of two scans is intended to reduce noise and to be consistent with methods from other MESA papers using the AS [11,15]. Further details on the Agatston score can be found in previously published reports [17,24]. Participants were notified of their scores on the scale of no coronary calcification, less than average, average, and greater than average.

Calculation of the spatially weighted calcium score

In developing the SWCS, an important property was for the SWCS to quantify CAC in a manner comparable to the AS for those with AS > 0, while providing meaningful non-zero scores for those with AS = 0. Calculation of the SWCS started with the set of voxels identified by the reader as representing the coronary arteries. First, we assigned a weight to each voxel using a weighting function with parameters derived from the scan's phantom. The goal of the first step was to calibrate and weight each voxel according to the phantom so that scores across the images were comparable. Second, each voxel was then assigned a score depending on the weight assigned to it and its neighbors. The goal of the second step was to use the surrounding information of each voxel to obtain a more accurate value, and to reduce the impact of noise by upweighting those voxels with neighboring voxels that had high attenuation levels and downweighting those whose neighbors had low attenuation levels. The detailed algorithm appears in the Additional file 1: Appendix with illustrations of the weighting scheme.

Statistical analysis

Distributions of participant characteristics were described using means and standard deviations. Comparisons of these characteristics across groups were made using the *t*-test. Distributions of the CAC scores were described graphically using kernel density estimators and scatter-plots with loess smoothers.

We used Cox proportional hazards regression models similar to those used by Detrano et al. [11] to estimate hazard ratios for hard CHD and any CHD events as they relate to the SWCS and AS in all participants and the subset with AS > 0. The models were all adjusted for race, age, sex, smoking, diabetes, cholesterol, blood pressure, lipid-lowering medication use, and antihypertensive medication use. The AS and SWCS were transformed by taking the base-2 logarithm after adding 1 to the score ($\log_2$[score + 1]).

Kaplan-Meier survival curves for all CHD events were estimated and plotted for both the SWCS and the AS. The AS K-M curves were stratified into the following percentiles: 0-50%, 50–62.5%, 62.5-75%, 75–87.5%, and 87.5-100%. The SWCS K-M curves were stratified similarly, but with additional 0-25% and 25-50% stratifications to further evaluate any additional ordering the SWCS may provide for participants with levels of CAC that are undetectable by the AS.

To summarize the association between the CAC scores and traditionally recognized CHD risk factors, we first summarized the risk factors in a linear predictor (LP) based on MESA data. The LP for each participant was the sum of their covariate values multiplied by the fitted coefficients from a Cox proportional hazards model. The Cox proportional hazards model was fitted using all CHD events as the outcome and baseline age, systolic blood pressure, diastolic blood pressure, total cholesterol, HDL, diabetes, smoking, and sex as covariates. The covariates were chosen based on the Framingham risk variables [25,26]. We used linear regression models to estimate the relationship of the LP with the SWCS and AS in all participants and the subset with AS > 0. The models were all adjusted for weight, height, and site to accommodate different scanners across sites and different settings used for participants over 100 kg scanned using multi-detector CT scanners. The SWCS and AS were transformed by taking the natural logarithm after adding 1 to the score (log[score + 1]).

We used methods similar to those used by Callister et al. [19] to assess the reproducibility of the scores. We calculated the absolute difference between the scores of each scan relative to their mean: $|x_1 - x_2|/[(x_1 + x_2)/2] \times 100$ where x_1 is the score from the first scan and x_2 is the score from the second scan. This was used as the primary measure of reproducibility and referred to as the percent difference for both the SWCS and AS. We also used the intraclass correlation coefficients to assess the reproducibility of the SWCS and the AS. Analyses were all done in R version 2.11.1 [27].

Results

Demographics

We compared demographics and risk factors between those with AS = 0 and AS > 0 (Table 1). The two groups were significantly different with respect to age, sex, hypertension, and treated diabetes, but not for status as a current smoker. We also bifurcated those with AS = 0 into those above and below the median based on their SWCS, comparing demographics and risk factors between these two subgroups. The two subgroups were significantly different with respect to sex, hypertension, treated diabetes, and Framingham 10-year risk, but not for age and current smoking status. As expected, the SWCS of participants with AS = 0 tend to be lower than those with AS > 0, with medians of 0.78 (range, 0.00-284.48) versus 58.99 (range, 0.22-4262.70), respectively. We note that while some participants had very small SWCS, all participants had positive SWCS. A visual representation of the relationship of the AS and SWCS among participants with AS > 0 is shown in the Figure 1. As suggested by the scatterplot, there is a high correlation of 0.99 and the linear relationship can be summarized by the equation $y = 0.52 + 0.67x$.

CT image data was available in 6568 of the 6814 participants. Of these, 6253 (91.8%) had image data available for both CT scans and 315 (4.6%) for one scan. The distribution of the SWCS was quite skewed; thus we present the smoothed density of the SWCS plus a constant of 1, on the natural log scale in Figure 2. For the 6568 participants who received at least one scan, we show the smoothed density for all participants, participants with AS > 0, and participants with AS = 0.

Association of SWCS with CHD events

There were 6508 participants with available measures of all the variables used for the events analysis. The average follow-up time was 6.0 years, during which 291 participants experienced a CHD event of which 171 were hard CHD events. Among those with AS = 0, 34 participants experienced a CHD event, of which 22 were hard CHD events.

An increase in the SWCS was associated with an increase in risk of CHD events (Table 2). A statistically significant relationship was observed when the model was applied to all participants, and when restricted to participants with AS > 0. Furthermore, the relationships were similar to those seen when the SWCS was replaced by the AS in the same models.

A twofold increase in the SWCS or the AS was associated with a 23% (95% CI, 16 to 30) or 19% (95% CI, 14 to 26) increase in risk of hard CHD events, respectively.

Table 1 Demographics and risk factors

	AS = 0 (n = 3299)				AS > 0 (n = 3269)
Characteristic	SWCS 0–0.78 <50%tile (n = 1649)	SWCS 0.78-284.48 >50%tile (n = 1650)	P*	All	SWCS 0.22-4262.70
Age (year)	57.88	58.06	0.56	57.97	66.40
Male Sex (%)	30.38% (501)	42.73% (705)	<0.001	36.56% (1206)	57.63% (1884)
Hypertension (%)	30.38% (501)	40.24% (664)	<0.001	35.31% (1165)	54.70% (1788)
Treated Diabetes (%)	4.44% (73)	10.23% (168)	<0.001	7.33% (241)	12.83% (418)
Current Smoker (%)	14.20% (233)	12.78% (210)	0.25	13.49% (443)	12.84% (419)
Framingham 10-yr Risk (Mean [SD])	0.080 (0.062)	0.102 (0.073)	<0.001	0.083 (0.063)	0.137 (0.094)

P-value is for difference between SWCS <50th percentile and SWCS >50th percentile. Calculated using *t*-test for age, and chi-squared tests for other characteristics. Framingham 10-yr Risk calculated using Circulation 1998 method.

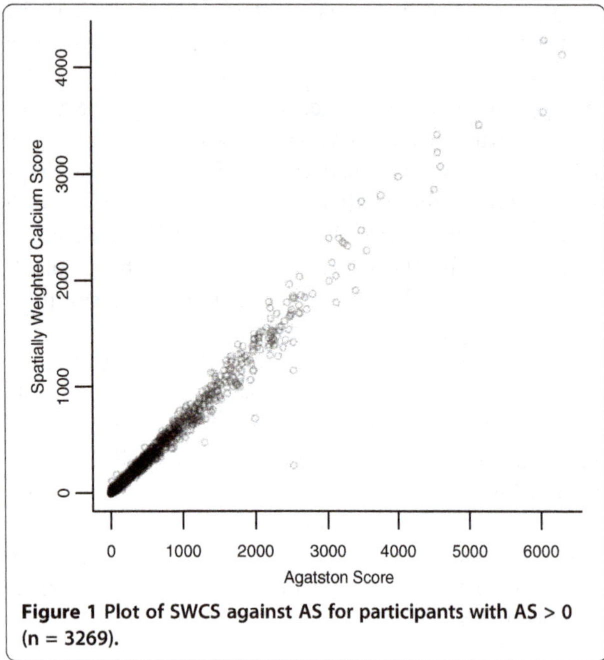

Figure 1 Plot of SWCS against AS for participants with AS > 0 (n = 3269).

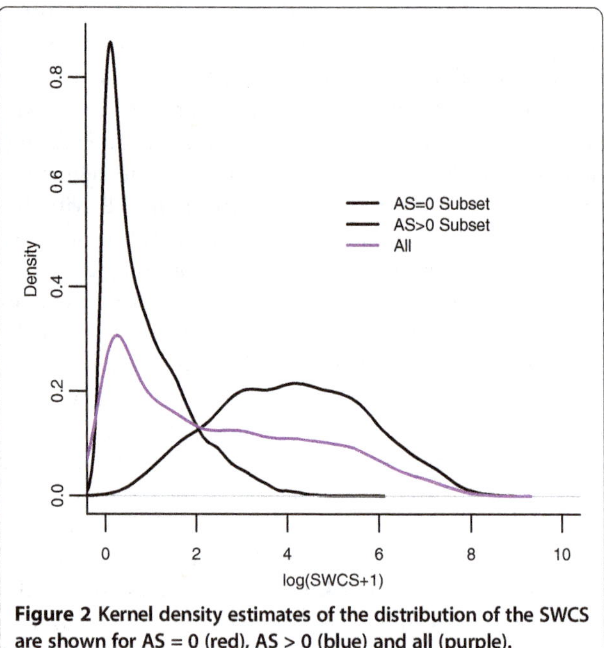

Figure 2 Kernel density estimates of the distribution of the SWCS are shown for AS = 0 (red), AS > 0 (blue) and all (purple).

Furthermore, among participants with AS > 0, a twofold increase in the SWCS or AS was associated with an 18% (95% CI, 9 to 27) or 16% (95% CI, 8 to 25) increase in risk of hard CHD events, respectively.

When we restricted the model to only participants with AS = 0, a twofold increase in the SWCS was associated with a hazard ratio of 1.11 (95% CI, 0.79 to 1.51) for hard CHD events.

The cumulative event rate and number of all CHD events among participants grouped by different percentile stratifications of the scores is shown in Figure 3. An ideal risk score would have Kaplan-Meier curves that are well separated and ordered across the quantile-based strata. For the 75–87.5 and 87.5-100 percentile stratifications, the SWCS and AS appear to do equally well at differentiating the quantiles in terms of event risk. The 50–62.5 and 62.5-75 percentile stratifications of the SWCS separate appropriately over time, while those of the AS appear in the incorrect order throughout most of follow-up. That is, that the higher quantile group has lower risk. Finally, the 0–25 and 25–50 percentile stratifications of the SWCS appear to demonstrate some separation, suggesting the SWCS provides a degree of meaningful ordering of CAC in terms of risk in the lower quantiles as well.

Association of SWCS with CHD risk factors

Among the 6510 participants with complete data for the risk factors, an increase in the SWCS was associated with an increase in the LP (Table 3). For all participants, on the log(CAC + 1) scale, each unit increase in the SWCS and AS was associated with an increase in the mean of the LP of 0.23 (95% CI, 0.22 to 0.24) and 0.18 (95% CI, 0.17 to 0.19), respectively. For participants with AS > 0, on the log(CAC + 1) scale, each unit increase in the SWCS and AS was associated with an increase in the mean of the LP of 0.18 (95% CI, 0.16 to 0.20) and 0.16 (95% CI, 0.15 to 0.18),

Table 2 Hazard ratios for hard and all CHD events for twofold increase in AS and SWCSs

		Hard Coronary Event		Any Coronary Event	
Participants	CAC	No. Events/No. At Risk	Hazard Ratio (95% CI)	No. Events/No. At Risk	Hazard Ratio (95% CI)
All	Log_2(AS + 1)	171/6508	1.19 (1.14-1.26)	291/6508	1.25 (1.20-1.30)
	Log_2(SWCS + 1)		1.23 (1.16-1.30)		1.28 (1.22-1.35)
AS > 0	Log_2(AS + 1)	149/3243	1.16 (1.08-1.25)	257/3243	1.24 (1.17-1.31)
	Log_2(SWCS + 1)		1.18 (1.09-1.27)		1.25 (1.18-1.33)
AS = 0	Log_2(SWCS + 1)	22/3265	1.11 (0.79-1.55)	34/3265	1.04 (0.79-1.38)

Each unit increase in Log_2(Score+1) represents doubling of CAC. All regressions adjusted for race, age, sex, smoking, diabetes, cholesterol, blood pressure, lipid-lowering medication use, and antihypertensive medication use.

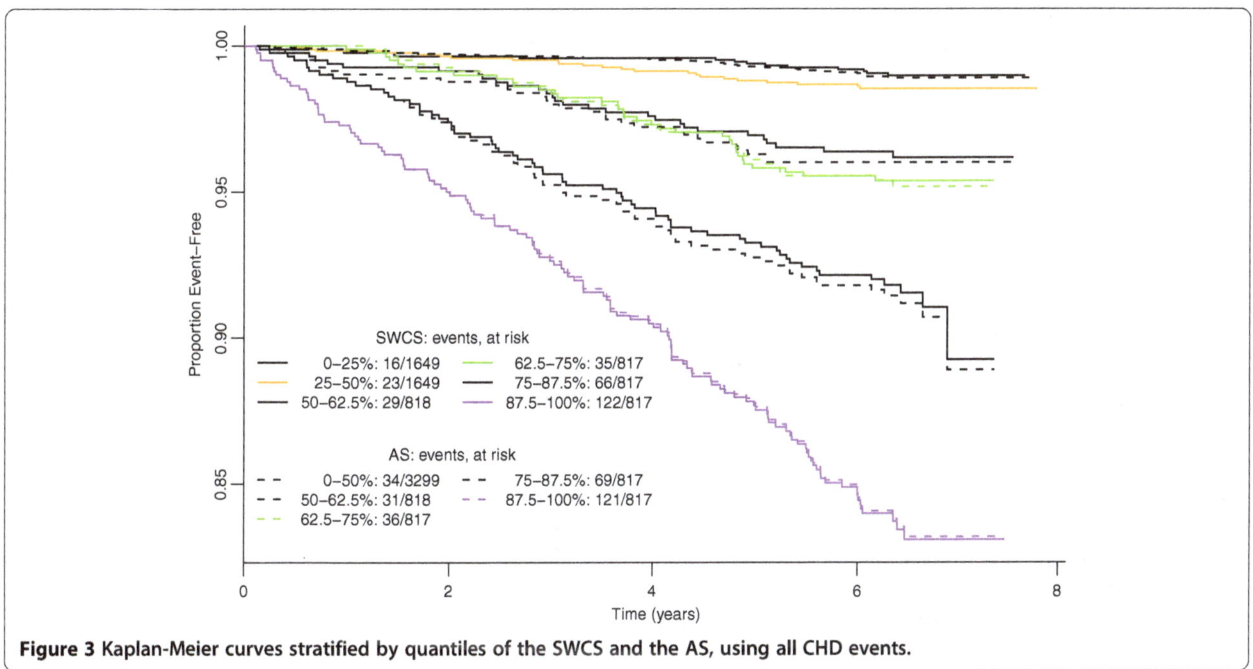

Figure 3 Kaplan-Meier curves stratified by quantiles of the SWCS and the AS, using all CHD events.

respectively. For participants with AS = 0, each unit increase in the log of the SWCS plus one was associated with an increase in the mean of the LP of 0.18 (95% CI, 0.14 to 0.22).

For all participants, and participants with AS > 0, the R^2 values for the SWCS and AS are comparable. For participants with AS = 0, the R^2 value is 0.12. A scatterplot of the LP against the log(SWCS + 1) for all participants is shown in Figure 4. The dot colors represent participants with AS = 0 or AS > 0. Smoothed curves through the points for all participants, and the subsets of participants with AS = 0 and participants with AS > 0 are also shown in different colors. The vertical lines at the bottom and top of the plot are visual aids indicating the distributions of log(SWCS + 1) for participants with AS = 0 or AS > 0.

Reproducibility

After excluding scans judged by the scan readers to have unacceptable levels of noise, there were 3102 participants who had at least one scan with AS > 0. The median percent difference across participants was 16.87% and 18.29% for the SWCS and AS, respectively (Table 4). The median of the percent difference in AS minus the percent difference in SWCS was 2.02% (95% CI, 1.66 to 2.40; P < 0.001).

When we performed the same analysis on the subset of 2849 participants with AS > 0 for both scans, the SWCS still showed better reproducibility compared to the AS.

Table 3 Results of linear regression of linear predictor on SWCS and AS

Participants	CAC	Slope	95% CI	P	R^2
All	Log(AS + 1)	0.182	(0.174-0.190)	<0.001	0.32
	Log(SWCS + 1)	0.226	(0.216-0.235)	<0.001	0.32
AS > 0	Log(AS + 1)	0.164	(0.149-0.179)	<0.001	0.19
	Log(SWCS + 1)	0.178	(0.162-0.195)	<0.001	0.19
AS = 0	Log(SWCS + 1)	0.181	(0.138-0.224)	<0.001	0.12

All regressions adjusted for site, weight, and height.

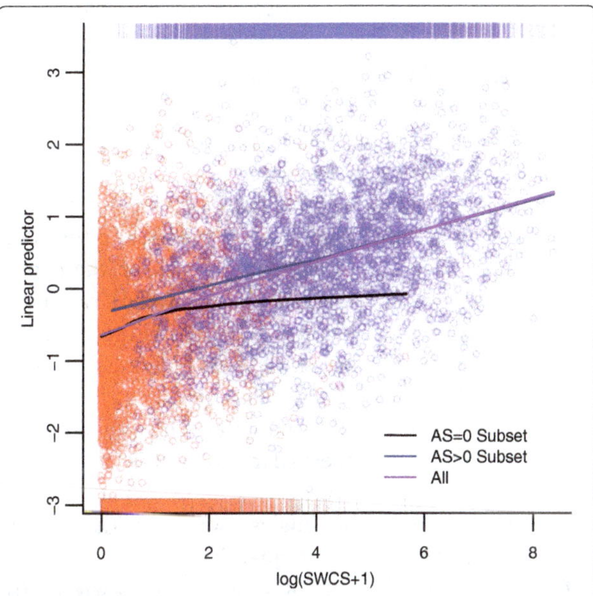

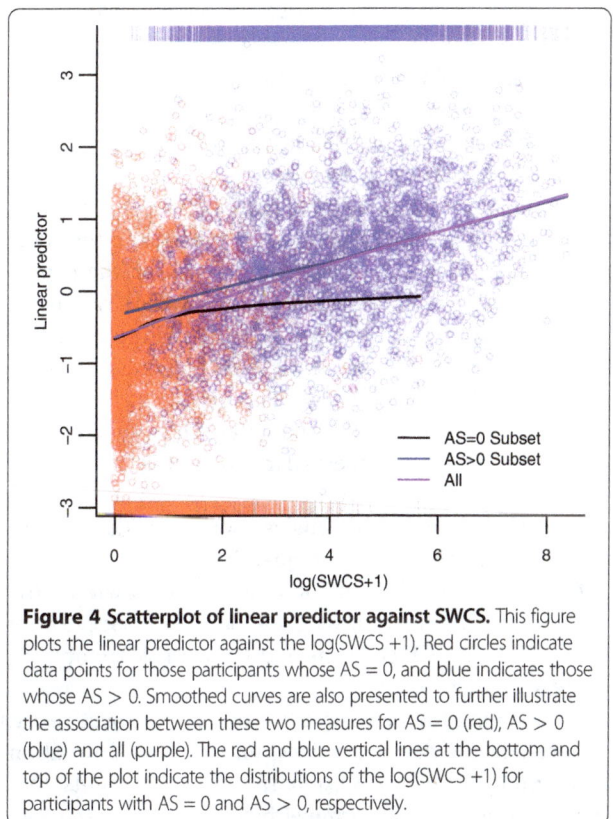

Figure 4 Scatterplot of linear predictor against SWCS. This figure plots the linear predictor against the log(SWCS +1). Red circles indicate data points for those participants whose AS = 0, and blue indicates those whose AS > 0. Smoothed curves are also presented to further illustrate the association between these two measures for AS = 0 (red), AS > 0 (blue) and all (purple). The red and blue vertical lines at the bottom and top of the plot indicate the distributions of the log(SWCS +1) for participants with AS = 0 and AS > 0, respectively.

Table 4 Reproducibility of SWCS and AS

	Participants with AS > 0 for at least one scan (n = 3102)		Participants with AS > 0 for both scans (n = 2849)	
Variable	Median	Mean	Median	Mean
% Change in SWCS	16.87	31.23	15.30	24.71
% Change in AS	18.29	41.52	16.26	27.38
% Change in AS minus % Change in SWCS	2.02 (1.66-2.40)*	10.31 (9.05, 11.56)*	1.05 (0.74-1.51)*	2.68 (1.99-3.36)*

*P<0.001. P-values based on paired *t*-test for mean and Wilcoxon test for median.

We also performed the same analysis further restricted to participants with AS < 50 (n = 892) for both scans and AS < 100 (n = 1307) for both scans. Among these subsets of participants with low but non-zero AS, SWCS still showed better reproducibility.

For the participants for whom we had CT image data for both scans (n = 6253), the intraclass correlation coefficients for the SWCS and AS were 0.988 and 0.989, respectively. For those with AS > 0 for both scans (n = 2849), the intraclass correlation coefficients for the SWCS and AS were both 0.986. For those with AS = 0 for both scans (n = 3151), the intraclass correlation coefficient for the SWCS was 0.406.

Discussion

In this paper, we present a method for quantifying coronary artery calcification as measured by CT that is independent of a threshold and instead calibrated to the phantom where the attenuation levels represent known densities. We adjust for noise in an automated way using spatial information in the image. The SWCS is shown to be highly related to both risk of CHD events and traditional CHD risk factors. In fact, it retains its strong relationship to traditional risk factors even when the AS equals zero.

Historically, interest in CAC has largely focused on its ability as a predictor of clinical CHD events, and the AS is an effective method of quantifying CAC for these purposes. However, our approach is motivated by studies where the primary interest in CAC is its ability to measure atherosclerotic burden across all levels of disease. In these cases, the AS is less suitable. Specifically, a continuous score for CAC would be more tractable in situations where the extent of atherosclerosis itself is of primary interest.

The primary goal of our analysis was to validate the effectiveness of the SWCS at quantifying CAC. Unfortunately, the "true" burden of CAC is unknown in the MESA patients. Instead, we examined the association of the SWCS with CHD events and known risk factors (via a linear predictor).

In validating the new score, we had three objectives: 1. Ensure that the new score does not lose any information about subclinical disease and risk of CHD events that the AS provides. 2. Determine that a positive score given to participants with AS = 0 is not merely noise, but rather measures lower levels of true subclinical disease. 3. Determine that the new score is at least as reproducible as the AS. We next address how we assessed these three points.

For Point 1, we compared the relationship of the AS and events to that of the SWCS and events. We observed statistically significant and strong relationships between the SWCS and CHD events and risk factors. For the subset of participants with AS > 0, the relationships between the LP and risk of events and CAC scores was similar for both CAC scores, suggesting that the SWCS is replicating the information in the AS in those participants with AS > 0. Furthermore, a simple visual examination of the plot (Figure 1) of each non-zero AS against its corresponding SWCS suggests very strong correlation between the two scores. For all participants, and participants with AS > 0, the R^2 values for the SWCS and AS are comparable. We emphasize that since the goal of our analysis is validation of the SWCS, the focus should be on R^2 as a descriptive statistic comparing the SWCS and AS rather than as a measure of predictive accuracy. Nonetheless, the relatively low R^2 values make sense, as the linear regression model only includes CAC, site, weight, and height. In particular, when we consider that CAC has been demonstrated to provide additional predictive information in addition to the traditional cardiovascular risk factors [8,10,15,16,28,29] (which were used to construct the linear predictor), it is unsurprising that the R^2 values are not high.

Examining these relationships in participants with AS = 0 addresses Point 2. For all CHD events, a doubling of SWCS was associated with a hazard ratio of 1.11 (95% CI, 0.79 to 1.55). For CHD risk, we observed a significant association between the SWCS and the LP; each unit increase in the log(SWCS + 1) was associated with an increase in the mean LP of 0.18 (95% CI, 0.14 to 0.22). The Kaplan-Meier curves for the first two quartiles of the SWCS show a distinct separation. Furthermore, the 50–62.5 and 62.5-75.0 percentile curves for the SWCS appear to be better separated than those of the AS. This suggests that the SWCS algorithm was in fact detecting additional useful information, and that the continuous scale represents a meaningful ordering of CAC suitable for measuring atherosclerotic burden and the attendant risk of CHD events.

To address Point 3, we assessed the reproducibility of the SWCS in comparison with the AS. Using the percent difference as a measure of reproducibility, we found that the median percent difference was 16.87% and 18.29% for the SWCS and AS, respectively. The intraclass correlations were 0.988 and 0.989 for the SWCS and AS, respectively. Our results suggest that the SWCS is at least as reproducible as the Agatston score.

There are two main limitations for the SWCS. One limitation was the lack of a true gold standard for validating the SWCS. The MESA study is composed of a large population of asymptomatic individuals and thus cardiac catheterization (with either angiography or intravascular ultrasound) was not a practical validation method, as it is restricted to studies of symptomatic populations or in treatment trials [18,30-32]. Of course, histologic validation [1,2] was not an option either. We instead used prediction of events and risk of events as a surrogate for a true gold standard, which in itself was limited by the small number of events in those participants with AS = 0. Furthermore, the emergence of models combining CAC measures with traditional risk summaries such as the Framingham risk [28,29] suggests potential for using alternative, potentially richer models for validation. Regardless of the validation used, it would be useful to perform further validation using an independent but comparable dataset. In particular, separate in vitro experimental studies to validate SWCS would be highly desirable. Another limitation involves the applicability of the results outside of the MESA. The SWCS was designed to be a cost-effective approach to rescoring the MESA CT images in a less conservative manner than the original approach to reduce the number of false negatives (when the CAC score is zero but subclinical disease is in fact present). To use the approach presented here in other large studies where comparable calibration phantoms were not scanned or tracing the coronary arteries was not done is not possible.

Conclusions

In conclusion, we have developed a new continuous method of quantifying coronary artery calcium that may provide a continuous and improved measure of atherosclerosis compared to existing coronary artery calcium scoring methods. This new method is anticipated to be advantageous in research applications, especially in the evaluation of genetic and environmental risk factors.

Competing interests

The authors declare that they have no competing interests.

Acknowledgements

We thank the other investigators, the staff, and the participants of the MESA study for their valuable contributions. A full list of participating MESA investigators and institutions can be found at http://www.mesa-nhlbi.org [23]. Although the research described in this presentation has been funded wholly or in part by the United States Environmental Protection Agency through RD831697 to the University of Washington, it has not been subjected to the Agency's required peer and policy review and therefore does not necessarily reflect the views of the Agency and no official endorsement should be inferred. C. Jason Liang receives support from the Biostatistics, Epidemiologic & Bioinformatic Training in Environmental Health Training Grant (ES015459). This research was supported by contracts N01-HC-95159 through N01-HC-95169 from the National Heart, Lung, and Blood Institute.

Author details

[1]Department of Biostatistics, University of Washington, Seattle, WA, USA. [2]Division of Cardiology, Los Angeles Biomedical Research Institute at Harbor-UCLA Medical Center, Torrance, CA, USA. [3]Environmental & Occupational Health Sciences, Medicine, and Epidemiology, University of Washington, Seattle, WA, USA. [4]Vaccine and Infectious Disease and Public Health Sciences Divisions, Fred Hutchinson Cancer Research Center, Seattle, WA, USA.

Authors' contributions

CJL performed the statistical analysis and drafted the manuscript. MJB provided clinical expertise and contributed to the design of the reproducibility analysis. JDK provided epidemiological expertise and contributed to the overall design and coordination of the study. RAK provided input on the technical development of the score and helped with the design of the validation analysis. ERB conceived the study, led its overall design and coordination, and helped to draft the manuscript. All authors read and approved the final manuscript.

References

1. Mautner GC, Mautner SL, Froehlich J, Feuerstein IM, Proschan MA, Roberts WC, Doppman JL: **Coronary Artery Calcification: Assessment with Electron Beam CT and Histomorphometric Correlation.** *Radiology* 1994, **192**:619–623.
2. Rumberger JA, Simons DB, Fitzpatrick LA, Sheedy PF, Schwartz RS: **Coronary Artery Calcium Area by Electron-Beam Computed Tomography and Coronary Atherosclerotic Plaque Area: A Histopathologic Correlative Study.** *Circulation* 1995, **92**:2157–2162.
3. Budoff MJ, Achenbach S, Blumenthal RS, Carr JJ, Goldin JG, Greenland P, Guerci AD, Lima JAC, Rader DJ, Rubin GD, Shaw LJ, Wiegers SE: **Assessment of Coronary Artery Disease by Cardiac Computed Tomography A Scientific Statement From the American Heart Association Committee on Cardiovascular Imaging and Intervention, Council on Cardiovascular Radiology and Intervention, and Committee on Cardiac Imaging, Council on Clinical Cardiology.** *Circulation* 2006, **114**:1761–1791.
4. Greenland P, Bonow RO, Brundage BH, Budoff MJ, Eisenberg MJ, Grundy SM, Lauer MS, Post WS, Raggi P, Redberg RF, Rodgers GP, Shaw LJ, Taylor AJ, Weintraub WS: **ACCF/AHA 2007 clinical expert consensus document on coronary artery calcium scoring by computed tomography in global cardiovascular risk assessment and in valuation of patients with chest pain: a report of the American College of Cardiology Foundation Clinical Expert Consensus Task Force (ACCF/AHA Writing Committee to Update the 2000 Expert Consensus Document on Electron Beam Computed Tomography).** *J Am Coll Cardiol* 2007, **49**:378–402.
5. Taylor AJ, Cequeira M, Hodgson JM, Mark D, Min J, O'Gara P, Rubin GD: **ACCF/SCCT/ACR/AHA/ASE/ASNC/NASCI/SCAI/SCMR 2010 appropriate use criteria for cardiac computed tomography: a report of the American College of Cardiology Foundation Appropriate Use Criteria Task Force, the Society of Cardiovascular Computed Tomography, the American College of Radiology, the American Heart Association, the American Society of Echocardiography, the American Society of Nuclear Cardiology, the Society for Cardiovascular Angiography and Interventions, and the Society for Cardiovascular Magnetic Resonance.** *J Am Coll Cardiol* 2010, **56**:1864–1894.
6. O'Malley PG, Taylor AJ, Jackson JL, Doherty TM, Detrano RC: **Prognostic**

Value of Coronary Electron-Beam Computed Tomography for Coronary Heart Disease Events in Asymptomatic Populations. *Am J Cardiol* 2000, **85**:945–948.

7. Shaw LJ, Raggi P, Schisterman E, Berman DS, Callister TQ: **Prognostic Value of Cardiac Risk Factors and Coronary Artery Screening for All-Cause Mortality.** *Radiology* 2003, **228**:826–833.
8. Greenland P, LaBree L, Azen SP, Doherty TM, Detrano RC: **Coronary Artery Calcium Score Combined With Framingham Score for Risk Prediction in Asymptomatic Individuals.** *JAMA* 2004, **291**:210–215.
9. Arad Y, Goodman KJ, Roth M, Newstein D, Guerci AD: **Coronary Calcification, Coronary Disease Risk Factors, C-Reactive Protein, and Atherosclerotic Cardiovascular Disease Events - The St. Francis Heart Study.** *J Am Coll Cardiol* 2005, **46**:158–165.
10. Budoff MJ, Shaw LJ, Liu ST, Weinstein SR, Mosler TP, Tseng PH, Flores FR, Callister TQ, Raggi P, Berman DS: **Long-Term Prognosis Associated With Coronary Calcification.** *J Am Coll Cardiol* 2007, **49**:1860–1870.
11. Detrano R, Guerci AD, Carr JJ, Bild DE, Burke G, Folsom AR, Liu K, Shea S, Szklo M, Bluemke DA, O'Leary DH, Tracy R, Watson K, Wong ND, Kronmal RA: **Coronary Calcium as a Predictor of Coronary Events in Four Racial or Ethnic Groups.** *N Engl J Med* 2008, **358**:1336–1345.
12. Bluemke DA, Achenback S, Budoff M, Gerber TC, Gersh B, Hillis LD, Hundley WG, Manning WJ, Printz BF, Stuber M, Woodard PK: **Noninvasive Coronary Artery Imaging Magnetic Resonance Angiography and Multidetector Computed Tomography Angiography A Scientific Statement From the American Heart Association Committee on Cardiovascular Imaging and Intervention of the Council on Cardiovascular Radiology and Intervention, and the Councils on Clinical Cardiology and Cardiovascular Disease in the Young.** *Circulation* 2008, **118**:586–606.
13. Raggi P, Gongora MC, Gopal A, Callister TQ, Budoff M, Shaw LJ: **Coronary Artery Calcium to Predict All-Cause Mortality in Elderly Men and Women.** *J Am Coll Cardiol* 2008, **52**:17–23.
14. Blaha M, Budoff MJ, Shaw LJ, Khosa F, Rumberger JA, Berman D, Callister T, Raggi P, Blumenthal RS, Nasir K: **Absence of Coronary Artery Calcification and All-Cause Mortality.** *J Am Coll Cardiol* 2009, **2**:692–700.
15. Budoff MJ, Nasir K, McClelland RL, Detrano R, Wong N, Blumenthal RS, Kondos G, Kronmal RA: **Coronary Calcium Predicts Events Better With Absolute Calcium Scores Than Age-Sex-Race/Ethnicity Percentiles.** *J Am Coll Cardiol* 2009, **53**:345–352.
16. Polonsky TS, McClelland RL, Jorgensen NW, Bild DE, Burke GL, Guerci AD, Greenland P: **Coronary Artery Calcium Score and Risk Classification for Coronary Heart Disease Prediction.** *JAMA* 2010, **303**:1610–1616.
17. Agatston AS, Janowitz WR, Hildner FJ, Zusmer NR, Viamonte M, Detrano R: **Quantification of coronary-artery calcium using ultrafast computed-tomography.** *J Am Coll Cardiol* 1990, **15**:827–832.
18. Hong C, Becker CR, Schoepf UJ, Ohnesorge B, Bruening R, Reiser MF: **Coronary Artery Calcium: Absolute Quantification in Nonenhanced and Contrast-enhanced Multi-Detector Row CT Studies.** *Radiology* 2002, **223**:474–480.
19. Callister TQ, Cooil B, Raya SP, Lippolis NJ, Russo DJ, Raggi P: **Coronary Artery Disease: Improved Reproducibility of Calcium Scoring with an Electron-Beam CT Volumetric Method.** *Radiology* 1998, **208**:807–814.
20. Hong C, Bae KT, Pilgram TK: **Coronary Artery Calcium: Accuracy and Reproducibility of Measurements with Multi-Detector Row Ct – Assessment of Effects of Different Thresholds and Quantification Methods.** *Radiology* 2003, **227**:795–801.
21. Cohen MA, Adar SD, Allen RW, Avol E, Curl CL, Gould T, Hardie D, Ho A, Kinney P, Larson TV, Sampson P, Sheppard L, Stukovsky KD, Swan SS, Liu LJS, Kaufman JD: **Approach to Estimating Participant Pollutant Exposures in the Multi-Ethnic Study of Atherosclerosis and Air Pollution (MESA Air).** *Environ Sci Technol* 2009, **43**:4687–4693.
22. Bild DE, Bluemke DA, Burke GL, Detrano R, Roux AVD, Folsom AR, Greenland P, Jacobs DR Jr, Kronmal R, Liu K, Nelson JC, O'Leary D, Saad MF, Shea S, Szklo M, Tracy RP: **Multi-Ethnic Study of Atherosclerosis: Objectives and Design.** *Am J Epidemol* 2002, **156**:871–881.
23. MESA - Multi-Ethnic Study of Atherosclerosis:, . http://www.mesa-nhlbi.org].
24. Carr JJ, Nelson JC, Wong ND, McNitt-Gray M, Arad Y, Jacobs DR, Sidney S, Bild DE, Williams OD, Detrano RC: **Calcified Coronary Artery Plaque Measurement with Cardiac CT in Population based Studies: Standardized Protocol of Multi-Ethnic Study of Atherosclerosis (MESA) and Coronary Artery Risk Development in Young Adults (CARDIA) Study.** *Radiology* 2005, **234**:35–43.
25. Wilson PW, D'Agostino RB, Levy D, Belanger AM, Silbershatz H, Kannel WB: **Prediction of Coronary Heart Disease Using Risk Factor Categories.** *Circulation* 1998, **97**:1837–1847.
26. D'Agostino RB Sr, Grundy S, Sullivan LM, Wilson P: **Validation of the Framingham Coronary Heart Disease Prediction Scores: Results of a Multiple Ethnic Groups Investigation.** *JAMA* 2001, **286**:180–187.
27. R Development Core Team: *R: A Language and Environment for Statistical Computing*. Vienna, Austria: R Foundation for Statistical Computing; 2010. http://www.R-project.org. ISBN 3-900051-07-0.
28. Chironi G, Simon A, Megnien JL, Sirieix ME, Mousseaux E, Pessana F, Armentano R: **Impact of coronary artery calcium on cardiovascular risk categorization and lipid-lowering drug eligibility in asymptomatic hypercholesterolemic men.** *International Journal of Cardiology* 2011, **151**:200–204.
29. Pessana F, Armentano R, Chironi G, Megnien JL, Mousseaux E, Simon A: **Subclinical atherosclerosis modeling: integration of coronary artery calcium score to Framingham equation.** In *31st Annual International Conference of the IEEE EMBS: 2–6 September 2009*. Minneapolis: 31st Annual International Conference of the IEEE EMBS; 2009:5348–5351.
30. Broderick LS, Shemesh J, Wilensky RL, Eckert GJ, Zhou XH, Torres WE, Balk MA, Rogers WJ, Conces DJ Jr, Kopecky KK: **Measurement of Coronary Artery Calcium with Dual-Slice Helical CT Compared with Coronary Angiography: Evaluation of CT Scoring Methods, Interobserver Variations, and Reproducibility.** *AJR* 1996, **167**:439–444.
31. Mintz GS, Nissen SE, Anderson WD, Bailey SR, Erbel R, Fitzgerald PJ, Pinto FJ, Rosenfield K, Siegel RJ, Tuzcu EM, Yock PG: **ACC Clinical Expert Consensus Document on Standards for the acquisition, measurement and reporting of intravascular ultrasound studies: a report of the American College of Cardiology Task Force on Clinical Expert Consensus Documents (Committee to Develop a Clinical Expert Consensus Document on Standards for Acquisition, Measurement and Reporting of Intravascular Ultrasound Studies [IVUS]).** *J Am Coll Cardiol* 2001, **37**:1478–1492.
32. Nicholls SJ, Hsu A, Wolski K, Hu B, Bayturan O, Lavoie A, Uno K, Tuzcu EM, Nissen SE: **Intravascular Ultrasound-Derived Measures of Coronary Atherosclerotic Plaque Burden and Clinical Outcome.** *J Am Coll Cardiol* 2010, **55**:2399–2407.

Integration of 3D anatomical data obtained by CT imaging and 3D optical scanning for computer aided implant surgery

Gianni Frisardi[1,2*†], Giacomo Chessa[2†], Sandro Barone[3†], Alessandro Paoli[3†], Armando Razionale[3†], Flavio Frisardi[1†]

Abstract

Background: A precise placement of dental implants is a crucial step to optimize both prosthetic aspects and functional constraints. In this context, the use of virtual guiding systems has been recognized as a fundamental tool to control the ideal implant position. In particular, complex periodontal surgeries can be performed using preoperative planning based on CT data. The critical point of the procedure relies on the lack of accuracy in transferring CT planning information to surgical field through custom-made stereo-lithographic surgical guides.

Methods: In this work, a novel methodology is proposed for monitoring loss of accuracy in transferring CT dental information into periodontal surgical field. The methodology is based on integrating 3D data of anatomical (impression and cast) and preoperative (radiographic template) models, obtained by both CT and optical scanning processes.

Results: A clinical case, relative to a fully edentulous jaw patient, has been used as test case to assess the accuracy of the various steps concurring in manufacturing surgical guides. In particular, a surgical guide has been designed to place implants in the bone structure of the patient. The analysis of the results has allowed the clinician to monitor all the errors, which have been occurring step by step manufacturing the physical templates.

Conclusions: The use of an optical scanner, which has a higher resolution and accuracy than CT scanning, has demonstrated to be a valid support to control the precision of the various physical models adopted and to point out possible error sources. A case study regarding a fully edentulous patient has confirmed the feasibility of the proposed methodology.

Background

Over the last few years, dental prostheses supported by osseointegrated implants have progressively replaced the use of removable dentures in the treatment of edentulous patients. The restoration of missing teeth must provide a patient with aesthetical, biomechanical and functional requirements of natural dentition, particularly concerning chewing functions. When conventional implantation techniques are used, the clinical outcome is often unpredictable, since it greatly relies on skills and experience of dental surgeons.

The placement of endosseous implants is based on invasive procedures which require a long time to be completed. Recently, many different implant planning procedures have been developed to support oral implant positioning. Number, size, position of implants must be related to bone morphology, as well as to the accompanying vital structures (e.g. neurovascular bundles). Complex surgical interventions can be performed using preoperative planning based on 3D imaging. The developments in computer-assisted surgery have brought to the definition of effective operating procedures in dental implantology. Several systems have been designed to guide treatment-planning processes: from simulation environments to surgical fields [1]. The guided approaches are generally based on three-dimensional reconstructions of patient anatomies processing data obtained by either Computed Tomography (CT) or Cone-Beam Computed Tomography (CBCT) [2]. These methodologies allow more accurate assessments of

* Correspondence: frisardi@tin.it
† Contributed equally
[1]"Epochè" Orofacial Pain Center, Nettuno (Rome), Italy
Full list of author information is available at the end of the article

surgical difficulties through less invasive procedures and operating time reductions. In particular, radiographic data (depth and proximity to anatomical landmarks) and restorative requirements are crucial for a complete transfer of implant planning (positioning, trajectory and distribution) to surgical field [3]. Virtual planning processes provide digital models of drill guides, which are typically manufactured by stereo-lithography and used as surgical guidance in the preparation of implant receptor sites.

In the past decade, a methodology based on the use of two different guides and a double CT scan procedure, has been introduced [4] and later commercialized as NobelGuide® by NobelBiocare (Zurich, Switzerland). This procedure involves an intermediate template (*radiographic template*) that is used to refer the soft tissues with respect to the bone structure derived from patient CT scan data. The guide is manufactured on the basis of diagnostic wax-up reproducing the desired prosthetic end result. The diagnostic wax-up is obtained starting from the dental cast, produced from the impression of the patient's mouth, and helps in the definition of a proper dental prosthesis design. Moreover, the radiographic template is made of a non radio-opaque material, usually acrylic resin, to avoid image disturbs when CT scans of patients are carried. Then, the template is separately scanned changing radiological parameters in order to visualize the acrylic resin. The computer-based alignment of the prosthetic model with respect to the maxillofacial structure is obtained by small radio-opaque gutta-percha spheres inserted within the radiographic template. These gutta-percha markers are visible in both the different CT scans and can be used as references to register the two data sets through point-based rigid registration techniques [5].

Specific 3D image-based software programs for implant surgery planning, based on CT scan data, have been recently developed and clinically approved by many manufacturers. These software applications allow surgeons to locate implant receptor sites and simulate implant placement [6]. The planned implant positions are then transferred to the surgical field by means of a surgical guide made by stereo-lithographic techniques. Surgical guides can be bone-supported, tooth-supported or mucosa-supported depending on the specific patient's conditions. Bone-supported guides are designed to fit on the jawbone and can be used for partially or fully edentulous cases, while tooth-supported guides are tailored to fit directly on the teeth. The latters are mostly effective for single tooth and partially edentulous cases. Mucosa-supported surgical guides are rather designed for placement on soft tissues and are recommended for fully edentulous patients when minimally invasive surgery is required.

The surgical guide is then placed within the patient's mouth and can be anchored, especially when mucosa-supported guides are used, to the jawbone by stabilizing pins (Anchor Pins).

The weak point of the whole procedure relies on the accuracy in transferring information deriving from CT data into surgical planning. Geometrical deviations of implant positions between planning and intervention stages could cause irreversible damages of anatomical structure, such as sensory nerves. The surgical guide should closely fit with the hard and/or soft tissue surface in a unique and stable position in order to accurately transfer the pre-operative treatment plan. If the surgical template is not accurate, the fit will be improper, compromising the implant placement. Even small angular errors in the placement of perforation guides can, indeed, propagate in considerable horizontal deviations due to the depth of the implant.

A previous in ex vivo study to assess the accuracy of 10-15 mm-long implant positioning using CBCT, revealed a mean angular deviation of 2° (*SD* ± 0.8, range 0.7° ÷ 4°) and a mean linear deviation of 1.1 mm (*SD* ± 0.7 mm, range 0.3 ÷ 2.3 mm) at the hexagon and 2 mm (*SD* ± 0.7 mm, range 0.7 ÷ 2.4 mm) at the tip [7].

Sarment *et al.* [8] compared the accuracy of a stereolithographic surgical template to conventional surgical template *in vitro*. An average linear deviation of 1.5 mm at the entrance, and 2.1 mm at the apex for the conventional template, as compared with 0.9 and 1.0 mm for the stereo-lithographic surgical template was reported.

Di Giacomo *et al.* [9] published a preliminary study involving the placement of 21 implants using a stereolithographic surgical template, showing an angular deviation of 7.25° between planned and actual implant axes, whereas the linear deviation was 1.45 mm.

In a recent study [10], the accuracy of a surgical template in transferring planned implant position to the real patient surgery has been assessed. The mean mesiodistal angular deviation of the planned to the actual was 0.17° (*SD* ± 5.02°) ranging from 0.262° to 12.2°, though, the mean bucco-lingual angular deviation was 0.46° (*SD* ± 4.48°) ranging from 0.085° to 7.67°.

These studies confirm that the error could be high, especially in neurovascular anatomical districts, such as the mandibular nerve. In this anatomical area, a moderate damage may also result in severe symptoms. For example, the lesion of the mandibular nerve is of the Wallerian degenerative type [11], which is a slow degenerative process and the diagnosis by laser-evoked potentials and trigeminal reflexes would allow early decompression [12].

Deviations between planning and postoperative outcome may reflect the sum of many error sources. For instance, CT scan quality and processing of DICOM

(*Digital Imaging and Communication in Medicine*) images affect the creation of the corresponding 3D digital models. Misalignment errors can also be introduced during the arrangement of the radiographic template within the maxillofacial structures by the gutta-percha markers. Moreover, further inaccuracies can be introduced in manufacturing physical models by stereo-lithographic techniques.

This paper concerns the development of an innovative methodology to evaluate the accuracy in transferring CT based implant planning into surgical fields for oral rehabilitation.

Methods

The proposed methodology is based on the combined use of CT scan data and a structured light vision system. In particular, the data acquisition phase regards two different scanning technologies: radiological scanning and optical scanning.

A clinical case, relative to a fully edentulous patient, has been used as test case to assess the feasibility of the proposed methodology. The ethics approval was obtained by Human Research Ethics Committee at the Sassari Hospital (n° 971) and written form approval was obtained by the patient.

Optical scanning

The 3D optical scanner used in this work is based on a stereo vision approach with structured coded light projection [13]. The optical unit is composed of a monochrome digital camera (CCD - 1280 × 960 pixels) and a multimedia white light projector (DLP - 1024 × 768 pixels) that are used as active devices for a triangulation process. The digitizer is integrated with a rotary axis, automatically controlled by a stepper motor with a resolution of 400 steps per round (Figure 1). The scanner is capable of measuring about 1 million 3D points within the field of view (100 mm × 80 mm), with a spatial resolution of 0.1 mm and an overall accuracy of 0.01 mm [13].

CT scan data

CT scanning of maxillofacial region is based on the acquisition of several slices of the jaw bone at each turn of a helical movement of an x-ray source and a reciprocating area detector. The acquired data can be stored in DICOM format.

In this work, CT scanning has been performed using a system Toshiba Aquilion by Toshiba Medical Systems, Japan, with 0.5 mm slice thickness. 3D models have been reconstructed processing DICOM images by means of 3D Slicer (version 3.2), a freely available open source software initially developed as a joint effort between the Surgical Planning Lab at Brigham and

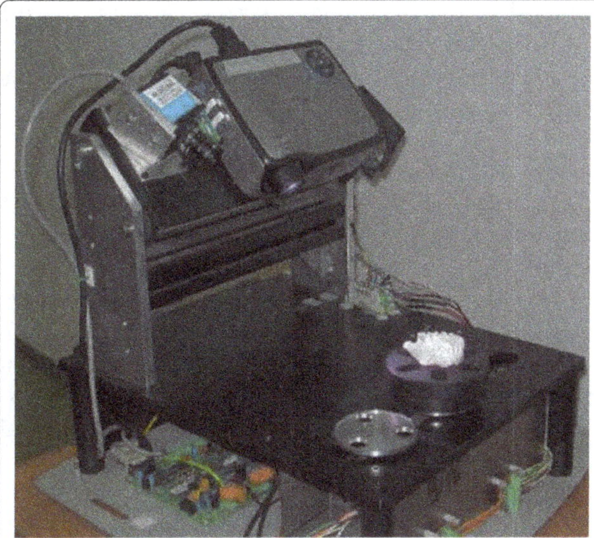

Figure 1 Optical scanner. 3D optical scanner used to capture dental models.

Women's Hospital and the MIT Artificial Intelligence Lab. The software has now evolved into a national platform supported by a variety of federal funding sources [14]. 3D Slicer is an end-user application to process medical images and to generate 3D volumetric data set, which can be used to provide primary reconstruction images in three orthogonal planes (axial, sagittal and coronal). 3D models of anatomical structure can be generated through a powerful and robust segmentation tool on the basis of a semi-automated approach. The displayed gray level of the voxels representing hard tissues can be dynamically altered to provide the most realistic appearance of the bone structure, minimizing soft tissues and the superimposition of metal artifacts (Figure 2). Initial segmentation of CT data can then be

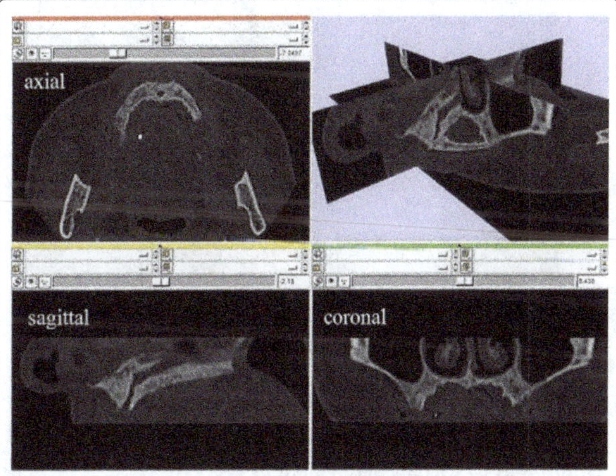

Figure 2 CT data. Maxilla CT data in the axial, sagittal and coronal planes and a fully 3D vision.

obtained by threshold segmentation. This involves the manual selection of a threshold value that can be dynamically adjusted to provide the optimal filling of the interested structure in all the slices acquired.

3D reconstructions

The accuracy of 3D reconstruction based on CT data analysis may be affected by several factors that should be considered in surgical treatment planning. A reduction of image quality may be caused by metallic artifacts and/or patient motions. Moreover, the influence of an appropriate segmentation on the final 3D representation is a matter of utmost importance [15]. The segmentation process typically relies on the adopted mathematical algorithm, on spatial and contrast resolution of the slice images, on technical skills of the operator in selecting the optimal threshold value. Metal restorations as well as tissues not belonging to the structure of interest (i.e. antagonistic teeth) must be carefully cleaned up from the CT scan images when models for interactive planning are prepared. This process can lead to different volume reconstructions due to the operator's selection of threshold values, even if proved and patented software is used. In particular, the detection of the optimal threshold value is not straightforward when images presenting smooth intensity distributions are processed (Figure 3). For this reason, a methodology to verify the accuracy of the 3D reconstruction of CT derived images would be necessary for clinical applications.

In this work, a validation process for 3D reconstructions of radiographic templates used in implant guided surgery has been developed using the optical scanner. As previously illustrated, the radiological template (Figure 4A) is manually manufactured on the basis of the diagnostic wax-up to take into account prosthesis design, and on the gypsum dental cast (Figure 4B) to assure the optimal fitting of the mating surfaces. The 3D model of the radiographic template is reconstructed processing the DICOM images (Figure 5A). The radiographic template is also acquired by the optical scanner. The 3D model as obtained by the structured light scanning system (Figure 5B) is used as the gold standard to improve the accuracy of the CT reconstruction. The comparison between the CT reconstructed and the optically captured models gives the information to optimize the parameters of the DICOM images segmentation process. The data acquired by the optical scanner are aligned to the model obtained by the CT reconstruction through a point-based registration technique. Correspondent pairs of points are manually selected on the two different models and the rigid transformation between the two objects is determined by applying the singular value decomposition (SVD) method [5]. The alignment is then refined by applying a surface-based registration technique through best fitting algorithms [16].

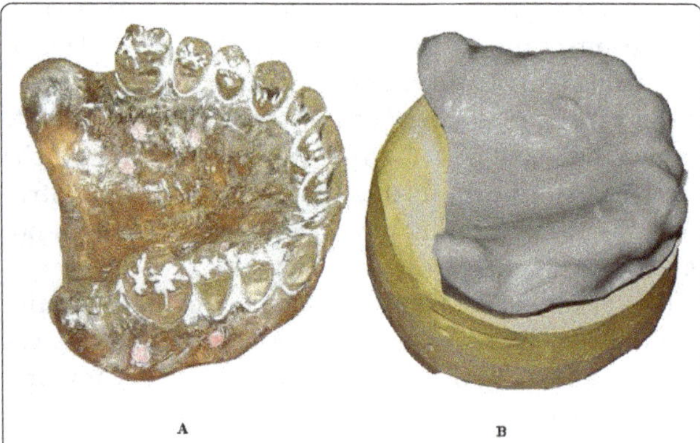

Figure 4 (A-B) Preoperative and anatomical dental models. (A) Radiographic template with gutta-percha markers, (B) gypsum dental cast.

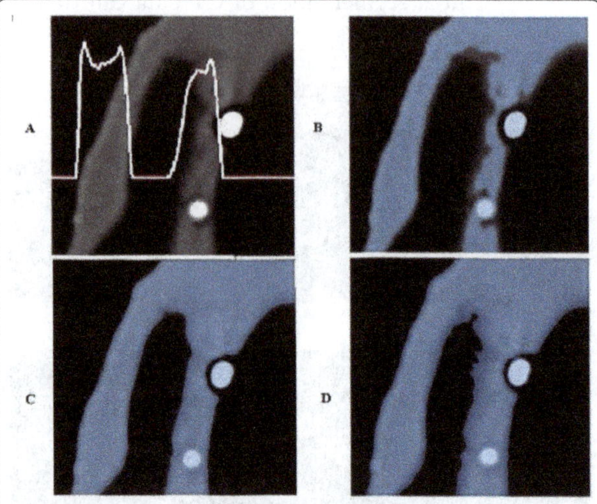

Figure 3 (A-D) CT data segmentation process. (A) DICOM image of the radiographic template with associated a row grey intensity level, (B-D) segmentation with three different threshold values.

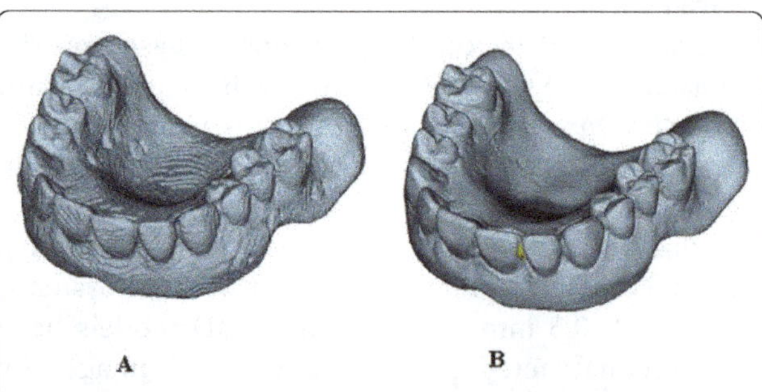

Figure 5 (A-B) Digital models of the radiographic template. 3D digital models of the radiographic template obtained by CT data (A) and by the optical scanner (B).

Figure 6 shows the full-field 3D compare of three different reconstructions of the radiological guide, obtained varying the threshold values, with respect to the model obtained by the optical scanner. The distribution of discrepancies between the datasets obtained using the two scanning technologies, with both positive and negative deviations, quantifies the dimensional difference of the CT based reconstruction that can turn out to be smaller (Figure 6A) or greater (Figure 6C). The search of the optimal threshold value can therefore be made by minimizing the absolute mean of the distances between the two models (Figure 6B). Histogram plots of these distributions are reported in Figure 6D, whereas Table 1 reports the associated statistical data (mean and standard deviation).

Results

In the present work, a clinical case, relative to a fully edentulous patient, has been used as test case to assess the accuracy of the various steps concurring in manufacturing surgical guides. A study surgical template (Figure 7B), called Duplicate Radiographic Template (D.R.T) and based on the same CT data used to fabricate the mucosa-supported surgical guide, has been manufactured by a stereo-lithographic process. This template does not present the holes to hold the drill guides since the first requirement was just the reproduction of the only functional areas to wearing the guide. All the physical models (impression, cast, radiographic template, study surgical template) have been acquired by the optical scanner. The 3D digital models have been realigned by best fitting techniques in order to evaluate the discrepancies between the different shapes. The virtual alignments have been conducted by only referring the mating surfaces of the various models, since the crucial problem regards the proper fit between the final surgical guide and the patient's mucosa.

Table 1 Statistical data relative to different DICOM reconstructions

3D Compare	*Mean value* [mm]	*SD* [mm]
A	-0.224	0.226
B	-0.008	0.200
C	0.185	0.179

Mean and standard deviation of the discrepancies in the three different cases reported in Figure 6 and relative to the threshold values used in Figure 3 (B-D).

Figure 8 shows the 3D compare between the patient mouth's impression (Figure 7A) and the relative study cast (*mean value* -0.004 mm, *SD* 0.067 mm). The manufacturing of the gypsum cast is the first critical step of the whole process that can be verified, since the accuracy in detecting the impression is not measurable. Mismatch between the impression and the gypsum cast may cause improper fitting of the radiographic template, which could result stable on the cast, but floating or not wearable in the patient's mouth.

In Figure 9, the distributions of the optical measurement discrepancies between corresponding points of the gypsum cast and, respectively, the radiological guide (Figure 9B) (*mean value* -0.009 mm, *SD* 0.069 mm) and the surgical guide or Duplicate Radiographic Template (Figure 9C) (*mean value* 0.013 mm, *SD* 0.141 mm) are reported. Moreover, the fitting of the radiological guide model, obtained by processing DICOM images on the gypsum cast has been verified (Figure 9A) (*mean value* -0.004 mm, *SD* 0.082 mm). Table 2 summarizes the same results in terms of mean value and standard deviation of the misalignments. Histogram plots relative to these distributions are reported in Figure 9D.

Discussion

The analysis of the results allows the detection of possible errors occurred in manufacturing surgical guides.

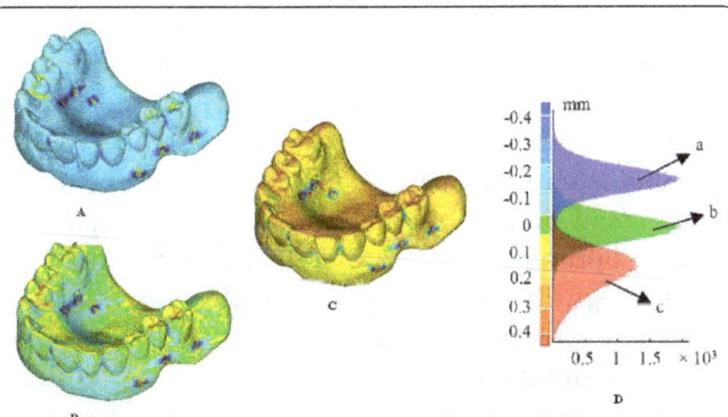

Figure 6 (A-D) Full-field 3D comparisons of three different reconstructions of the radiographic template. Full-field 3D compare of three different DICOM reconstructions of the radiographic template with respect to the model obtained by the optical scanner and relative histogram plots (D). The DICOM model (Figure 5A) results smaller (A), comparable (B) and greater (C) than the one obtained by the optical scanner (Figure 5B).

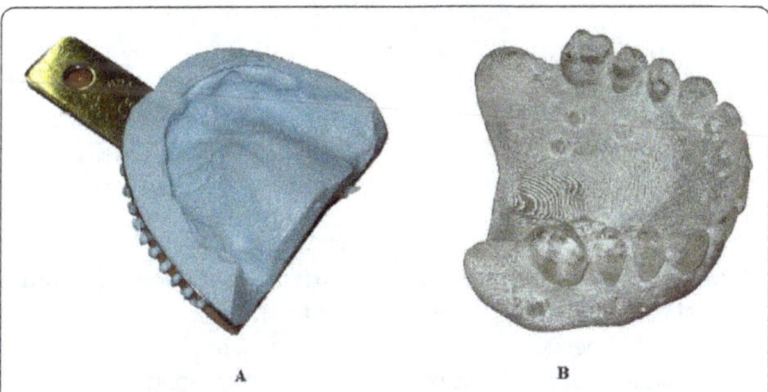

Figure 7 (A-B) Impression and radiographic template. Patient's mouth impression (A) and Duplicate Radiographic Template (B).

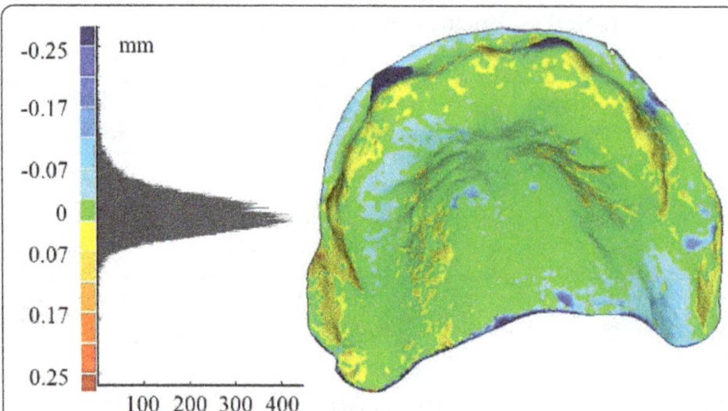

Figure 8 Full-field 3D comparison between impression and cast. 3D compare between the impression and the gypsum cast models obtained by optical scanning.

Low discrepancy values between the impression and cast models prove the correctness in the manufacturing process of the gypsum cast. The almost perfect superimposition between the radiological template and the study cast should have been expected since the radiological template is customized by manually fitting it on the cast. The transfer from the radiological to the surgical guides involves two distinct processes: the reconstruction of the radiological guide model by CT scanning and the manufacturing of the surgical guide starting from this digital model. The accuracy of the first step has been verified aligning the model obtained by processing the DICOM images with the gypsum cast. The fine adjustment of the threshold value in the segmentation process, using the model obtained by optical scanning as the anatomical truth, has allowed the minimization of the deviations with respect to the cast. For this reason, the high misalignment errors regarding the surgical template can be attributed to the stereo-lithographic process, which has been used to manufacture the surgical guide. The geometrical differences of the surfaces mating with the gypsum cast, certainly affect the overall accuracy in the implant placement positions. As a further proof, the surgical guide has demonstrated to improperly fit the physical model of the dental gypsum cast. This could lead the surgeon to anchor the template in the wrong way, compromising the desired implant placement.

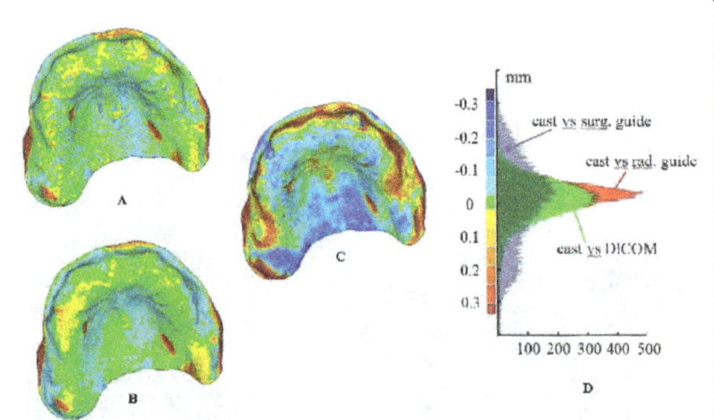

Figure 9 (A-D) Full-field 3D comparisons between cast and dental models. Full-field distributions of the measurements discrepancies between gypsum cast model and, respectively, the radiological guide model as obtained by DICOM processing (A), the radiological guide model (B) and the Duplicate radiographic Template "D.R.T." (C) as obtained by the optical scanner. (D) Relative histogram plots.

Table 2 Statistical data relative to discrepancies between cast and dental models

3D Compare	Impression		Gypsum cast	
	Mean value [mm]	*SD* [mm]	*Mean value* [mm]	*SD* [mm]
DICOM	-	-	-0.004	0.082
Gypsum cast	-0.004	0.067	-	-
Radiological template	-	-	-0.009	0.069
Surgical template	-	-	0.013	0.141

Mean and standard deviation of the discrepancies reported in Figure 8 and Figure 9.

A thorough study of the effect of these discrepancies on the maximum deviations obtained between the planned positions of the implants and the postoperative result should be done.

Conclusions

In this paper, a methodology to evaluate the transfer accuracy of CT dental information into periodontal surgical field has been proposed. The procedure is based on the integration of a structured light vision system within the CT scan based preoperative planning process. The use of the optical scanner, having a higher resolution and accuracy than CT scanning, has demonstrated to be a valid support to evaluate the precision of the various physical models adopted and to point out possible error sources. Optical scanning of the radiological guide, mounted on the gypsum cast, could be furthermore helpful for the integration of the prosthetic data within the bone structure. In case of not fully edentulous patients, the acquisition of teeth's shape could be used, in addition to gutta-percha markers, to optimize or verify the positioning of the radiological guide with respect to the maxillofacial structure. Moreover, the accurate digital model of the mouth impression could be the base for the direct design of the radiological guide using CAD/CAM technologies, without passing through manufacturing the gypsum cast, drastically reducing errors and planning time.

Acknowledgements

Written consent was obtained from the patient for publication of present study.

Author details
[1]"Epochè" Orofacial Pain Center, Nettuno (Rome), Italy. [2]Department of Prosthetic Rehabilitation, University of Sassari, Italy. [3]Department of Mechanical, Nuclear and Production Engineering, University of Pisa, Italy.

Authors' contributions
GF, GC, SB, AP, AR and FF participated to the conception and design of the work, to the acquisition of data, wrote the paper, participated in the analysis and interpretation of data and reviewed the manuscript. All the authors read and approved the final manuscript.

Competing interests
The authors declare that they have no competing interests.

References

1. Vercruyssen M, Jacobs R, Van Assche N, van Steenberghe D: **The use of CT scan based planning for oral rehabilitation by means of implants and its transfer to the surgical field: a critical review on accuracy.** *J Oral Rehabil* 2008, **35**:454-474.
2. Scarfe WC, Farman AG, Sukovic P: **Clinical applications of cone-beam computed tomography in dental practice.** *J Can Dent Assoc* 2006, **72**:75-80.
3. Tardieu PB, Vrielinck L, Escolano E: **Computer-assisted implant placement. A case report: treatment of the mandible.** *Int J Oral Maxillofac Implants* 2003, **18**:599-604.
4. Verstreken K, Van Cleynenbreugel J, Martens K, Marchal G, van Steenberghe D, Suetens P: **An image-guided planning system for endosseous oral implants.** *IEEE Trans Med Imaging* 1998, **17**:842-852.
5. Eggert DW, Lorusso A, Fischer RB: **Estimating 3-D rigid body transformations: a comparison of four major algorithms.** *Mach Vis Appl* 1997, **9**:272-290.
6. Azari A, Nikzad S: **Computer-assisted implantology: historical background and potential outcomes - a review.** *Int J Med Robotics Comput Assist Surg* 2008, **4**:95-104.
7. Van Assche N, van Steenberghe D, Guerrero ME, Hirsch E, Schutyser F, Quirynen M, Jacobs R: **Accuracy of implant placement based on pre-surgical planning of three-dimensional cone-beam images: a pilot study.** *J Clin Periodontol* 2007, **34**:816-821.
8. Sarment DP, Sukovic P, Clinthorne N: **Accuracy of implant placement with a stereolithographic surgical guide.** *Int J Oral Maxillofac Implants* 2003, **18**:571-577.
9. Di Giacomo GA, Cury PR, de Araujo NS, Sendyk WR, Sendyk CL: **Clinical application of stereolithographic surgical guides for implant placement: preliminary results.** *J Periodontol* 2005, **76**:503-507.
10. Al-Harbi SA, Sun AY: **Implant placement accuracy when using stereolithographic template as a surgical guide: preliminary results.** *Implant Dent* 2009, **18**:46-56.
11. Mi W, Beirowski B, Gillingwater TH, Adalbert R, Wagner D, Grumme D, Osaka H, Conforti L, Arnhold S, Addicks K, *et al*: **The slow Wallerian degeneration gene, WldS, inhibits axonal spheroid pathology in gracile axonal dystrophy mice.** *Brain* 2005, **128**:405-416.
12. Romaniello A, Cruccu G, Frisardi G, Arendt-Nielsen L, Svensson P: **Assessment of nociceptive trigeminal pathways by laser-evoked potentials and laser silent periods in patients with painful temporomandibular disorders.** *Pain* 2003, **103**:31-39.
13. Barone S, Paoli A, Razionale AV: **An Innovative Methodology for the Design of Custom Dental Prostheses by Optical Scanning.** In *Proceedings of XXI INGEGRAF: 10-12 June 2009; Lugo.* Edited by: INGEGRAF. Lugo; 2009:264-272.
14. **3D Slicer (version 3.2).** [http://www.slicer.org].
15. Brown AA, Scarfe WC, Scheetz JP, Silveira AM, Farman AG: **Linear accuracy of cone beam CT derived 3D images.** *Angle Orthod* 2009, **79**:150-157.
16. Besl PJ, McKay ND: **A Method for Registration of 3D Shapes.** *IEEE Trans Pattern Anal Mach Intell* 1992, **14**:239-256.

21

The effect of a manual instrumentation technique on five types of premolar root canal geometry assessed by microcomputed tomography and three-dimensional reconstruction

Ke-Zeng Li[1], Yuan Gao[1], Ru Zhang[1], Tao Hu[1*] and Bin Guo[2*]

Abstract

Background: Together with diagnosis and treatment planning, a good knowledge of the root canal system and its frequent variations is a necessity for successful root canal therapy. The selection of instrumentation techniques for variants in internal anatomy of teeth has significant effects on the shaping ability and cleaning effectiveness. The aim of this study was to reveal the differences made by including variations in the internal anatomy of premolars into the study protocol for investigation of a single instrumentation technique (hand ProTaper instruments) assessed by microcomputed tomography and three-dimensional reconstruction.

Methods: Five single-root premolars, whose root canal systems were classified into one of five types, were scanned with micro-CT before and after preparation with a hand ProTaper instrument. Instrumentation characteristics were measured quantitatively in 3-D using a customized application framework based on MeVisLab. Numeric values were obtained for canal surface area, volume, volume changes, percentage of untouched surface, dentin wall thickness, and the thickness of dentin removed. Preparation errors were also evaluated using a color-coded reconstruction.

Results: Canal volumes and surface areas were increased after instrumentation. Prepared canals of all five types were straightened, with transportation toward the inner aspects of S-shaped or multiple curves. However, a ledge was formed at the apical third curve of the type II canal system and a wide range in the percentage of unchanged canal surfaces (27.4-83.0%) was recorded. The dentin walls were more than 0.3 mm thick except in a 1 mm zone from the apical surface and the hazardous area of the type II canal system after preparation with an F3 instrument.

Conclusions: The 3-D color-coded images showed different morphological changes in the five types of root canal systems shaped with the same hand instrumentation technique. Premolars are among the most complex teeth for root canal treatment and instrumentation techniques for the root canal systems of premolars should be selected individually depending on the 3-D canal configuration of each tooth. Further study is needed to demonstrate the differences made by including variations in the internal anatomy of teeth into the study protocol of clinical RCT for identifying the best preparation technique.

Keywords: Manual instruments, Microcomputed tomography, Root canal preparation, Root canal system, Three-dimensional imaging

* Correspondence: acomnet@263.net; guobin0408@126.com
[1]State Key Laboratory of Oral Diseases, West China College of Stomatology, Sichuan University, Chengdu, P.R. China
[2]Institute of Stomatology, Chinese PLA General Hospital, Beijing, P.R. China
Full list of author information is available at the end of the article

Background

The study of dental and root canal morphology is a critical theme in endodontic education, training, and treatment [1-5]. Together with diagnosis and treatment planning, a good knowledge of the root canal system and its frequent variations is an absolute necessity for successful root canal therapy [6]. Hess (1921) reported on the wide variation and complexity of root canal systems, establishing that a root with a tapering canal and a single foramen was the exception rather than the rule [7]. Weine (2004) categorized the canal systems in any one root into types I-IV [8] and Yoshioka et al. [9] (2004) added type V to Weine's classification. Vertucci (2005) described a much more complex canal system and identified eight different pulp space configurations [4].

Among these classifications, Weine's classification does not consider the possible positions for large auxiliary canals or the position at which the apical foramina exit the root. Any combination of these factors could be present in any dimension of the canals, regardless of any specific configuration. Thus, Weine's classification uses a simple, direct, and clinically oriented approach [8].

In addition, a number of conventional techniques have been used for evaluating root canal morphology and the shaping ability and cleaning effectiveness of various instruments [5,10-14]. Using the modified muffle system, the exposure of radiographs under reproducible conditions in two directions (buccolingual and mesiodistal) was guaranteed to take radiographs before, during and after root canal preparation [14]. Tooth decalcification allowed effective histological evaluation of the preparation [13], but the destruction of the specimens by the muffle system and decalcification may impede the simultaneous investigation of different parameters of root canal preparation. In addition, periapical radiographs provide only two-dimensional information about root canal morphology [12].

Recently, microcomputed tomography (micro-CT) has emerged as a powerful tool for the evaluation of root canal morphology [15]. Micro-CT technology allows noninvasive evaluation of both the external and internal morphology of a tooth in a detailed and accurate manner [2,3]. Though micro-CT is expensive and time-consuming and not suitable for clinical use, it would be an effective way to examine the shape of the root canal after preparation [16,17] and obturation [18]. In comparison, the cone-beam computed tomography (CBCT) designed for dental use can provide the clinician with an imaging modality that is capable of providing a 3D representation of the maxillofacial region with minimal distortion, and it can also enhance detection and mapping the root canal system with the potential to improve the quality of root canal therapy [5,19,20].

Preparation of root canal systems includes both enlargement and shaping of the complex endodontic space together with its disinfection. A variety of instruments and techniques have been developed and described for this critical stage of root canal treatment [10]. Studies of the efficacy of various instruments for root canal preparation have typically been performed in simulated canals with simple anatomy [21,22] or in extracted human teeth with different curvatures [5,10,12-14,23,24].

Nickel-titanium (NiTi) rotary instruments were introduced to improve root canal preparation. Hand NiTi instruments can also be selected instead of rotary instruments in teeth with difficult canal anatomy and/or problematic handpiece access [25]. The ProTaper for hand use (HPT) appeared as an alternative NiTi instrument to the rotary ProTaper, embodying the same philosophy, indications, and sequence, but at a lower cost. The instrumentation is entirely manual, dispensing with the use of an electric motor [26]. The HPT instruments are recommended for use in reaming or "modified balanced forces" motion, differing from the motor-driven NiTi instruments [27]. Some limited studies of HPT instruments have been carried out [26-28]. An evaluation of preparation efficacy that integrates the canal system classification with various instruments has not been performed.

Therefore, the object of this study was to demonstrate the difference made by including variations in internal anatomy of premolars into the study protocol for investigation of a single instrumentation technique (HPT) using micro-CT and 3-D reconstruction. This is an observational report with limited numbers of teeth and techniques. And further study with large sample size is needed to obtain the clinically relevant conclusions.

Methods

Specimen selection and preparation

Thirty single-root premolars were randomly selected from a collection of extracted human teeth from a Chinese population sample based on mature apices without visible apical resorption and no prior endodontic treatment. These teeth were extracted because of periodontitis or orthodontic need. After understanding and written consent was obtained from patients, the extracted teeth were collected by the West China Hospital of Stomatology for teaching and research. The present study was approved by the Ethics Committee of the West China Hospital of Stomatology, and the premolars were selected from the teeth bank of the hospital. After extraction, tissue fragments and calcified debris were removed from the teeth by scaling and the teeth were stored in 0.1% thymol until used.

Preoperative radiographs of each selected tooth were first taken from the buccolingual and mesiodistal directions, then their canal system classifications were evaluated by an endodontist. After the radiographic evaluation and without probing the canals for patency so as to avoid modifying the canals' apical anatomy, premolars whose canal systems were classified into one of four categories (types I, II, III, IV) according to Weine's classification [8] were scanned using a micro-CT system (μCT-80; Scanco Medical, Bassersdorf, Switzerland) with an isotropic voxel size of 36 μm. Images were acquired from 622 slices of each tooth. From these images, a 3-D model of the tooth and canal system was constructed with a framework system (MeVisLab 2.0, MeVis Research, Bremen, Germany) on a personal computer (Athlon II X2, 2.8 GHz CPU, 2 Gbyte RAM, Windows XP) according to a customized application framework using MeVisLab [29]. The reconstructed 3-D model of the root canal system in each premolar was carefully examined. Unexpectedly, in addition to the four categories of Weine's classification [8], we found one mandibular first premolar whose canal system was classified as type V based on the system of Yoshioka *et al.* [9], which was not recognized by the professional endodontist from the preoperative periapical radiographs. Finally, five representative single-root premolars (teeth A, B, C, D, and E), each of whose canal system was classified into one of five categories (types I, II, III, IV, and V), were included in this study. In addition to the reconstruction of the tooth and canal, we also calculated the root canal diameter and showed its morphology with a 3-D color-coded image of the prepreparation canal systems.

After preparing a standard access cavity with #2 and #4 high-speed round carbide burs, using ample water cooling, each root canal was passively negotiated with a #10 K-file to the apical foramen. The working length of the canal was determined by observing the tip of the file protruding through the apical foramen and subtracting 1 mm from the recorded length.

In tooth E, however, the entrance of the lingual canal formed a perpendicular angle with the buccal canal, so we could not directly explore this canal with a #10 K-file. To find the lingual canal orifice, we adjusted the procedure: based on the length and location of the canal identified through the 3-D tooth model, a #40 K-file was used to remove the overhanging dentin above the orifice of the lingual canal, filing toward the occlusal surface. Chelating agents were also used to soften the overhanging dentin during this procedure. After the overhanging dentin was cleared, we explored the lingual canal with #8 and #10 K-files, then the working length was determined as per the aforementioned method.

According to the manufacturer's instructions, all root canals were explored with a #15 K-file after exploring with a #10 K-file, then the canals were prepared using a set of new HPT instruments (Dentsply Maillefer). Instrumental sequences followed the manufacturer's instructions: first, canals were flared coronally with S1 (followed by SX if necessary), then their working lengths were measured and confirmed with a #15 K-file, after which they were prepared with S1, S2, F1, F2, and F3 at the working length, using a "modified balanced forces" motion.

During preparation, RC-Prep (Premier Products, Plymouth Meeting, PA) was used as the lubricant. Irrigation was performed with 2 ml of 1% sodium hypochlorite (NaOCl) solution after each instrument and canal patency was ascertained with a #10 K-file for each canal. All root canals were prepared by a single operator.

Micro-CT measurement and 3-D evaluation

After preparation with each HPT instrument at the working length, canals were dried with sterile paper points, then the teeth were scanned using the same micro-CT system. A series of micro-CT images were again obtained with the same isotropic voxel size of 36 μm.

To evaluate the efficacy of root canal preparation, volumes of interest were selected extending from the cemento-enamel junction to the apex of the roots. Using the customized application framework MeVisLab [29], the canal models (pre- and postpreparation) were reconstructed and superimposed and the instrumentation characteristics were quantitatively measured in 3-D. Numeric values were obtained for canal surface area, volume, volume changes, percentage of untouched surface, dentin wall thickness, and the thickness of dentin removed. The location of dentin removed or a lack of change during preparation were also demonstrated using the 3-D color images. Preparation errors such as canal straightening, ledging, elbow formation, or zipping were also evaluated using the color-coded reconstruction.

Results

Noninstrumented specimens

For the five single root premolars whose root canal systems were classified into one of five types, volume rendering revealed detailed 3-D images of the root canal system, dentin, and enamel (Figure 1) and the various curves of the root canal were also shown in the 3-D model of the prepreparation canal (Figure 1, 2).

The 3-D-coded images of the canal diameter and its distribution are shown in Figure 2. The canal diameter of the main root canals of all teeth is greater than 100

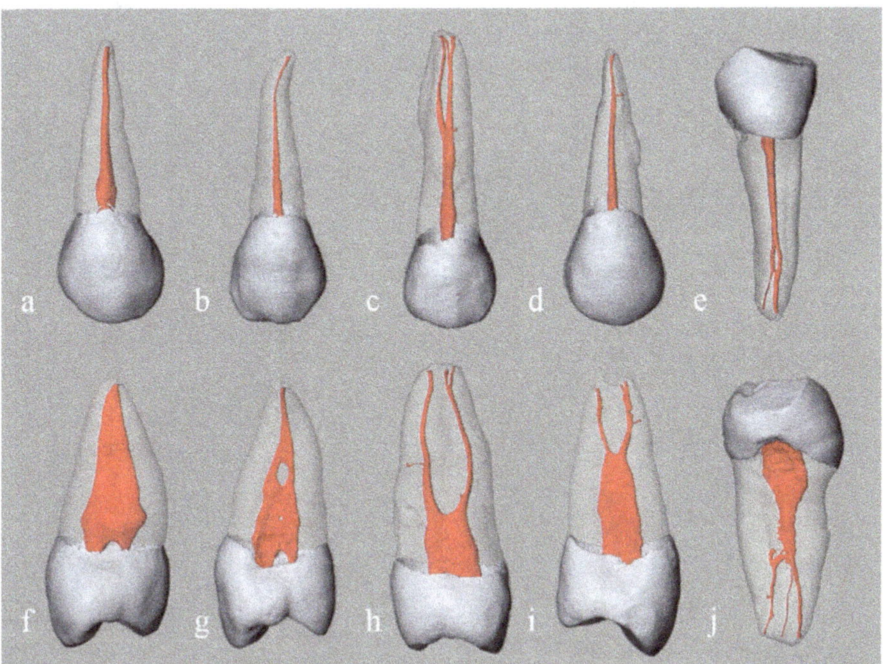

Figure 1 3-D image shows the enamel, dentin, and root canal with surface rendering. Root canal system classification: (a, f) type I of Tooth A, (b, g) type II of Tooth B, (c, h) type III of Tooth C, (d, i) type IV of Tooth D, (e, j) type V of Tooth E. Except for mandibular premolar E, teeth were maxillary premolars. The images in the top and bottom row are viewed from buccolingual and mesiodistal directions, respectively.

μm, except that the entrance of the additional canal in Tooth E is less than 60 μm.

Effect after instrumentation

The gross canal anatomy of all teeth was substantially changed after root canal preparation with F3 (Figure 3). A gradual increase in the diameter along the length of the canal was noted. The canal volumes and surface areas were increased after instrumentation in all teeth. Superposition images of noninstrumented and instrumented canals reveal a wide range (27.4-83.0%) in the proportion of surfaces unchanged during preparation. Table 1 shows the increases in canal volume (ΔV in mm^3) and surface area (ΔA in mm^2) and the percentages of unchanged surface (ΔP) for the five types canal systems. The type I canal system of Tooth A showed the least increases of canal volume and surface area (less than 5%) and largest unchanged surface (83%). The type II canal system of Tooth B and the type V canal system of Tooth E revealed the highest increases of canal volume and surface area (more than 146%), and least unchanged surface (less than 29%), and the additional canal of Tooth E remained untouched. In addition, the type III canal system of Tooth C and the type IV canal system of Tooth D had the middle increases of canal volume, surface area, and unchanged surface.

In the mesiodistal direction, all main canals were straightened after preparation with an F3 instrument and the straightening tended to occur toward the inner aspects of the curved parts of the root canal of teeth B, C, D and E (Figure 3). However, when viewed from the buccolingual direction, there was a transportation toward the outer aspects of the root canal and ledge formation at the apical third curve of Tooth B. Corresponding with the trend in canal transportation, more dentin was removed at the inner aspects of the curved parts and the outer aspect at the apical third curve of Tooth B (Figure 4).

The dentin wall thicknesses of canals after they were prepared with an F3 instrument are presented in Figure 5. Except for the mesial side of the lingual canal of Tooth D, all the dentin wall thicknesses were more than 0.3 mm. However, in a 1 mm zone near the apical foramen most of the dentin wall thicknesses were less than 0.3 mm. A hazardous zone was noted that was caused by the ledge formation in tooth B. No other preparation error or HPT instrument fractures occurred during the preparation of any canal.

Discussion

The present study aimed to reveal the differences made by including variations in internal anatomy of premolars into the study protocol for investigation of a single

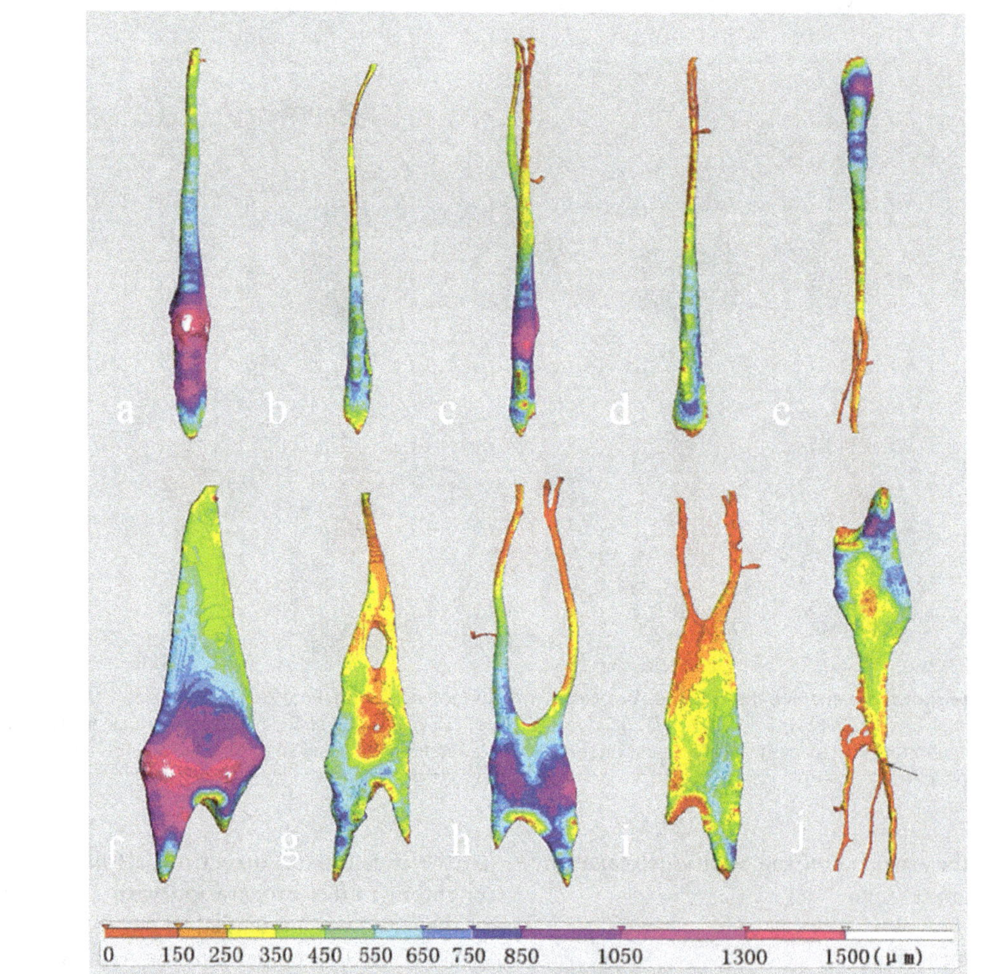

Figure 2 3-D color-coded image shows the canal diameter distribution of prepreparation canals. The bar indicates the diameter expressed in μm. The images in the top and bottom row are viewed from buccolingual and mesiodistal directions, respectively. Letters indicate the same teeth as in Figure 1. The arrow indicates the entrance of the additional canal of Tooth E.

instrumentation technique (HPT) using micro-CT and 3-D reconstruction technology. Because of the diversity of clinical cases in endodontic therapy, we wanted to develop a study protocol that integrates the canal system classification with various instruments to evaluate the preparation efficacy using 3-D reconstruction techniques. As a pilot study, only five teeth of different categories of root canal configuration (one each of types I, II, III, IV and V) were selected. The results showed the difference of morphological changes in the five types of root canal systems shaped with the same hand instrumentation technique. However, because of the limited numbers of teeth and techniques, no statistical evaluation could be made concerning the instrumentation technique.

In the current study, color-coded images obtained by 3-D reconstruction gave insight into the morphological changes in different types of root canal systems shaped with the same instrumentation technique.

In tooth A, there is a single flattened and straight root canal that was classified as type I canal system. After F3 instrumentation, 83% of the canal surface still remained unchanged. A similar result was also found for the widened canal after it was prepared by rotary ProTaper instruments [17].

In the type II canal system of tooth B, there are multiple or S-shaped curves in the canals and an isthmus communication between two root canals localized in the coronal third. After it was prepared with F3, the volume of the canal system increased by 150.2% and a ledge was formed in the apical curved part. The ledge was possibly caused by the additive effects of instrumentation to the working length for both the buccal and lingual canals, but the use of chelating agents [30] and the much more

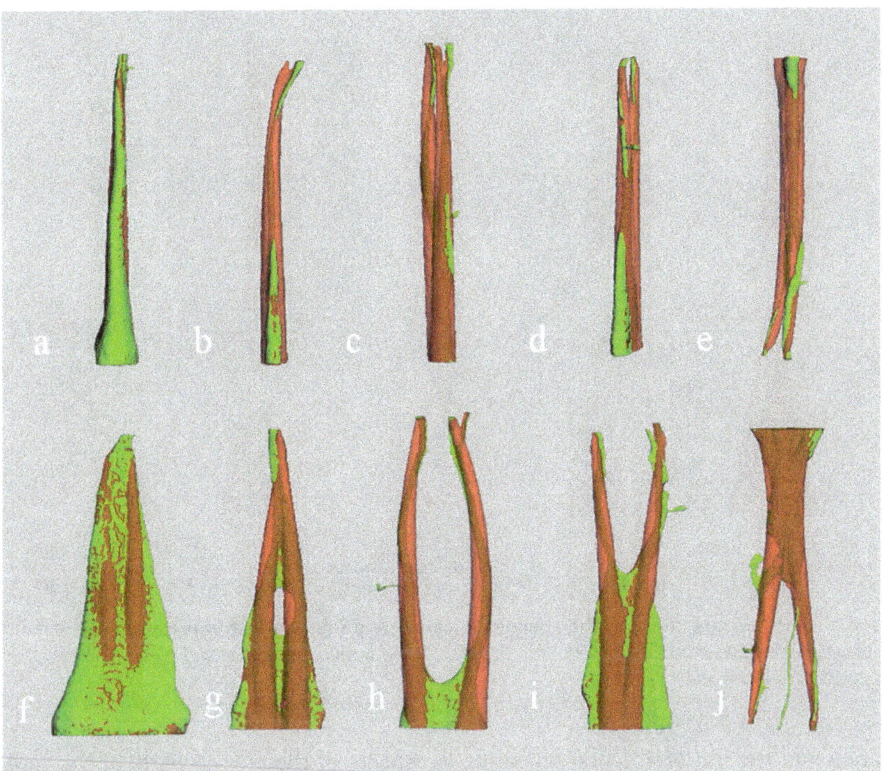

Figure 3 3-D color compound images showing the pre- and postpreparation effects. Prepreparation canal systems (green); the change in canal shapes post preparation (red). Mixed colors indicate superposition; green color alone shows the surfaces untouched during shaping. The images in the top and bottom row are viewed from buccolingual and mesiodistal directions, respectively. Letters indicate the same teeth as in Figure 1.

complicated root canal anatomy with curves in multiple positions and planes could also have contributed [15]. When the morphology of the root canals after preparation with S1, S2, F1, and F2 were also evaluated from 3-D canal models (data not shown), we found that significant transportation was created after the use of F1 and a ledge was formed after the use of F2. These results may suggest that the working length needs to be reconfirmed after instrumentation of a type II canal system as in Tooth B using F1 [31].

Table 1 Changes in canal volumes, surface areas, and the percentages of surface unchanged after preparation

	Tooth (canal system classification)				
	A (type I)	B (type II)	C (type III)	D (type IV)	E (type V)
Δ Volume (mm^3) *	0.84	5.67	7.30	4.05	4.16
	+4.8%	+150.2%	+96.7%	+85.6%	+146.3%
Δ Area (mm^2) *	2.95	19.99	28.26	15.59	17.57
	+3.4%	+42.9%	+42.4%	+32.9%	+49.0%
Δ Percentage (%)	83.0%	28.9%	41.1%	40.7%	27.4%

*Absolute scores (upper lines) and relative findings (lower lines), expressed as percentages of the initial values.

Although there were multiple or S-shaped curves in the type III canal system of Tooth C and the type IV canal system of Tooth D, we achieved a good instrumentation effect in the coronal and middle third after the use of F3. However, there was an additional untouched canal surface caused by apical transportation in the apical third and we found it impossible to prepare the accessory canal in the apical third using HPT instruments, except by exploring it with small, pre-curved K-files. In clinical cases where the canal systems are like those in Tooth C and Tooth D, these unchanged surfaces may harbor microorganisms and allow for the presence of residual infection post treatment [32].

In the type V canal system of Tooth E, it is regrettable that we could not accomplish the instrumentation of the additional canal after preparing the other two canals with F3. The volume increased up to 146.3%, mainly caused by the removal of the dentin protuberance. In clinical cases that have type V canal systems like Tooth E, CT data and 3-D canal models could be useful to

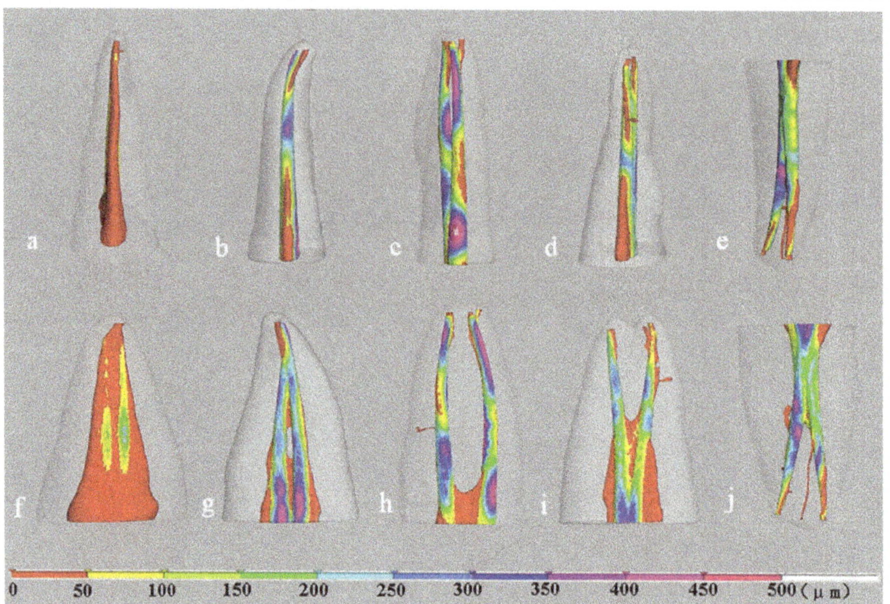

Figure 4 Color-coded distance images showing the changes in canal shape during instrumentation. The distance also indicates the amount of dentin removed. The images in the top and bottom row are viewed from buccolingual and mesiodistal directions, respectively. Letters indicate the same teeth as in Figure 1.

guide instrumentation and the use of a dental operating microscope and ultrasonic technique would be suitable for more efficiently exploring and finding the unusual canal access [1,33].

In the mesiodistal direction, all main canals were straightened after preparation with an F3 instrument and the straightening tended to occur toward the inner aspects of the curved parts of the root canal of teeth B, C, D and E (Figure 3). Our results are consistent with those of Yang [34]. In previous studies [35,36], the ProTaper Universal instruments with noncutting tips showed better performance than the conventional ProTaper instruments for root canal transportation. However, Özer reported that all three rotary systems

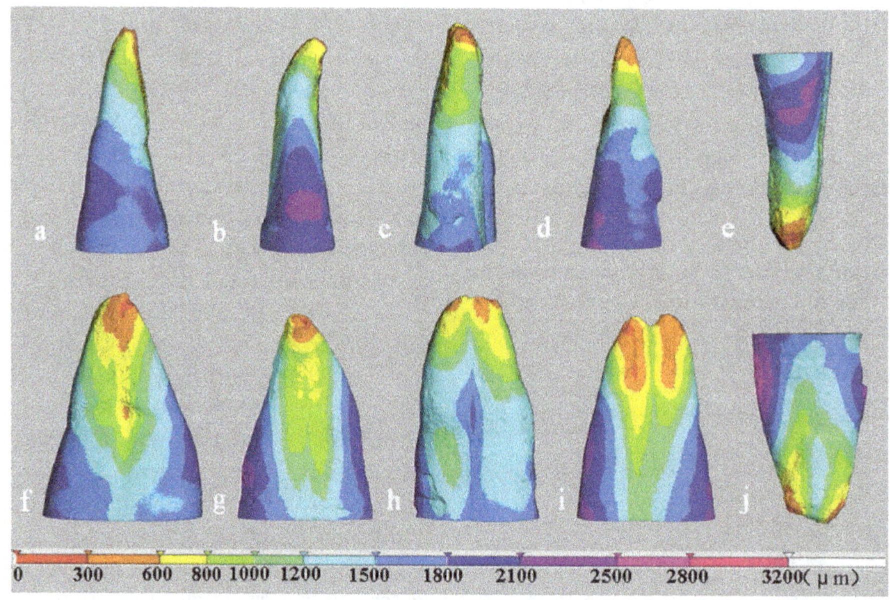

Figure 5 Color-coded images showing the distribution of thickness between the root external surface and canal surface. The images in the top and bottom row are viewed from buccolingual and mesiodistal directions, respectively. Letters indicate the same teeth as in Figure 1.

(ProTaper Universal, Hero 642 Apical, FlexMaster) showed similar results during preparation of curved root canals and for transportation despite their noncutting tips [37].

For the five types of canal systems in this study, there was a wide range (27.4-83.0%) in the percentage of surface unchanged during preparation. The untouched area was distributed in the recesses of the flattened canal, the isthmus of the type II canal system, the outer aspects of multiple or S-shaped curves, lateral and accessory canals, and the additional canal of Tooth E. It has been shown that frequent and copious irrigation with sodium hypochlorite not only flushes out debris from the canal lumen, but also dissolves organic tissue in the noninstrumented areas and the predentin layer [38]. More dentin debris can be removed from the isthmus, oval extensions in the root canal, and irregularities of the root canal wall by the use of ultrasonic irrigation with NaOCl as the irrigant [39,40]. Furthermore, in the mid-1990s, a method and device was presented that allowed cleansing of root canals without the need for manual instrumentation, and this noninstrumental hydrodynamic technique (NIT) showed an equal or even better cleanliness in all root sections than hand instrumentation [41,42]. Thus, the untouched area within each type of canal system configuration, although not amenable to mechanical debridement, might be cleaned by these means.

In daily clinical practice, there are some cases in which conventional intraoral radiography and/or panoramic radiography alone do not provide enough information on the pathologic condition [43]. It is important to visualize and to have knowledge of the internal tooth anatomy before undertaking endodontic therapy [4]. Micro-CT has emerged as a powerful tool for evaluation of root canal morphology. Unfortunately, this technique is not suitable for clinical use, but cone-beam computed tomography (CBCT) systems have now been introduced for 3-D imaging of hard tissues of the maxillofacial region, with minimal distortion [44]. When encountering a case with a complicated canal system (such as type II or V) by radiographic evaluation, CBCT may be a good choice to allow appropriate management of the endodontic problem for endodontists [19,44].

Conclusions

From 3-D color-coded images, we discovered obviously different morphological changes in the five types of root canal systems shaped with the same hand instrumentation technique. These results provide further information that premolars are among the most difficult teeth to be treated endodontically and that instrumentation techniques for the root canal systems of premolars should be judged individually depending on the 3-D canal configuration of each tooth. Further study is needed to demonstrate the differences made by including variations in internal anatomy of teeth into the study protocol for investigation of various instrumentation techniques.

Acknowledgements

This work was supported by the Key Clinical Program of the Ministry of Health of China. The funder had no role in study design, data collection and analysis, decision to publish, or preparation of the manuscript. The authors also wish to thank Hong-
Bing Wu for his help with the acquisition of the raw data.

Author details

[1]State Key Laboratory of Oral Diseases, West China College of Stomatology, Sichuan University, Chengdu, P.R. China. [2]Institute of Stomatology, Chinese PLA General Hospital, Beijing, P.R. China.

Authors' contributions

KZL, YG, RZ, TH and BG participated in the design of the experiment and wrote the manuscript. KZL and YG participated in the acquisition, analysis and interpretation of data. All authors read and approved the final manuscript.

Competing interests

The authors declare that they have no competing interests.

References

1. Al-Fouzan KS: **The microscopic diagnosis and treatment of a mandibular second premolar with four canals.** *Int Endod J* 2001, **34**:406-410.
2. Plotino G, Grande NM, Pecci R, Bedini R, Pameijer CN, Somma F: **Three-dimensional imaging using microcomputed tomography for studying tooth macromorphology.** *J Am Dent Assoc* 2006, **137**:1555-1561.
3. Rhodes JS, Pitt Ford TR, Lynch JA, Liepins PJ, Curtis RV: **Micro-computed tomography: a new tool for experimental endodontology.** *Int Endod J* 1999, **32**:165-170.
4. Vertucci FJ: **Root canal morphology and its relationship to endodontic procedures.** *Endod Topics* 2005, **10**:3-29.
5. de Alencar AH, Dummer PM, Oliveira HC, Pécora JD, Estrela C: **Procedural errors during root canal preparation using rotary NiTi instruments detected by periapical radiography and cone beam computed tomography.** *Braz Dent J* 2010, **21**:543-549.
6. Friedman S: **Prognosis of initial endodontic therapy.** *Endod Topics* 2002, **2**:59-88.
7. Hess W: **Formation of root canals in human teeth.** *J Natl Dent Assoc* 1921, **3**:704-725.
8. Weine FS: **Initiating endodontic treatment.** In *Endodontic Therapy..* 6 edition. Edited by: Weine FS. St. Louis, MO, USA: Mosby; 2004:106-110.
9. Yoshioka T, Villegas JC, Kobayashi C, Suda H: **Radiographic evaluation of root canal multiplicity in mandibular first premolars.** *J Endod* 2004, **30**:73-74.
10. Hülsmann M, Peters OA, Dummer PMH: **Mechanical preparation of root canals: shaping goals, techniques and means.** *Endod Topics* 2005, **10**:30-76.
11. Gekelman D, Ramamurthy R, Mirfarsi S, Paqué F, Peters OA: **Rotary nickel-titanium GT and ProTaper files for root canal shaping by novice operators: a radiographic and micro-computed tomography evaluation.** *J Endod* 2009, **35**:1584-1588.
12. Bürklein S, Hiller C, Huda M, Schäfer E: **Shaping ability and cleaning effectiveness of Mtwo versus coated and uncoated EasyShape instruments in severely curved root canals of extracted teeth.** *Int Endod J* 2011, **44**:447-457.
13. Fornari VJ, Silva-Sousa YT, Vanni JR, Pécora JD, Versiani MA, Sousa-Neto MD: **Histological evaluation of the effectiveness of increased apical**

enlargement for cleaning the apical third of curved canals. *Int Endod J* 2010, **43**:988-994.
14. Vaudt J, Bitter K, Neumann K, Kielbassa AM: **Ex vivo study on root canal instrumentation of two rotary nickel-titanium systems in comparison to stainless steel hand instruments.** *Int Endod J* 2009, **42**:22-33.
15. Peters OA: **Current challenges and concepts in the preparation of root canal systems: a review.** *J Endod* 2004, **30**:559-567.
16. Bergmans L, Van Cleynenbreugel J, Wevers M, Lambrechts P, Bergmans L: **A methodology for quantitative evaluation of root canal instrumentation using microcomputed tomography.** *Int Endod J* 2001, **34**:390-398.
17. Peters OA, Peters CI, Schönenberger K, Barbakow F: **ProTaper rotary root canal preparation: effects of canal anatomy on final shape analysed by micro CT.** *Int Endod J* 2003, **36**:86-92.
18. Jung M, Lommel D, Klimek J: **The imaging of root canal obturation using micro-CT.** *Int Endod J* 2005, **38**:617-626.
19. Zhang R, Yang H, Yu X, Wang H, Hu T, Dummer PMH: **Use of CBCT to identify the morphology of maxillary permanent molar teeth in a Chinese subpopulation.** *Int Endod J* 2011, **44**:162-169.
20. Özer SY: **Comparison of root canal transportation induced by three rotary systems with noncutting tips using computed tomography.** *Oral Surg Oral Med Oral Pathol Oral Radiol Endod* 2011, **111**:244-250.
21. Garip Y, Günday M: **The use of computed tomography when comparing nickel-titanium and stainless steel files during preparation of simulated curved canals.** *Int Endod J* 2001, **34**:452-457.
22. Schirrmeister JF, Strohl C, Altenburger MJ, Wrbas KT, Hellwig E: **Shaping ability and safety of five different rotary nickel-titanium instruments compared with stainless steel hand instrumentation in simulated curved root canals.** *Oral Surg Oral Med Oral Pathol Oral Radiol Endod* 2006, **101**:807-813.
23. Moore J, Fitz-Walter P, Parashos P: **A micro-computed tomographic evaluation of apical root canal preparation using three instrumentation techniques.** *Int Endod J* 2009, **42**:1057-1064.
24. Paqué F, Ganahl D, Peters OA: **Effects of root canal preparation on apical geometry assessed by micro-computed tomography.** *J Endod* 2009, **35**:1056-1059.
25. Saunders EM: **Hand instrumentation in root canal preparation.** *Endod Topics* 2005, **10**:163-167.
26. Aguiar CM, Câmara AC: **Radiological evaluation of the morphological changes of root canals shaped with ProTaper for hand use and the ProTaper and RaCe rotary instruments.** *Aust Endod J* 2008, **34**:115-119.
27. Pasqualini D, Scotti N, Tamagnone L, Ellena F, Berutti E: **Hand-operated and rotary ProTaper instruments: a comparison of working time and number of rotations in simulated root canals.** *J Endod* 2008, **34**:314-317.
28. Huang DM, Luo HX, Cheung GS, Zhang L, Tan H, Zhou XD: **Study of the progressive changes in canal shape after using different instruments by hand in simulated S-shaped canals.** *J Endod* 2007, **33**:986-989.
29. Gao Y, Peters OA, Wu H, Zhou X: **An application framework of three-dimensional reconstruction and measurement for endodontic research.** *J Endod* 2009, **35**:269-274.
30. Bramante CM, Betti LV: **Comparative analysis of curved root canal preparation using nickel-titanium instruments with or without EDTA.** *J Endod* 2000, **26**:278-280.
31. Garg N, Garg A: **procedural accidents.** In *Textbook of endodontics.*. 1 edition. Edited by: Garg N & Garg A. New Delhi, India: Jaypee Brothers Medical Publishers; 2007:262.
32. Nair PN, Henry S, Cano V, Vera J: **Microbial status of apical root canal system of human mandibular first molars with primary apical periodontitis after "one-visit" endodontic treatment.** *Oral Surg Oral Med Oral Pathol Oral Radiol Endod* 2005, **99**:231-252.
33. Alaçam T, Tinaz AC, Genç O, Kayaoglu G: **Second mesiobuccal canal detection in maxillary first molars using microscopy and ultrasonics.** *Aust Endod J* 2008, **34**:106-109.
34. Yang GB, Zhou XD, Zhang H, Wu HK: **Shaping ability of progressive versus constant taper instruments in simulated root canals.** *Int Endod J* 2006, **39**:791-799.
35. Guelzow A, Stamm O, Martus P, Kielbassa AM: **Comparative study of six rotary nickel titanium systems and hand instrumentation for root canal preparation.** *Int Endod J* 2005, **38**:743-752.
36. Javaheri HH, Javaheri GH: **A comparison of three Ni-Ti rotary instruments in apical transportation.** *J Endod* 2007, **33**:284-286.
37. Özer SY: **Comparison of root canal transportation induced by three rotary systems with noncutting tips using computed tomography.** *Oral Surg Oral Med Oral Pathol Oral Radiol Endo* 2011, **111**:244-250.
38. Cheung LH, Cheung GS: **Evaluation of a rotary instrumentation method for C-shaped canals with micro-computed tomography.** *J Endod* 2008, **34**:1233-1238.
39. Lee SJ, Wu MK, Wesselink PR: **The effectiveness of syringe irrigation and ultrasonics to remove debris from simulated irregularities within prepared root canal walls.** *Int Endod J* 2004, **37**:672-678.
40. Lumley PJ, Walmsley AD, Walton RE, Rippin JW: **Cleaning of oval canals using ultrasonic or sonic instrumentation.** *J Endod* 1993, **19**:453-457.
41. Lussi A, Nussbächer U, Grosrey J: **A novel noninstrumented technique for cleansing the root canal system.** *J Endod* 1993, **19**:549-553.
42. Lussi A, Portmann P, Nussbächer U, Imwinkelried S, Grosrey J: **Comparison of two devices for root canal cleansing by the noninstrumentation technology.** *J Endod* 1999, **25**:9-13.
43. Velvart P, Hecker H, Tillinger G: **Detection of the apical lesion and the mandibular canal in conventional radiography and computed tomography.** *Oral Surg Oral Med Oral Pathol Oral Radiol Endod* 2001, **92**:682-688.
44. Patel S: **New dimensions in endodontic imaging: Part 2. Cone-beam computed tomography.** *Int Endod J* 2009, **42**:463-475.

22

Novel computed tomographic chest metrics to detect pulmonary hypertension

Andrew L Chan[1*], Maya M Juarez[1], David K Shelton[2], Taylor MacDonald[2], Chin-Shang Li[3], Tzu-Chun Lin[4] and Timothy E Albertson[1]

Abstract

Background: Early diagnosis of pulmonary hypertension (PH) can potentially improve survival and quality of life. Detecting PH using echocardiography is often insensitive in subjects with lung fibrosis or hyperinflation. Right heart catheterization (RHC) for the diagnosis of PH adds risk and expense due to its invasive nature. Pre-defined measurements utilizing computed tomography (CT) of the chest may be an alternative non-invasive method of detecting PH.

Methods: This study retrospectively reviewed 101 acutely hospitalized inpatients with heterogeneous diagnoses, who consecutively underwent CT chest and RHC during the same admission. Two separate teams, each consisting of a radiologist and pulmonologist, blinded to clinical and RHC data, individually reviewed the chest CT's.

Results: Multiple regression analyses controlling for age, sex, ascending aortic diameter, body surface area, thoracic diameter and pulmonary wedge pressure showed that a main pulmonary artery (PA) diameter ≥29 mm (odds ratio (OR) = 4.8), right descending PA diameter ≥19 mm (OR = 7.0), true right descending PA diameter ≥ 16 mm (OR = 4.1), true left descending PA diameter ≥ 21 mm (OR = 15.5), right ventricular (RV) free wall ≥ 6 mm (OR = 30.5), RV wall/left ventricular (LV) wall ratio ≥0.32 (OR = 8.8), RV/LV lumen ratio ≥1.28 (OR = 28.8), main PA/ascending aorta ratio ≥0.84 (OR = 6.0) and main PA/descending aorta ratio ≥ 1.29 (OR = 5.7) were significant predictors of PH in this population of hospitalized patients.

Conclusion: This combination of easily measured CT-based metrics may, upon confirmatory studies, aid in the non-invasive detection of PH and hence in the determination of RHC candidacy in acutely hospitalized patients.

Background

Pulmonary hypertension (PH) is characterized by the presence of increased pulmonary vascular resistance caused by a combination of vasoconstriction, vascular remodeling, and thrombosis. Unfortunately, it can be potentially life-threatening as progressive right ventricular dilatation and hypertrophy may lead to heart failure within a few years [1,2]. As the treatment of PH has advanced dramatically over the past decade [3], early diagnosis may be key to its optimal treatment. While right heart catheterization (RHC) remains the "gold standard" for the measurement of pulmonary arterial pressure (PAP) [4], its invasive nature confers both risk and expense, and hence can delay diagnosis. Echocardiography as a noninvasive means of estimating PAP is limited in patients with obesity, lung hyperinflation and pulmonary fibrosis [5-7]. Magnetic resonance imaging methods have unfortunately also not been shown to accurately estimate PAP [8].

Other noninvasive PH screening tools include a prediction formula for estimating mean PAP using standard pulmonary function measurements in patients with idiopathic pulmonary fibrosis [9]. In addition, computed tomography (CT)-determined main pulmonary artery diameter has been shown to have excellent diagnostic value in the detection of PH in patients with parenchymal lung disease [10]. Such noninvasive approaches towards the detection of PH can reduce patient risk and expense, and may allow earlier patient screening towards a confirmatory RHC [11] or perhaps even obviate its necessity. This study retrospectively reviewed the records of inpatients who had

* Correspondence: alchan@ucdavis.edu
[1]Division of Pulmonary/Critical Care and Sleep Medicine, University of California, Davis Medical Center, Sacramento, CA and VA Northern California Health Care System, USA
Full list of author information is available at the end of the article

undergone a RHC together with a CT chest. A pre-defined set of CT chest-based metrics was then measured, and the relationship of these metrics to RHC-demonstrated PH was assessed.

Methods

Patients

The medical records of 101 hospitalized adult patients who consecutively underwent chest CT with or without contrast and a resting RHC during the same hospitalization were retrospectively reviewed. These patients had been admitted to this tertiary care teaching institution between January 2006 and July 2006. Approval for this review was obtained from the University of California, Davis Institutional Review Board with waiver of consent.

Measurements

Non-ECG-gated CT scans of the chest were performed using GE Lightspeed 16 scanners (GE Medical Systems; Milwaukee, Wisconsin). Our standard reconstruction protocol utilized helical technique, 5 mm slice every 5 mm with 1.25 mm every 1.25 mm reconstruction as well. The lung windows were also reconstructed with a "bone algorithm" and the soft tissue windows were reconstructed with a standard soft tissue smoothing algorithm. Standard lung windows (Width 1850, Level -740) on bone reconstruction algorithms and standard soft tissue windows (Width 400, Level 80) were used.

Two separate teams, each consisting of a radiologist and a pulmonologist, blinded to the clinical and hemodynamic data, independently reviewed the chest CT's. Pre-defined radiographic metrics corresponding to possible predictors of PH and to potential indicators of body habitus (to standardize predictors of PH) were measured by each team member and then averaged (Table 1).

Cardiac catheterization was performed at rest for clinical indications. Hemodynamic measurements, including mean pulmonary arterial pressure (mPAP), pulmonary wedge pressure (PWP), patient diagnoses and demographics (sex, age, height, and weight) were recorded. Body surface area (BSA) was calculated using the formula $BSA = (W^{0.425} \times H^{0.725}) \times 0.007184$, and body mass index (BMI) was calculated using the formula $BMI = weight (kg)/(height (cm))^2$.

PH was defined as a resting mPAP of 25 mmHg or greater; "no-PH" was defined as mPAP <25 mmHg.

Statistical Analyses

Summary statistics are reported as mean ± standard deviation (median; range). A two-sided Wilcoxon rank-sum test was used to compare each of the quantitative hypothesized predictors of PH and various demographics between the PH and no-PH groups. A two-sided Fisher's exact test was used to compare gender, obesity (BMI ≥30), and proportion of mechanical ventilation between the PH and no-PH groups. Statistical analyses involving the RV wall, RV lumen, LV wall, LV lumen, or interventricular septum were performed using only data derived from CT's that were contrast-enhanced.

Simple logistic regression was used to study the relationship between each hypothesized predictor of PH and the outcome PH vs. no-PH. The optimal cutoff point or upper limit of normal (ULN) for the quantitative hypothesized predictor of PH was determined using receiver operating characteristic (ROC) analysis, where the ULN was deemed to be the value that yielded the best trade off between sensitivity and specificity for each PH predictor. Multiple logistic regression was used to assess the relationship between each of the dichotomous hypothesized predictors of PH (i.e. variables dichotomized at the ULN cutoff) and the outcome PH vs. no-PH in order to control for sex, ascending aorta diameter (AA), BSA, thoracic diameter (TD), and pulmonary wedge pressure (PWP) >15. A p-value ≤ 0.05 was considered statistically significant. Statistical analyses were performed with SAS v 9.2 (SAS Institute Inc., Cary, NC, USA).

Results

101 consecutive hospitalized patients (46 women, 55 men) who underwent both CT chest and RHC were included. Their mean age was 61.4 ± 15.6 years (median = 60; range 23 to 91 years). Fifty-three patients had PH. Fifty-seven percent of patients with PH, and 52% of the no-PH patients were male. The underlying patient primary diagnoses reflect the reason for hospitalization, and were heterogeneous (Table 2).

The RHC's and chest CT's were performed a mean of 3 days apart (median = 1 day, range = 0-16 days); 46% of RHC's were performed on the same day as the chest CT's, and most within 2 days (60%). A majority of CT's were contrast-enhanced (36/48 in the no-PH group and 41/53 in the PH group). Overall, 43% (43/101) of patients had an elevated PWP (>15 mmHg), and most were in the PH group (40/53 = 75%).

There was no significant difference in age, height, or sex between the PH and no-PH groups. However, PH patients had a significantly higher mean weight, BSA, and BMI than no-PH patients (Table 3). 41% of PH patients were obese (BMI≥30) compared to 18% of no-PH patients (p = 0.0175).

A comparison of the predictors of PH revealed significantly higher measurements of PA, RDPA, true RDPA, and hilar diameters in the PH group. The RV free wall thickness, RV wall/LV wall ratio, hilar diameter, and

Table 1 Radiographic metrics

Hypothesized predictors of PH	How measured
Main pulmonary artery diameter (PA)	Widest lumen at or near level of PA bifurcation *
Right pulmonary artery diameter (RPA)	Widest lumen caudal to ascending aorta
Left pulmonary artery diameter (LPA)	Widest lumen
Right descending pulmonary artery (RDPA)	Distance from lateral wall of right bronchus intermedius to lateral wall of RDPA (equivalent to the RDPA measurement on a chest x-ray)
True right descending pulmonary artery (true RDPA)	RDPA lumen diameter only *
True left descending pulmonary artery (true LDPA)	Lumen diameter distal to left upper lobe bronchus takeoff
Right ventricular free wall (RV wall)	Mid-ventricle *
Right ventricular lumen diameter (RV lumen)	Mid-ventricle *
Left ventricular free wall (LV wall)	Mid-ventricle *
Left ventricular lumen diameter (LV lumen)	Mid-ventricle *
IV septum bowing into LV	Yes or no
Left apical artery to corresponding bronchus ratio	Most apical bronchovascular pair
Hilar diameter (HD)	At level of right middle lobe bronchus takeoff
Hilar/Thoracic ratio	HD/Inner thoracic diameter (TD) measured at same level as HD
Landmarks used to standardize predictors of PH	
Ascending aorta diameter (AA)	Widest diameter at the level of the PA measurement *
Descending aorta diameter (DA)	At same level as AA *

* Also see Figure 1.

main PA/AA ratio were also significantly increased in this group (Table 4). Inter-observer variability in measurements within each team was less than 5%.

Relationship of hypothesized predictors of PH to the dichotomous outcome PH vs. no-PH

The seven significant predictors of PH in Table 4 were also found to be significantly correlated to the outcome (PH vs. no-PH) when using logistic regression. An OR and ULN for each predictor of PH was determined from these regression analyses. The optimal cutoff point or ULN was determined by the ROC analysis to be the value that yielded the best tradeoff between sensitivity and specificity for each PH quantitative predictor (Table 5).

Table 2 Patient primary diagnoses

	N
Coronary arterial disease	27
Congestive heart failure	22
Valvular disease	12
Pulmonary embolism	5
Cardiac arrhythmia	4
Pulmonary infection	4
Aortic aneurysm or dissection	3
Idiopathic PH	3
Interstitial lung disease	3
ARDS	2
Cardiac tamponade	2
COPD	2
Obstructive sleep apnea	2
Other *	10

*Other includes: cancer, anorexigen drug use, cerebrovascular accident, end-stage renal disease, hepatopulmonary syndrome, kyphoscoliosis, prior history of lung transplant, malignant hypertension, scleroderma, and trauma.

Controlling for body size, age, sex and PWP

Each dichotomous CT-derived predictor of PH (e.g. PA diameter ≥ 29 mm) and potential confounders (age, sex, AA, BSA, thoracic diameter, and PWP category (>15 or ≤ 15 mmHg)) were regressed to the outcome, PH vs. no-PH, using multiple logistic regression models. In addition to the parameters in Table 5, two additional predictors of PH (interventricular (IV) septum bowing into LV and main PA/AA ratio > 1) were included in these analyses. Several predictors of PH were found to be statistically significant when controlling for age, sex, PWP, and indicators of body size (Table 6). Diagrammatic representations of the significant predictors of PH from Table 6 are represented in Figure 1.

Discussion

A National Institutes of Health Registry found that the mean time from onset of symptoms (dyspnea 60%, fatigue 19%, syncope 8%, and chest pain 7%) to correct diagnosis of PH was 2 years [12]. Early diagnosis is key to effective treatment and potential prevention of further vascular remodeling. When ineffectively treated, the median survival of patients with idiopathic PH is

Table 3 Patient demographics

	PH mean ± SD	No-PH mean ± SD	P
Age (yrs)	59.5 ± 15.4	63.5 ± 15.8	0.1948
Sex (% men)	56.6	52.1	0.6923
Height (cm)	169.8 ± 10.9	167.4 ± 10.8	0.3395
Weight (kg)	**85.4 ± 22.1**	**71.7 ± 18.5**	**0.0029**
BSA	**1.9 ± 0.3**	**1.8 ± 0.3**	**0.0085**
BMI	**29.6 ± 7.1**	**25.3 ± 4.9**	**0.0024**
Mechanical ventilation (%)	15.1	8.3	0.3650

Table 4 Comparison of hypothesized predictors of PH in the PH and no-PH groups

	PH mean ± SD	No-PH mean ± SD	P
Main PA diameter (mm)	**32.2 ± 5.3**	**29.0 ± 3.9**	**0.0021**
Left PA diameter (mm)	24.2 ± 4.6	22.9 ± 3.2	0.1225
Right PA diameter (mm)	24.0 ± 4.3	23.4 ± 3.7	0.4618
RDPA diameter (mm)	**19.4 ± 4.4**	**17.0 ± 2.6**	**0.0072**
True RDPA diameter (mm)	**15.3 ± 3.7**	**13.4 ± 2.4**	**0.0027**
True LDPA diameter (mm)	19.4 ± 3.8	18.1 ± 3.4	0.0509
RV free wall thickness (mm)	**5.4 ± 2.4**	**4.0 ± 1.2**	**0.0023**
RV lumen diameter (mm)	36.9 ± 10.1	35.3 ± 7.9	0.4293
LV free wall (mm)	11.6 ± 3.6	11.1 ± 3.3	0.4820
LV lumen (mm)	44.0 ± 15.5	42.9 ± 9.5	0.9942
Hilar diameter (mm)	**127.1 ± 13.7**	**118.2 ± 12.0**	**0.0018**
RV wall/LV wall ratio	**0.51 ± 0.25**	**0.38 ± 0.14**	**0.0214**
RV lumen/LV lumen ratio	1.02 ± 0.85	0.85 ± 0.26	0.9796
L apical artery/bronchus ratio	1.33 ± 0.43	1.27 ± 0.35	0.6023
Hilar/thoracic ratio	0.51 ± 0.04	0.49 ± 0.04	0.0687
Main PA/AA ratio	**0.97 ± 0.2**	**0.86 ± 0.13**	**0.0014**
Main PA/DA ratio	1.24 ± 0.27	1.15 ± 0.17	0.2023
	PH %	no-PH %	
IV septum bowed into LV	16.7	2.7	0.0608

See table 1 for definitions of radiographic metrics.

2.8 years [13]. However over the past 2 decades, PH treatment options have evolved to improve both survival and quality of life [14]. This retrospective analysis suggests that CT-based metrics can help detect PH, potentially enabling earlier treatment.

Although no significant differences in age, height or gender were found between PH and no-PH patients in this study, patients in the PH group demonstrated significantly greater body weight, BMI and BSA. There were significantly more obese patients in the PH group (41%) compared to the no-PH group (18%). Nevertheless, most patients in both groups were not obese. The presence of obesity, though, may contribute to PH, as Hague et al [15] found pulmonary hypertensive changes in 72% of obese subjects, a statistically higher proportion than when compared to the control group ($p < 0.001$).

Despite the heterogeneity of the primary diagnoses of patients in this study, the commonest diagnoses of coronary arterial disease (CAD) and congestive heart failure (CHF) were approximately equal in preponderance in both the PH group and the no-PH group (47% vs. 50%, respectively). A majority of patients (76%) demonstrated an elevated PWP in the PH group, compared to 6% in the no-PH group. This may be due in part to the higher rate of obesity in the PH group, and possible development of obesity cardiomyopathy, in the absence of other risk factors such as CAD [16].

The current study not only confirmed a significant difference in the PA diameter between PH and no-PH patients, but also showed significant differences in measurement of the RDPA, True RDPA, RV free wall thickness, RV Wall/LV Wall ratio, Hilar Diameter, and Main PA/AA ratio (Table 4). These pre-defined CT-based parameters had been previously selected at least in part on the basis of the existing published literature [17-20], modified and augmented using straightforward to

Table 5 Simple logistic regression of hypothesized predictors of PH to outcome (PH vs. no-PH)

	P	OR	Lower 95% CI	Upper 95% CI	ROC AUC	Sensitivity (%)	Specificity (%)	Upper limit of normal (ULN) cutoff
Main PA diameter (mm)	**0.0020**	**1.2**	**1.1**	**1.3**	**0.68**	**67.9**	**56.3**	**29 mm**
Left PA diameter (mm)	0.1158	1.1	1.0	1.2	0.59	47.2	62.5	24 mm
Right PA diameter (mm)	0.4187	1.0	0.9	1.1	0.54	37.7	64.6	25 mm
RDPA diameter (mm)	**0.0031**	**1.2**	**1.1**	**1.4**	**0.66**	**43.4**	**79.2**	**19 mm**
True RDPA diameter (mm)	**0.0053**	**1.2**	**1.1**	**1.4**	**0.67**	**32.1**	**83.3**	**16 mm**
True LDPA diameter (mm)	0.0814	1.1	1.0	1.2	0.61	32.1	77.1	21 mm
RV Free Wall thickness (mm)	**0.0070**	**1.5**	**1.1**	**2.1**	**0.69**	**21.4**	**91.9**	**6 mm**
RV Lumen diameter (mm)	0.4248	1.0	1.0	1.1	0.55	66.7	18.9	30 mm
LV Free Wall (mm)	0.5105	1.0	0.9	1.2	0.55	9.5	78.4	15 mm
LV Lumen (mm)	0.7136	1.0	1.0	1.0	0.50	0.0	83.3	57 mm
Hilar diameter (mm)	**0.0017**	**1.1**	**1.0**	**1.1**	**0.68**	**54.7**	**68.8**	**124 mm**
RV wall/LV wall ratio	**0.0152**	**22.8**	**1.8**	**283.4**	**0.64**	**61.9**	**64.9**	**0.32**
RV lumen/LV lumen ratio	0.2942	1.8	0.6	5.3	0.50	19.0	94.4	1.28
L apical artery/broncus ratio	0.4379	1.5	0.5	4.2	0.53	11.3	87.5	1.75
Hilar/thoracic ratio	0.0785	>5000	0.4	>5000	0.61	35.8	79.2	0.52
Main PA/AA ratio	**0.0035**	**58.7**	**3.8**	**900.7**	**0.68**	**79.2**	**50.0**	**0.84**
Main PA/DA ratio	0.0626	6.7	0.9	50.3	0.57	30.2	83.3	1.29

See table 1 for definitions of radiographic metrics.

Table 6 Multiple logistic regression to control for potential confounders

	P	OR	AUC	Sensitivity (%)	Specificity (%)
Main PA diameter ≥29 mm	**0.0196**	**4.8**	**0.93**	**77.4**	**89.6**
Left PA diameter ≥24 mm	0.2160	2.6	0.92	77.4	87.5
Right PA diameter ≥25 mm	0.4461	1.9	0.91	73.6	93.8
RDPA diameter ≥19 mm	**0.0059**	**7.0**	**0.93**	**83.0**	**85.4**
True RDPA diameter ≥16 mm	**0.0487**	**4.1**	**0.92**	**83.0**	**87.5**
True LDPA diameter ≥21 mm	**0.0075**	**15.5**	**0.93**	**79.2**	**91.7**
RV free wall ≥6 mm	**0.0303**	**30.5**	**0.95**	**81.0**	**91.9**
RV lumen ≥30 mm	0.0915	5.8	0.95	92.9	73.0
LV free wall ≥15 mm	0.1607	5.2	0.95	85.7	83.8
LV lumen ≥57 mm	0.3945	3.0	0.94	76.2	88.9
Hilar diameter ≥124 mm	0.2968	2.2	0.92	81.1	75.0
RV wall/LV wall ratio ≥0.32	**0.0141**	**8.8**	**0.96**	**78.6**	**83.8**
RV lumen/LV lumen ratio ≥1.28	**0.0196**	**28.8**	**0.95**	**85.7**	**86.1**
L apical artery/bronchus ratio ≥1.75	0.2851	3.5	0.92	75.5	87.5
Hilar/thoracic ratio ≥0.52	0.0757	3.7	0.92	75.5	87.5
Main PA/AA ratio ≥0.84	**0.0208**	**6.0**	**0.93**	**73.6**	**91.7**
Main PA/DA ratio ≥1.29	**0.0269**	**5.7**	**0.93**	**77.4**	**89.6**
IV septum bowing into LV (yes or no)	0.1053	11.6	0.95	81.0	89.2
Main PA/AA ratio >1	**0.0085**	**9.1**	**0.93**	**86.8**	**79.2**

Regression of the outcome variable (PH vs. no-PH) to the predictors:

ULN for each hypothesized predictor of PH, age, sex, ascending aorta diameter (AA), BSA, thoracic diameter (TD), and pulmonary wedge pressure (PWP) >15 mmHg.

Note: one logistic regression model was created for each hypothesized predictor of PAH. For example, the analysis in the first row above included the predictors: Main PA diameter ≥29, age, sex, AA, BSA, TD, and PWP >15. See table 1 for definitions of radiographic metrics.

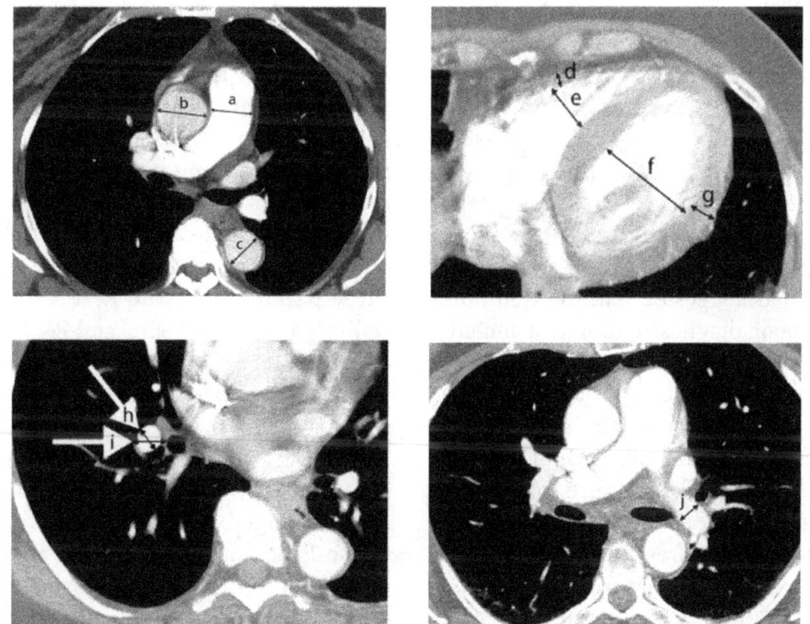

Figure 1 Radiographic measurements. The radiometric measurements used to derive the predictors of PH that were found to be significant in Table 6 included: main PA (a), AA (b), DA (c), RV free wall (d), RV lumen (e), LV lumen (f), LV free wall (g), true RDPA (h), RDPA as would be seen on chest x-ray (i), and true LDPA (j).

measure CT-based metrics. For example, the width of the RDPA has been shown to be a significant predictor for PH [18,20], as has the diastolic RV outflow tract wall thickness [21]. In addition to this, this study novelly found a significant difference between the PH group and no-PH group in terms of the true RDPA diameter. Certainly, the presence of significant abnormalities in the measurements above ought to promptly engender further investigation as to the presence of pulmonary hypertension.

Modeling to control for the potential confounders [22-24] of age, sex, AA, BSA, thoracic diameter, and especially PWP (>15 or ≤15 mmHg) using multiple logistic regression, showed that 10 parameters were significant predictors of PH, despite the fact that 76% of patients in the PH group had an elevated PWP, and 30.7% of all patients were obese (Table 6).

Beiderlinden et al, in a study of ARDS patients with at least moderate PH (mean PA pressure of >30 mmHg), reported a sensitivity of 54% and a specificity of 63% utilizing a pulmonary artery trunk diameter ≥29 mm [25]. They also suggested that CT chest parameters were an unreliable tool in the detection of PH in ARDS patients; speculating that pulmonary vascular changes in chronic rather than acute PH may lead to remodeling of the PA and hence enlargement of its diameter. While it is difficult to ascertain the proportion of patients in the current study with chronic PH, controlling for age, sex, AA, BSA, thoracic diameter, and PWP category yielded a superior sensitivity and specificity for prediction of PH of 77.4% and 89.6%, respectively using an ULN value for PA diameter of ≥29 mmHg.

The current study also found that an ULN cutoff of 1.29 for the main PA/DA ratio and an ULN cutoff of >0.84 for the main PA/AA ratio could both be used to predict PH. While this main PA/AA ratio had been demonstrated in a previous study to strongly correlate with mPAP in a patient population under 50 years of age also with heterogenous diagnoses [23], a more recent study however has suggested that the traditional PA/AA ratio >1 is a poor diagnostic tool as it includes normal patients and is negatively affected by age [26]. In contrast, our study found significance using a main PA/AA ratio of ≥0.84 or >1 in acutely ill patients even after controlling for age in detecting the presence of PH.

Other novel predictors of PH that were found to be significant in this study included specific cardiac measurements, particularly the RV free wall of ≥6 mm, RV lumen/LV lumen ratio ≥1.28, and RV wall/LV wall ratio ≥0.32. Of these, the RV lumen/LV lumen ratio ≥1.28 showed high sensitivity (85.7%) and specificity (86.1%, OR = 28.8). Both the true LDPA diameter ≥21 mm and the true RDPA diameter ≥16 mm also afforded good sensitivities (79.2% and 83%, respectively) and high specificities (91.7% and 87.5%, respectively), with OR's of 15.5 and 4.1.

An ULN cutoff of ≥6 mm for the RV Free Wall showed significant promise as a predictor of PH (p = 0.0303) with a high OR of 30.5, and sensitivity of 81% and specificity of 91.9%. It has been suggested that the right ventricle adapts to the increased afterload in PH by increasing muscle mass and hence wall thickness, and by assuming a more rounded shape [27]. Other investigators [28] studied 16 patients with primary pulmonary hypertension and found an increase in resting right ventricular mass. Cardiovascular Magnetic Resonance Imaging may be helpful to further assess right ventricular structure and function in PH patients [29]. PA volume estimation utilizing CT-volumetry may also be useful in PH detection [30].

The current study has a number of limitations in part due to its retrospective nature. Selection bias may have been introduced by only including patients who underwent both RHC and chest CT. Nevertheless, a consecutive cohort of acutely hospitalized patients with heterogeneous diagnoses were studied, of whom about half had an acute primary diagnosis of CAD or CHF. While the majority of patients in the PH group were associated with an elevated PWP, controlling for this using multiple logistic regression models still resulted in statistical significance for eight pre-defined CT chest metrics for detecting PH.

Additional limitations include the fact that some patients underwent CT scanning breathing spontaneously, whilst others were on positive pressure ventilation. However, this was limited to a minority of patients (only 8.3% in the no-PH group and 15.1% in the PH group). Positive pressure ventilation may have affected end-expiratory PA diameter due to varying intrathoracic pressures and lung volumes, affecting transmural PA pressure. In a secondary analysis of the non-mechanically ventilated patient cohort (n = 89), all significant findings reported in Table 6 retained their significance, except for three parameters (true RDPA diameter ≥16 mm, RV wall/LV wall ratio ≥0.32, and RV lumen/LV lumen ratio ≥1.28). The loss of significance in these three parameters is unclear, and may have been related to a smaller sample size, a loss of power or physiological reasons.

The RHC's and chest CT's were performed a mean of 3 days apart (median = 1 day), another limitation. It is acknowledged that significant changes in PWP and hence PAP can occur even on an hourly or daily basis, depending on treatment. Nevertheless, relatively short delays between measurements are likely to only result in small and randomly distributed errors [25].

Standard CT window widths were used in this study, thus minimizing variability in anatomic measurements when compared to using non-standard window widths via a computer program using density profiles [22]. Clinician bias in measuring parameters was limited by using separate teams, blinded to the clinical and hemodynamic data, to independently review the chest CT's.

The high incidence of CT contrast enhancement in 75% of the no-PH group and in 77% of the PH group may have aided in metric measurement. Nevertheless, others have reported good inter-observer measurement accuracy in a study of a heterogeneous group of patients with PH, utilizing a mixture of enhanced and unenhanced CT scans of the chest [23]. Edwards et al also demonstrated that the measurement of the pulmonary artery diameter was extremely reproducible using unenhanced CT scans, with a standard deviation for the difference between 2 measurements of less than 0.08 cm and a mean difference of only 0.02 cm [22].

Conclusions

This study has shown that there is a group of CT chest-derived predictors of PH that shows significance, even after controlling for age, sex, AA, BSA, thoracic diameter, and especially PWP. Novel predictors including RV free wall ≥ 6 mm, RV lumen/LV lumen ratio ≥ 1.28, True LDPA diameter ≥ 21 mm and True RDPA diameter ≥ 16 mm amongst others, may serve as a template to detect PH in such patients with acute illnesses requiring hospitalization and aid in determining which patients require RHC. A confirmatory prospective multicentre study utilizing the significant CT chest metrics above, and large enough to enable pre-defined subset analysis on the various WHO Groups of PH, is needed.

Abbreviations

AA: ascending aorta; AUC: area under the curve; BMI: body mass index; BSA: body surface area; CAD: coronary arterial disease; CHF: congestive heart failure; CT: computed tomography; DA: descending aorta; IV: interventricular; LDPA: left descending pulmonary artery; LV: left ventricle; mPAP: mean pulmonary arterial pressure; OR: odds ratio; PA: pulmonary artery; PAP: pulmonary arterial pressure; PH: pulmonary hypertension; PWP: pulmonary wedge pressure; RDPA: right descending pulmonary artery; RHC: right-heart catheterization; ROC: receiver operating characteristic; RV: right ventricle; TD: thoracic diameter; TL: tracheal lumen; ULN: upper limit of normal.

Acknowledgements

Statistical support for this publication was made possible by Grant Number UL1 RR024146 from the National Center for Research Resources (NCRR), a component of the National Institutes of Health (NIH), and NIH Roadmap for Medical Research. Its contents are solely the responsibility of the authors and do not necessarily represent the official view of NCRR or NIH. Information on Re-engineering the Clinical Research Enterprise can be obtained from http://nihroadmap.nih.gov/clinicalresearch/overview-translational.asp

Author details

[1]Division of Pulmonary/Critical Care and Sleep Medicine, University of California, Davis Medical Center, Sacramento, CA and VA Northern California Health Care System, USA. [2]Department of Radiology, University of California, Davis Medical Center, Sacramento, CA, USA. [3]Department of Public Health Sciences, Division of Biostatistics, University of California, Davis, CA, USA. [4]Department of Statistics, University of California, Davis, CA, USA.

Authors' contributions

ALC: study concept and design; acquisition, analysis and interpretation of data; and drafting of manuscript. MMJ: study concept and design, coordination for the acquisition of data, analysis and interpretation of data, and drafting of manuscript. DKS: study concept and design; acquisition, analysis and interpretation of data; and critical revision of manuscript. TM: acquisition, analysis and interpretation of data; and critical revision of manuscript. CSL: analysis and interpretation of data; statistics expertise; and drafting of manuscript TCL: analysis and interpretation of data; statistics expertise; and drafting of manuscript. TEA: study concept and design; analysis and interpretation of data; and critical revision of manuscript.

Competing interests

The authors declare that they have no competing interests.

References

1. D'Alonzo GE, Barst RJ, Ayres SM, Bergofsky EH, Brundage BH, Detre KM, Fishman AP, Goldring RM, Groves BM, Kernis JT, *et al*: **Survival in patients with primary pulmonary hypertension. Results from a national prospective registry.** *Ann Intern Med* 1991, **115(5)**:343-349.
2. Wilkins MR, Paul GA, Strange JW, Tunariu N, Gin-Sing W, Banya WA, Westwood MA, Stefanidis A, Ng LL, Pennell DJ, *et al*: **Sildenafil versus Endothelin Receptor Antagonist for Pulmonary Hypertension (SERAPH) study.** *Am J Respir Crit Care Med* 2005, **171(11)**:1292-1297.
3. Rubin LJ: **Pulmonary arterial hypertension.** *Proc Am Thorac Soc* 2006, **3(1)**:111-115.
4. Devaraj A, Hansell DM: **Computed tomography signs of pulmonary hypertension: old and new observations.** *Clin Radiol* 2009, **64(8)**:751-760.
5. Perez-Enguix D, Morales P, Tomas JM, Vera F, Lloret RM: **Computed tomographic screening of pulmonary arterial hypertension in candidates for lung transplantation.** *Transplant Proc* 2007, **39(7)**:2405-2408.
6. Arcasoy SM, Christie JD, Ferrari VA, Sutton MS, Zisman DA, Blumenthal NP, Pochettino A, Kotloff RM: **Echocardiographic assessment of pulmonary hypertension in patients with advanced lung disease.** *Am J Respir Crit Care Med* 2003, **167(5)**:735-740.
7. Nathan SD, Noble PW, Tuder RM: **Idiopathic pulmonary fibrosis and pulmonary hypertension: connecting the dots.** *Am J Respir Crit Care Med* 2007, **175(9)**:875-880.
8. Roeleveld RJ, Marcus JT, Boonstra A, Postmus PE, Marques KM, Bronzwaer JG, Vonk-Noordegraaf A: **A comparison of noninvasive MRI-based methods of estimating pulmonary artery pressure in pulmonary hypertension.** *J Magn Reson Imaging* 2005, **22(1)**:67-72.
9. Zisman DA, Karlamangla AS, Kawut SM, Shlobin OA, Saggar R, Ross DJ, Schwarz MI, Belperio JA, Ardehali A, Lynch JP, *et al*: **Validation of a method to screen for pulmonary hypertension in advanced idiopathic pulmonary fibrosis.** *Chest* 2008, **133(3)**:640-645.
10. Tan RT, Kuzo R, Goodman LR, Siegel R, Haasler GB, Presberg KW: **Utility of CT scan evaluation for predicting pulmonary hypertension in patients with parenchymal lung disease. Medical College of Wisconsin Lung Transplant Group.** *Chest* 1998, **113(5)**:1250-1256.
11. Zisman DA, Ross DJ, Belperio JA, Saggar R, Lynch JP, Ardehali A, Karlamangla AS: **Prediction of pulmonary hypertension in idiopathic pulmonary fibrosis.** *Respir Med* 2007, **101(10)**:2153-2159.
12. Rich S, Dantzker DR, Ayres SM, Bergofsky EH, Brundage BH, Detre KM, Fishman AP, Goldring RM, Groves BM, Koerner SK, *et al*: **Primary pulmonary hypertension. A national prospective study.** *Ann Intern Med* 1987, **107(2)**:216-223.
13. McGoon MD, Kane GC: **Pulmonary hypertension: diagnosis and management.** *Mayo Clin Proc* 2009, **84(2)**:191-207.
14. Humbert M, Sitbon O, Simonneau G: **Treatment of pulmonary arterial hypertension.** *N Engl J Med* 2004, **351(14)**:1425-1436.
15. Haque AK, Gadre S, Taylor J, Haque SA, Freeman D, Duarte A: **Pulmonary and cardiovascular complications of obesity: an autopsy study of 76 obese subjects.** *Arch Pathol Lab Med* 2008, **132(9)**:1397-1404.
16. Dela Cruz CS, Matthay RA: **Role of obesity in cardiomyopathy and pulmonary hypertension.** *Clin Chest Med* 2009, **30(3)**:509-523, ix.

17. Kanemoto N, Furuya H, Etoh T, Sasamoto H, Matsuyama S: **Chest roentgenograms in primary pulmonary hypertension.** *Chest* 1979, **76(1)**:45-49.
18. Miller MR, Gorecka DM, Bishop JM: **Radiological prediction of pulmonary hypertension in chronic obstructive pulmonary disease.** *Eur Heart J* 1984, **5(7)**:581-587.
19. Chetty KG, Brown SE, Light RW: **Identification of pulmonary hypertension in chronic obstructive pulmonary disease from routine chest radiographs.** *Am Rev Respir Dis* 1982, **126(2)**:338-341.
20. Satoh T, Kyotani S, Okano Y, Nakanishi N, Kunieda T: **Descriptive patterns of severe chronic pulmonary hypertension by chest radiography.** *Respir Med* 2005, **99(3)**:329-336.
21. Revel MP, Faivre JB, Remy-Jardin M, Delannoy-Deken V, Duhamel A, Remy J: **Pulmonary hypertension: ECG-gated 64-section CT angiographic evaluation of new functional parameters as diagnostic criteria.** *Radiology* 2009, **250(2)**:558-566.
22. Edwards PD, Bull RK, Coulden R: **CT measurement of main pulmonary artery diameter.** *Br J Radiol* 1998, **71(850)**:1018-1020.
23. Ng CS, Wells AU, Padley SP: **A CT sign of chronic pulmonary arterial hypertension: the ratio of main pulmonary artery to aortic diameter.** *J Thorac Imaging* 1999, **14(4)**:270-278.
24. Karazincir S, Balci A, Seyfeli E, Akoglu S, Babayigit C, Akgul F, Yalcin F, Egilmez E: **CT assessment of main pulmonary artery diameter.** *Diagn Interv Radiol* 2008, **14(2)**:72-74.
25. Beiderlinden M, Kuehl H, Boes T, Peters J: **Prevalence of pulmonary hypertension associated with severe acute respiratory distress syndrome: predictive value of computed tomography.** *Intensive Care Med* 2006, **32(6)**:852-857.
26. Lin FY, Devereux RB, Roman MJ, Meng J, Jow VM, Jacobs A, Weinsaft JW, Shaw LJ, Berman DS, Callister TQ, *et al*: **Cardiac chamber volumes, function, and mass as determined by 64-multidetector row computed tomography: mean values among healthy adults free of hypertension and obesity.** *JACC Cardiovasc Imaging* 2008, **1(6)**:782-786.
27. Bogaard HJ, Abe K, Vonk Noordegraaf A, Voelkel NF: **The right ventricle under pressure: cellular and molecular mechanisms of right-heart failure in pulmonary hypertension.** *Chest* 2009, **135(3)**:794-804.
28. Nootens M, Wolfkiel CJ, Chomka EV, Rich S: **Understanding right and left ventricular systolic function and interactions at rest and with exercise in primary pulmonary hypertension.** *Am J Cardiol* 1995, **75(5)**:374-377.
29. Blyth KG, Peacock AJ: **Imaging the right ventricle in pulmonary hypertension.** *PVRI Review* 2009, **1**:180-185.
30. Froelich JJ, Koenig H, Knaak L, Krass S, Klose KJ: **Relationship between pulmonary artery volumes at computed tomography and pulmonary artery pressures in patients with- and without pulmonary hypertension.** *Eur J Radiol* 2008, **67(3)**:466-471.

23

Air column in esophagus and symptoms of gastroesophageal reflux disease

Alijavad Moosavi[1], Hanieh Raji[2], Mojtaba Teimoori[3] and Shadi Ghourchian[4*]

Abstract

Background: During imaging of the normal esophagus, air is often detected. The purpose of this study was to determine the correlation between the appearance of air bubbles on imaging and Gastroesophageal Reflux Disease (GERD) symptoms.

Methods: The cross-sectional imaging study was conducted at Rasole Akram Hospital, Tehran, Iran. A total of 44 patients underwent X-ray computed tomography (CT) scanning; the presence of air in the esophagus and visible on CT imaging was scrutinized.

Results: The average age of the subjects was 59 and the male to female ratio was 0.83. We found a significant relationship between the presence of GERD symptoms, the size of air bubbles and esophageal dilation (ED) on the CT scan.

Conclusions: Air bubbles in the esophagus may be seen frequently in CT scans, but their size and location can vary. The GERD symptoms can arise when a small diameter air column is present within the esophagus, especially in the middle and lower parts.

Keywords: Gastroesophageal Reflux Disease, chest computed tomography, radiographic anatomy

Background

Gastroesophageal Reflux Disease (GERD) is disruptive and places a great clinical and economic burden on patients and society as a whole [1]. A recent study estimated that 20% of the adult US population experience GERD-related symptoms at least once a week [2]. The disease is sometimes accompanied by extraluminal symptoms such as chronic cough, laryngitis, asthma and sinusitis [3]. GERD is one of the most common diseases that can be treated in many of those patients who suffer from it [4].

Air is usually seen in radiological exams of the normal esophagus, but the extent and distribution of air has not been well described, and there is a paucity of data [5]. Previously Proto showed air seen in 36% of normal chest radiograph and then in a study [6] reported that an air column is visible in 64% of CT scans of the normal esophagus. Bhalla and Silver [7] defined esophageal dilatation (ED) as an air column greater than 10 mm in the coronal plane. Ponce revealed that increase in esophageal diameter in is associated with greater disease evolution [8]. Halber have showed that air in the esophagus is a normal finding [9]. However, data to confirm these findings are scarce.

Therefore, the aim of this study is to identify and explore any relationships between GERD symptoms in the patients' history and the presence of air bubbles in the esophagus. We assessed the correlation between the size, number and position of any air bubbles, and the presence of GERD symptoms.

Methods

Study population

Our cross-sectional imaging study was conducted at Rasole Akram Hospital of Tehran University of Medical Sciences (TUMS), Tehran, Iran. The study was carried out in December of 2009 to May of 2010. A total of 44 patients underwent CT scanning as part of the clinical care of their pulmonary disease. Approval for the research was confirmed by the TUMS Ethics Committee.

* Correspondence: shadighourchian@yahoo.com
[4]Medical student, Scientific students' research center of Tehran University of Medical Sciences, DDRI of Rasoul hospital, Sattakhan street, Tehran (1445613131), Iran
Full list of author information is available at the end of the article

Study design

The study patients were selected from a group who were referred to the lung ward of our hospital. Since all of the cases were referred, it was expected that some of the patients' symptoms were caused by their main condition and so those patients were excluded. One exception was coughing, which was so prevalent that it could not be considered as an exclusion criterion in all patients; other investigated symptoms were all characteristic of upper gastrointestinal involvement. In addition, patients with a cough that was essentially related to lung disease were excluded as much as possible. Subsequently, the incidence of coughing related to respiratory disease was 30%. Because of the low prevalence of some symptoms in our study sample, e.g. nausea, some characteristics were omitted before performing the analysis.

Data collection

We designed a check list to include all major and minor symptoms of GERD, such as epigastric symptoms; chest pain; difficulty swallowing; chronic laryngitis and/or sore throat; a chronic cough, regurgitation, heartburn, toothache following the consumption of cold or hot food, frequent pulmonary problems, post-nasal discharge (PND), chronic sinusitis, frequent and resistant nausea, gastrointestinal bleeding, history of pregnancy, smoking or of taking *proton pump inhibitors (PPIs)* for a long time, a history of hiatal hernia (HH) or of any other diseases.

Definition

The CT images were reviewed by one of the authors, who is a trained pulmonologist in comparing the CT scans by unique criteria. The purpose of choosing different sizes and different numbers of axial images with air bubbles was to determine the presence or absence of bubbles in different parts of the esophagus with GERD symptoms. In addition, patients who had air columns in all axial images of CT were noted. The presence of air was characterized by its diameter, quantity, its location in the CT scan, and the presence or absence of ED. Because ED is not a recognized condition by standard clinical texts, we compared our findings with the criteria for a normal air column in the esophagus as determined by Dean [10]

Radiologic measurement

To match the sizes of air columns with the sizes determined in 2009, we used a c-100 scanner (cine-CT; C-100 Scanner, Imatron, San Francisco, CA), using 1 to 2 mm collimation. Images were reconstructed to a 512-pixel matrix using a sharp kernel and a 26 cm display field of view. The standard mediastinal window (width, 396 HU; level, 44 HU) and lung window (width, 1465 HU; level, -498 HU) were used. Following the guidelines given by Schraufnagel [10], the assessments were all limited to the thoracic esophagus. Because the normal air column was measured in separate parts of the esophagus by CT, we divided the esophagus into 3 sections including the supra ventricle (SV), ventricle (CV) and ventricle to lower esophageal sphincter (V-LES). ED was defined as the presence of air bubbles greater than 10 mm in the SV and CV. Furthermore, air bubbles > 15 mm were named ED in V-LES. [11], we considered presence of ED: yes/no question for a diameter greater than 15 mm, and their size: the exact quantitative size not yes/no question for ED of air bubbles.

Statistical analysis

Our analysis was done using SPSS software, version 17. We used frequency tests to quantify the frequency of men and women in our study population, and the frequency of symptoms among each gender.

To understand if there is any relationship between gender and the existence of ED in different segments of the esophagus, we used the chi-square test or Fisher's exact test when needed. Other qualitative variables were evaluated by a chi-square test as well, including epigastric symptoms such as chest pain, a chronic cough, regurgitation, heartburn, frequent pulmonary problems, frequent and resistant nausea, and a history of pregnancy, smoking, or a history of taking *PPIs* for two last weeks before imaging. Among all characteristics, the imminent presence of notable ED in V-LES was found in patients previously identified by means of endoscopy as suffering from HH. The expressed qualitative variables were also counted by a t-test, so that we could determine the correlation between symptoms and the sizes and number of bubbles in each segment, and in the whole esophagus. Some of these 9 variables had non-parametrical distributions, and were analyzed by the Mann-Whitney test. A P- Value > 0.05 was considered to be significant, and confidence interval (CI) was 95%.

Results

Demographic Data

Forty-four patients who had undergone a CT scan for their respiratory disease were evaluated. The average age of the patients was 59.31 ± 15.98 years and the male to female ratio was 0.83 (37 men and 8 women). Out of 44 patients, 11 (25%) had been taking omeprazole, and of these, 6 patients (54%) were female. In addition, of these patients, 5 (11.4%) were known by means of endoscopy to be HH cases, and 2 patients (40%) were female. Statistics showed that of the 20 patients (45.5%) with heartburn, 9 patients (45%) were female. Chronic cough was positive in 29 patients (65.9%), and of these, 11 patients

(37.9%) had a history of respiratory or other related diseases.

Air bubbles

The mean size of the bubbles was 11.44 ± 5.51 mm in SV, 8.53 ± 7.47 mm in VC, 10.70 ± 7.13 mm in V-LES and 30.88 ± 14.95 mm in the whole of the esophagus. (Figure 1, 2 and 3)

Of all the cases, 7 patients (16.3%) had ED in the whole esophagus. Of them, 71.4% (5 patients) were women. In other patients with sporadic involvement, however, the frequency of men and women was the same ($p > 0.05$).

There were no correlation test between the sizes of the bubbles in SV and CV ($p = 0.13$) but we see the significant correlation between SV and V-LES ($p = 0.006$), and between CV and V-LES ($p = 0.033$).

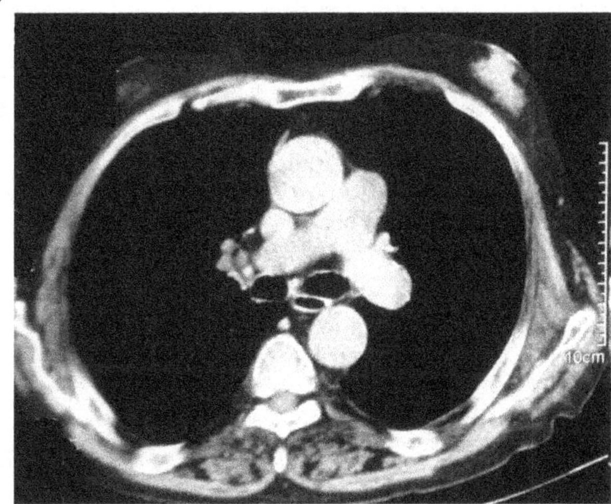

Figure 2 CT scan illustrate size taken at full length of esophagus in 75-year-old man. Greatest direct distance of air bubble of esophagus was measured. Recording line does not included soft tissue. The greatest space between its walls was measured. Scale is in millimeters.

Correlations of Air bubbles Upper Gastrointestinal symptoms

After analyzing all symptoms and relative characteristics, we found a significant relationship between the presence of ED in V-LES and heartburn (32.3% versus 76.9% in patients with and without ED, $p = 0.007$, Odds Ratio [OR] = 7). Heartburn in patients whose CT included an air column in all axial images was significantly more prevalent than in the group whose CT revealed just some sporadic bubbles ($P = 0.038$ and OR = 9.429), (Tables 1, 2, 3).

We found a significant relationship between main upper gastrointestinal symptoms accounting mainly for GERD and the sizes of bubbles, to the extent that they caused ED. Aside from the significant values of the qualitative characteristics, the relationship between heartburn and the appearance of ED > 15 mm in V-LES and also the presence of ED in all segments of the esophagus were highly significant. (Table 2, Table 3), Furthermore, a significant correlation was detected between the size of the air pockets in V-LES and heartburn ($p = 0.010$) (Table 1). The specific correlation between the two expressed characteristics was manifested by the prominent positive mean. The mean size of bubbles in patients who had heartburn was 13.67 ± 6.71 mm, and in patients who had no heartburn, it was 8.22 ± 6.62 mm. This confirmed the correlation between heartburn and an increase in the sizes of air pockets in V-LES ($p = 0.010$).

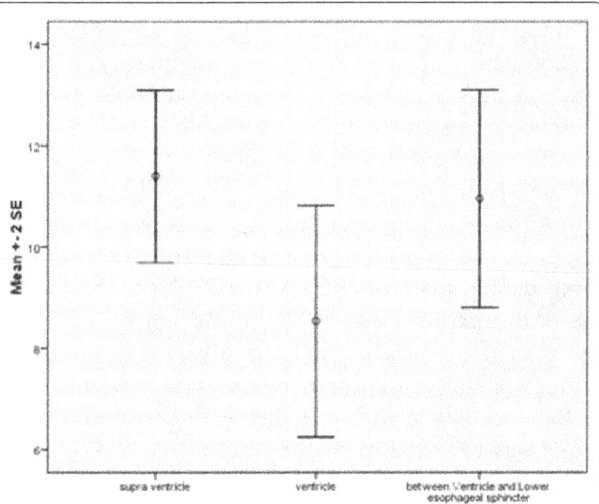

Figure 1 The correlation between sizes (mm) and location of the esophageal blobs.

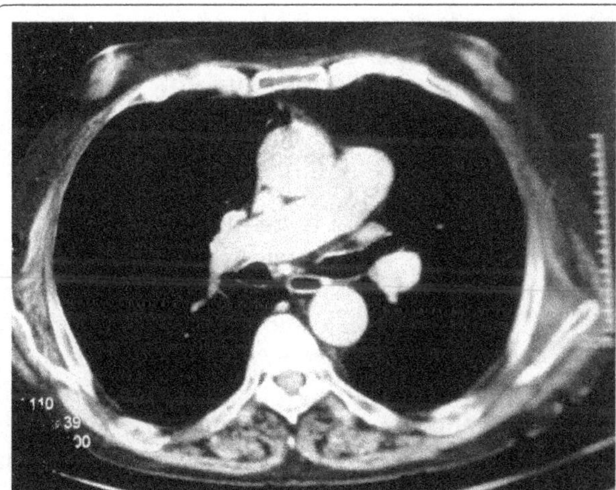

Figure 3 Lumina of air bubble going down thorax in previous patient as in Figure 1. This series of CT scans shows landmarks for distance down esophagus.

Table 1 Correlation between sizes of blobs and frequencies of characteristics

characteristics	SV	CV	V-LES	Total**
Chronic coughs	P = 0.119 *(mean of positives = 12.37 ± 5.52, mean of negatives = 9.63 ± 5.21)	P = 0.422 (mean of positives = 9.21 ± 7.40, mean of negatives = 7.26 ± 7.69)	P = 0.029 (mean of positives = 12.37 ± 6.69, mean of negatives = 7.46 ± 7.05)	P = 0.076 (mean of positives = 34.37 ± 14.37, mean of negatives = 24.36 ± 14.21)
Smoking	P = 0.94 (mean of positives = 13.30 ± 4.80, mean of negatives = 10.32 ± 5.72)	P = 0.780 (mean of positives = 8.30 ± 8.17, mean of negatives = 8.98 ± 7.15)	P = 0.151 (mean of positives = 13.06 ± 6.94, mean of negatives = 9.82 ± 6.92)	P = 0.253 (mean of positives = 34.66 ± 17.21, mean of negatives = 29.37 ± 13.45)
History of omeprazole	P = 0.214 (mean of positives = 9.63 ± 5.23, mean of negatives = 12.04 ± 5.55)	P = 0.493 (mean of positives = 7.181 ± 7.53, mean of negatives = 9.00 ± 7.51)	P = 0.710 (mean of positives = 10.00 ± 6.03, mean of negatives = 10.93 ± 7.54)	P = 0.537 (mean of positives = 26.81 ± 12.31, mean of negatives = 32.28 ± 15.68)
Hiatal hernia	P = 0.207 (mean of positives = 14.40 ± 4.33, mean of negatives = 11.06 ± 5.58)	P = 0.172 (mean of positives = 4.40 ± 6.06, mean of negatives = 9.07 ± 7.53)	P < 0.001(considered as a huge ED) (mean of positives = 20 ± 0.00, mean of negatives = 9.51 ± 6.69)	P = 0.869 (mean of positives = 38.80 ± 7.69, mean of negatives = 29.84 ± 15.41)
Heartburn	P = 0.040 (mean of positives = 13.30 ± 5.91, mean of negatives = 9.89 ± 4.75)	P = 0.920 (mean of positives = 8.5 ± 8.98, mean of negatives = 8.56 ± 6.07)	P = 0.010 (mean of positives = 13.67 ± 6.71, mean of negatives = 8.22 ± 6.62)	P = 0.230 (mean of positives = 35.47 ± 17.22, mean of negatives = 26.89 ± 11.60)
Epigastric pain	P = 0.665 (mean of positives = 11.97 ± 7.39, mean of negatives = 11.11 ± 4.05)	P = 0.905 (mean of positives = 8.80 ± 8.82, mean of negatives = 8.42 ± 6.62)	P = 0.023 (mean of positives = 12.97 ± 6.95, mean of negatives = 9.27 ± 7)	P = 0.688 (mean of positives = 33.64 ± 18.23, mean of negatives = 29.07 ± 12.41)
Regurgitation	P = 0.417 (mean of positives = 12.04 ± 5.76, mean of negatives = 10.65 ± 5.22)	P = 0.276 (mean of positives = 9.6 ± 7.90, mean of negatives = 7.05 ± 6.76)	P = 0.007 (mean of positives = 13.18 ± 6.12, mean of negatives = 7.44 ± 7.21)	P = 0.216 (mean of positives = 34.82 ± 15.78, mean of negatives = 25.41 ± 12.08)

*mean of positives shows the mean of blob size in the cases that had the characteristic and mean of negatives shows the mean of blob size in the cases that didn't have it.

**the summation of sizes of blobs in whole of esophagus.

Although the P-value of the correlation between regurgitation and the presence of ED in V-LES was not statistically significant (48.4% versus 76.9% in patient with and without ED, p = 0.081), there was a significant correlation between the sizes of the bubbles in V-LES and the presence of regurgitation (13.18 ± 6.12 mm versus 7.44 ± 7.21 mm air bubble size in patients with and without regurgitation, p = 0.007). Because of the predominantly positive findings of the presence of regurgitation, the correlation between the sizes of the bubbles and regurgitation was confirmed.

There was no significant correlation between regurgitation and the sizes of the bubbles in other parts of the esophagus, including CV and SV (12.04 ± 5.76 mm versus 9.60 ± 7.90 mm in SV and CV, p = 0.41 and p = 0.27 in SV and CV respectively).

Discussions and Conclusions

In a CT scan, air bubbles are frequently seen, and their sizes and locations may vary [10]. In this study, we found there was a relationship between the presence of air bubbles and some GERD symptoms such as heartburn.

As heartburn is considered to be the most prevalent problem in patients with recognized GERD, an increase in the probability of heartburn due to an increase in the diameter of air columns in most parts of the esophagus motivates widely different discussions. The dilation of the esophagus in V-LES can be ascribed to the probable concomitancy of lower esophageal sphincter (LES) dysfunction that can cause GERD symptoms. However, the presence of an air column in the whole esophagus and also the significant correlation between the sizes of bubbles and heartburn cannot be justified fully by our present knowledge, especially in SV. Furthermore in our study, there was no history of scleroderma or other diseases which can dilate the esophagus. While the average age of our patients was 59, ED could not be attributed to aging processes. A 2005 case report described a young woman who did not respond to twice-daily doses of Rabeprazole. Following further investigations, the cause was revealed to be air swallowing. Therefore, it may be that persistent heartburn can be caused by aerophagia. This is one hypothesis about the relationship between air bubbles and heartburn, as a major symptom of GERD [12].

Table 2 Frequencies and comparison between symptoms and relevant characteristics with the presence of esophageal dilation.

characteristics	presence of esophageal dilation comparing with the reference values/yes, no question					
	SV		CV		V-LES	
	ED-** 20.50%	ED+ 79.50%	ED- 41.90%	ED+ 70.50%	ED- 29.50%	ED+
Chronic coughs						
% *	44.4%	71.4%	55.6%	72%	58.1%	84.6%
P-value	0.235		0.264		0.162	
Smoking						
%	11.1%	41.2%	41.2%	32%	30%	46.2%
P-value	0.129		0.542		0.324	
History of taking proton						
pump inhibitors						
%	22.2%	25.7%	33.3%	20%	25.8%	23.1%
P-value	1		0.48		1	
Hiatal hernia						
%	0%	14.3%	16.7%	8%	0%	38.5%
P-value	0.566		0.634		0.01	
Heartburn						
%	22.1%	51.4%	61.1%	36%	32.3%	76.9%
P-value	0.15		0.103		0.007	
Epigastric pain						
%	33.3%	40%	44.4%	36%	35.5%	46.2%
P-value	1		0.576		0.507	
Regurgitation						
%	44.4%	60%	55.6%	60%	48.4%	76.9%
P-value	0.467		0.771		0.081	
History of pregnancy(in women)						
%	80%	63.2%	83.3%	58.8%	70.6%	57.1%
P-value	0.702		0.407		0.738	

* Percent of patients who presented symptom (positive symptom).

**- shows cases with no ED and + shows cases wi

Table 3 Frequencies of each characteristic in cases with sporadic air blobs and cases with air column in whole esophagus

characteristics		Chronic coughs %**	Smoking %	History of omeprazole %	Hiatal hernia %	Heartburn %	Epigastric pain %	Regurgitation %	History of pregnancy (in women) %
The presence of air column whole the esophagus (not necessarily ED in whole)	-*	61.1%	34.3%	25%	13.9%	38.9%	36.1%	52.8%	72.2%
	+	85.7%	42.9%	28.6%	0%	85.7%	57.1%	85.7%	40%
	P-value	0.391	0.686	1	0.572	0.038	0.407	0.209	1

*- shows cases with sporadic air blobs and + shows cases with air column in whole esophagus.

** Percent of patients who presented symptom (positive symptom).

As was previously noted, in our study, ED was defined as an air column greater than 10 cm in diameter in SV and CV and greater than 15 mm in diameter in V-LES. We observed that if the air bubbles were present in all sections of CT, regardless to their size, the risk for heartburn was greater than when there were only some sporadic air bubbles on CT (OR = 9.42). This finding requires further investigation.

Although there was no significant correlation between regurgitation and the presence of ED, there was a significant correlation between the size of air bubbles in V-LES and the presence of regurgitation. In a review of previous studies, Bredenoord and Weusten [13] showed that the rate of air swallowing was linked to the size of the intragastric air bubble. They also showed that the number of air swallows was linked to the size of the intragastric air.

Further, although there was no significant correlation between regurgitation and the size of bubbles in other parts of the esophagus, the notable differences between the average size of the air column in patients with regurgitation and patients with no regurgitation motivate the continued careful examination of more cases, especially because the average size in patients with regurgitation was higher. Szczesniak showed that regurgitation caused by GERD, and GERD itself can cause air bubbles in the esophagus, thus we can say that regurgitation can also cause air bubbles.

In our research, taking PPIs was considered a factor that confirmed the presence of previous upper gastrointestinal symptoms. Although there was a significant correlation between taking PPIs and the size of the air bubbles, scrutinizing the mean size of the bubbles in patients who used PPIs and those who didn't use the drug revealed some remarkable findings that suggest the need for repeating the study with more cases. In our study, the mean size of bubbles in patients who did not use PPIs was greater than the group who had previously used this drug. This suggests that taking PPIs decreases the size of the air bubbles and that a history of using PPIs could have an influence on some symptoms, which thus may have also had some influence on our results [14]. In a previous study, it was shown that some patients generated a distension-induced contractile response in the upper esophageal sphincter that was related to PPIs [15]. Therefore, it is reasonable to conclude that PPIs can decrease the size and incidence of air bubbles by treating GERD symptoms.

Limitations

Some minor symptoms of GERD were excluded from analysis, such as toothache that occurred following the consumption of cold or hot food. These minor symptoms were rare and would cause difficulties in a statistical analysis (because of the small amount of data in each group); therefore, we did not include them in our analysis. In a future study, the effects of air bubbles on all symptoms of GERD should be assessed.

Non-financial competing interests

There are not any non-financial competing interests (political, personal, religious, academic, ideological, intellectual, commercial or any other).

Abbreviations

GERD: Gastroesophageal Reflux Disease; CT: Computed tomography; ED: esophageal dilation; SV: supra ventricle; CV: cardiac ventricle; V-LES: ventricle to lower esophageal sphincter; OR: Odds Ratio; mm: millimeter.

Author details

[1]Department of pulmonary diseases, Rasoul-e-Akram Hospital, Tehran University of Medical Sciences, Sattakhan street, Tehran(1445613131), Iran. [2]Department of pulmonary diseases, Jundishopur University of Medical Sciences, Golestan boulevard, Ahvaz, Iran. [3]Nephrology and Urology Research Center, Medical Faculty, Baqyatallah University of Medical Sciences, Mollasadra street, Tehran, Iran. [4]Medical student, Scientific students' research center of Tehran University of Medical Sciences, DDRI of Rasoul hospital, Sattakhan street, Tehran (1445613131), Iran.

Authors' contributions

AM: study concept and design; acquisition, read and approved the final manuscript. HR: study concept and design, coordination for the acquisition of data, read and approved the final manuscript. MT: Critical drafting of manuscript and revision of manuscript, read and approved the final manuscript. Sh.Gh: Acquisition, Designing the study, analysis and interpretation of data, writing the manuscript, read and approved the final manuscript.

Competing interests

The authors declare that they have no competing interests.
Financial competing interests

- In the past five years we have not received reimbursements, fees, funding, or salary from an organization that may have any financial gains from the publication of this manuscript, either in now or in future.
- We do not hold any stocks or shares in an organization that may in any way gain or lose financially from the publication of this manuscript, either now or in the future.
- We do neither hold nor currently applying for any patents relating to the content of the manuscript. We have not received reimbursements, fees, funding, or salary from an organization that holds or has applied for patents relating to the content of the manuscript.
- We have not any financial competing interests.

References

1. Toghanian S, Wahlqvist P, Johnson DA, Bolge SC, Liljas B: **The burden of disrupting gastro-oesophageal reflux disease: a database study in US and European cohorts.** *Clin Drug Investig* 2010, **30(3)**:167-78.
2. Locke GR, Talley NJ, Fett SL, Zinsmeister AR, Melton LJ: **Prevalence and clinical spectrum of gastroesophageal reflux: a population-based study in Olmsted County, Minnesota.** *Gastroenterology* 1997, **112(5)**:1448-56.
3. Shaker R, Castell DO, Schoenfeld PS, Spechler SJ: **Nighttime heartburn is an under-appreciated clinical problem that impacts sleep and daytime function: the results of a Gallup survey conducted on behalf of the American Gastroenterological Association.** *Am J Gastroenterol* 2003, **98(7)**:1487-93.
4. Vakil N, van Zanten SV, Kahrilas P, Dent J, Jones R: **The Montreal definition and classification of gastroesophageal reflux disease: a global evidence-based consensus.** *Am J Gastroenterol* 2006, **101(8)**:1900-20, quiz 43.

5. Grainger RGAD: **Diagnostic radiology: a textbook of medical imaging.** UK: Churchill Livingstone; 2001.
6. Goldwin RLHE, Proto AV: **Computed tomography of the mediastinum: normal anatomy and indications for the use of CT.** *Radiology* 1977, **124**:235-41.
7. Bhalla M, Silver RM, Shepard JA, McLoud TC: **Chest CT in patients with scleroderma: prevalence of asymptomatic esophageal dilatation and mediastinal lymphadenopathy.** *AJR Am J Roentgenol* 1993, **161(2)**:269-72.
8. Ponce J, Garrigues V, Ramirez JJ, Pascual S, Arguello L, Berenguer J: **[The clinical significance of the magnitude of esophageal dilatation in idiopathic achalasia].** *Gastroenterol Hepatol* 1996, **19(5)**:235-9.
9. Halber MD, Daffner RH, Thompson WM: **CT of the esophagus: I. Normal appearance.** *AJR Am J Roentgenol* 1979, **133(6)**:1047-50.
10. Schraufnagel DE, Michel JC, Sheppard TJ, Saffold PC, Kondos GT: **CT of the normal esophagus to define the normal air column and its extent and distribution.** *AJR Am J Roentgenol* 2008, **191(3)**:748-52.
11. Vakil NB, Traxler B, Levine D: **Dysphagia in patients with erosive esophagitis: prevalence, severity, and response to proton pump inhibitor treatment.** *Clin Gastroenterol Hepatol* 2004, **2(8)**:665-8.
12. Zentilin P, Accornero L, Dulbecco P, Savarino E, Savarino V: **Air swallowing can be responsible for non-response of heartburn to high-dose proton pump inhibitor.** *Dig Liver Dis* 2005, **37(6)**:454-7.
13. Bredenoord AJ, Weusten BL, Timmer R, Akkermans LM, Smout AJ: **Relationships between air swallowing, intragastric air, belching and gastro-oesophageal reflux.** *Neurogastroenterol Motil* 2005, **17(3)**:341-7.
14. Dent J, Armstrong D, Delaney B, Moayyedi P, Talley NJ, Vakil N: **Symptom evaluation in reflux disease: workshop background, processes, terminology, recommendations, and discussion outputs.** *Gut* 2004, **53(Suppl 4)**:iv1-24.
15. Szczesniak MM, Williams RB, Brake HM, Maclean JC, Cole IE, Cook IJ: **Upregulation of the esophago-UES relaxation response: a possible pathophysiological mechanism in suspected reflux laryngitis.** *Neurogastroenterol Motil* 2010, **22(4)**:381-6, e89.

Influence of trigger type, tube voltage and heart rate on calcified plaque imaging in dual source cardiac computed tomography: phantom study

Tobias Penzkofer[1,2,3*], Eva Donandt[1], Peter Isfort[1,3], Thomas Allmendinger[4], Christiane K Kuhl[1], Andreas H Mahnken[1,3,5] and Philipp Bruners[1,3]

Abstract

Background: To investigate the impact of high pitch cardiac CT vs. retrospective ECG gated CT on the quantification of calcified vessel stenoses, with assessment of the influence of tube voltage, reconstruction kernel and heart rate.

Methods: A 4D cardiac movement phantom equipped with three different plaque phantoms (12.5%, 25% and 50% stenosis at different calcification levels), was scanned with a 128-row dual source CT scanner, applying different trigger types (gated vs. prospectively triggered high pitch), tube voltages (100-120 kV) and heart rates (50–90 beats per minute, bpm). Images were reconstructed using different standard (B26f, B46f, B70f) and iterative (I26f, I70f) convolution kernels. Absolute and relative plaque sizes were measured and statistically compared. Radiation dose associated with the different methods (gated vs. high pitch, 100 kV vs. 120 kV) were compared.

Results: Compared to the known diameters of the phantom plaques and vessels both CT-examination techniques overestimated the degrees of stenoses. Using the high pitch CT-protocol plaques appeared larger (0.09 ± 0.31 mm, 2 ± 8 percent points, PP) in comparison to the ECG-gated CT-scans. Reducing tube voltage had a similar effect, resulting in higher grading of the same stenoses by 3 ± 8 PP. In turn, sharper convolution kernels lead to a lower grading of stenoses (differences of up to 5%). Pairwise comparison of B26f and I26f, B46f and B70f, and B70f and I70f showed differences of $0–1 \pm 6–8$ PP of the plaque depiction. Motion artifacts were present only at 90 bpm high pitch experiments. High-pitch protocols were associated with significantly lower radiation doses compared with the ECG-gated protocols (258.0 mGy vs. 2829.8 mGy $CTDI_{vol}$, $p \leq 0.0001$).

Conclusion: Prospectively triggered high-pitch cardiac CT led to an overestimation of plaque diameter and degree of stenoses in a coronary phantom. This overestimation is only slight and probably negligible in a clinical situation. Even at higher heart rates high pitch CT-scanning allowed reliable measurements of plaque and vessel diameters with only slight differences compared ECG-gated protocols, although motion artifacts were present at 90 bpm using the high pitch protocols.

Background

Cardiac computed tomography (CT) is an established non-invasive method of assessing coronary artery morphology both in emergency and routine settings [1]. It is superior to magnetic resonance based methods of coronary angiography with respect to temporal and spatial resolution. However, continuous motion of the heart makes cardiac cross-sectional imaging a challenging task [1,2]. Different methods have been developed to overcome this problem, many of them rely on the uniformity of the cardiac cycle by imaging different sections of the heart over several consecutive heart beats. To date the vast majority of current CT systems uses either a prospectively ECG-triggered or retrospectively ECG-gated scanning protocol for this purpose. Since all these methods are associated with ionizing radiation applied to the patient, the risks and benefits need to be carefully weighted [3].

* Correspondence: tpenzkofer@ukaachen.de
[1]Department of Diagnostic and Interventional Radiology, Aachen University Hospital, RWTH Aachen University, Pauwelsstr. 30, 52074 Aachen, Germany
[2]Surgical Planning Laboratory, Department of Radiology, Brigham and Women's Hospital, 75 Francis Street, 02115 Boston, USA
Full list of author information is available at the end of the article

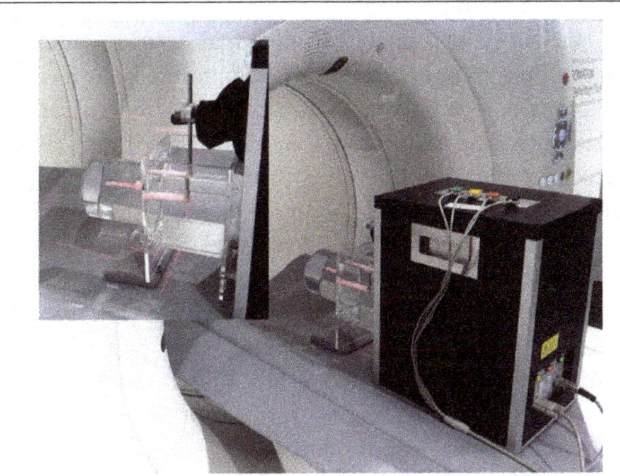

Figure 1 Cardiac movement phantom setting during the scans. (inlay) the coronary artery phantom (CAP) was placed in a water filled container. The cardiac phantom provides 4D motion with ECG-syncing over the scanners standard ECG-interface (ECGI).

Recent advances in CT technology led to the development of dual source based high pitch (pitch up to 3.4) scanning protocols with table speeds of up to 46 cm/sec [4-6], or even higher [7,8]. These protocols promise to image the heart within one heartbeat, obviating the need for gating or multi-step triggering, i.e. acquisition techniques that are inherently associated with redundant scan ranges leading to increased radiation doses.

The goal of this study was to evaluate the quantification of calcified stenosis in high pitch cardiac CT-scans versus an ECG-gated scan protocol in a controlled phantom environment. Secondary goal was to evaluate the influence of tube current, convolution kernel and heart rate on the different acquisition protocols.

Methods

Coronary movement phantom

A 4D coronary movement simulator (Sim4Dcardiac, QRM GmbH, Möhrendorf, Germany, Figure 1) was used for the study performing coronary artery movement patterns with heart rates of 50, 70 and 90 beats per minute (bpm). Three custom made dedicated coronary artery phantoms (QRM GmbH, Möhrendorf, Germany) each with defined calcified (high, medium and low calcification at 796, 401 and 197 mgHA/cm^3 at densities of 1.58, 1.30 and 1.16 g/cm^3) coronary stenoses of various degrees (50%, 25% and 12.5%) were used in a simulated 4.0 mm vessel. The absolute stenosis sizes were 0.5 mm (12.5%),

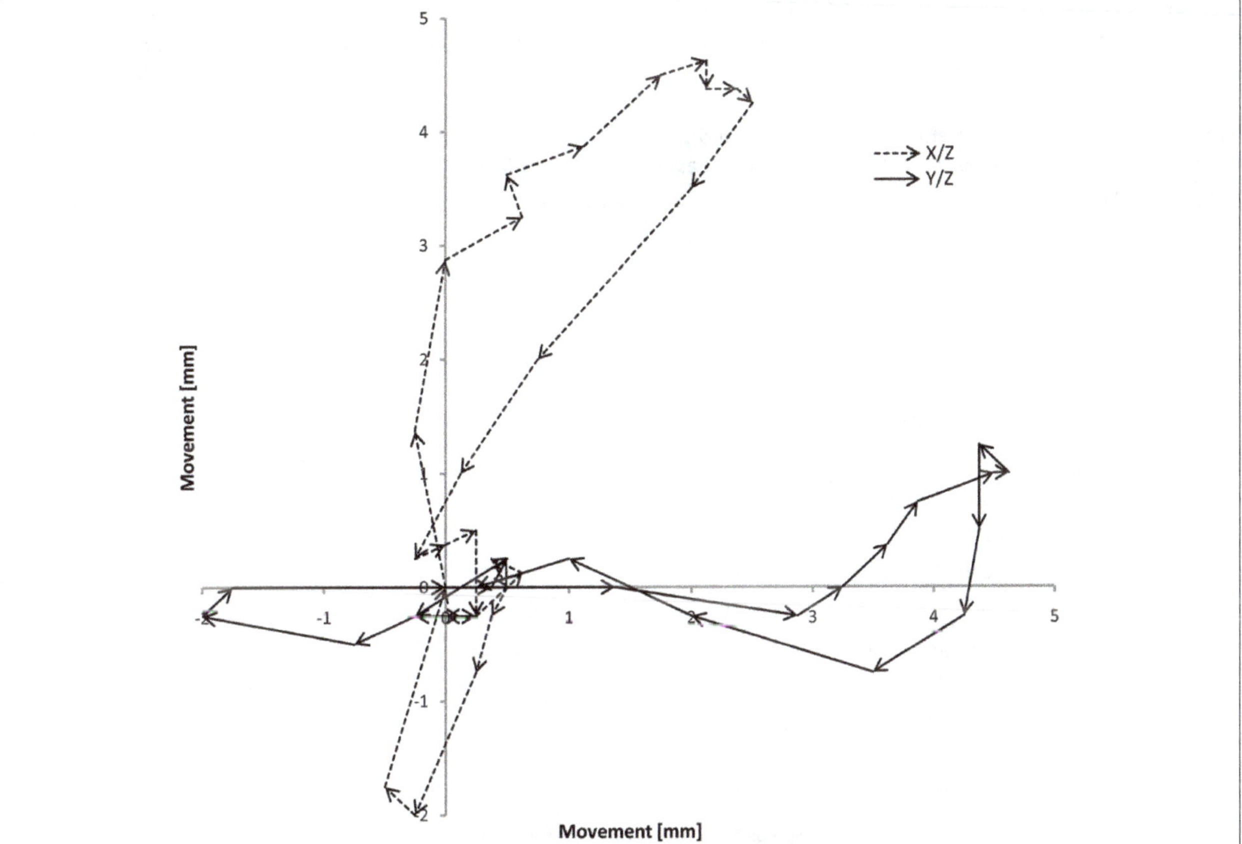

Figure 2 Cardiac movement as performed by the coronary movement simulator. The solid line represents the movement in the Y/Z plane, while the dashed line shows the path in the X/Z plane. Arrow length corresponds to movement speed.

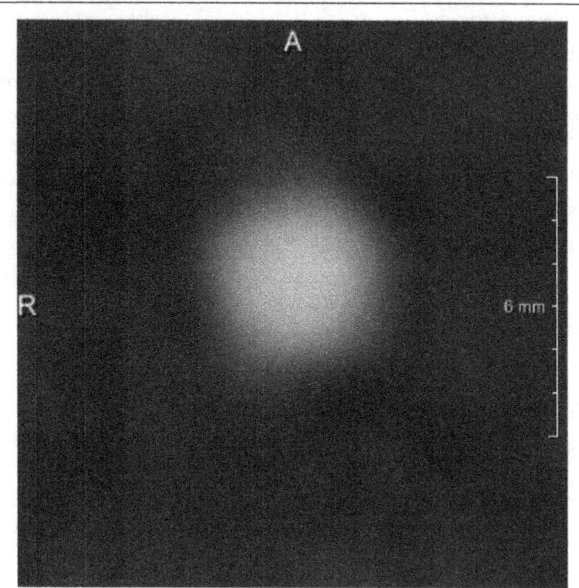

Figure 3 Low calcified stenosis (197 mmHA/cm^3) at the same position as Figure 8; the stenosis grade is not distinguishable due to insufficient contrast.

1 mm (25%) and 2 mm (50%). The movement protocol was derived from an electron beam scan (Figure 2) [9]. The coronary simulator provides an ECG output mapping the movement pattern to an ECG signal readable by the scanner's ECG analysis module.

CT examination protocols

A 128 slice high pitch capable dual source computed tomography scanner (Siemens Somatom Flash, Siemens Healthcare, Forchheim, Germany) was used for all experiments. The high pitch scans were performed using a dedicated high pitch cardiac protocol (dual source, 100 and 120 kV, 320 mAs/rot, pitch 3.4, prospective ECG trigger, collimation 128 × 0.6 mm, FoV 190 × 190 mm, scan length 90.0 mm, rotation time 0.28s) and a retrospectively ECG gated protocol (100 and 120 kV, 320 mAs/rot, retrospective ECG gating after pulsing at 50-100%, collimation 128 × 0.6 mm, pitch 0.19, rotation time 0.28s). Reconstructions were performed according to the vendor's specifications, identically for both modes with B26f, B46f, B70f standard kernels and iterative I26f and I70f kernels with a field of view of 190 × 190 mm and slice thicknesses of 0.6 mm (B26f, B46f, B70f) and 0.75 mm (I26f, I70f) avoiding undersampling of the acquired data.

Measurements

Measurements were performed manually using dedicated DICOM viewer software (Synedra View, Version 3.1, Synedra GmbH, Aachen, Germany) by one observer, and checked for validity by two others with 3 and 5 years of experience in thoracic imaging. For each combination of Kernel/Method/kV/plaque phantom three repeated measurements of plaque diameter and three repeated measurements of total vessel diameter were

Table 1 Absolute calcified stenosis diameters (true diameters: 12.5%: 0.5 mm, 25%: 1.0 mm, 50%: 2.0 mm), measured total vessel diameters (true diameter 4.0 mm) as measured for the different protocol types per phantom type

Density [mmHA/cm^3]	True stenosis size	Method	Plaque diameter [mm]	Vessel diameter [mm]	Measured stenosis [%]
197	12,5 %	High pitch	-	-	-
	(0.5 mm/4.0 mm)	Gating	-	-	-
	25%	High pitch	-	-	-
	(1.0 mm/4.0 mm)	Gating	-	-	-
	50%	High pitch	-	-	-
	(2.0 mm/4.0 mm)	Gating	-	-	-
401	12,5%	High pitch	0.97 ± 0.1	3.96 ± 0.1	24.6 ± 2.7
	(0.5 mm/4.0 mm)	Gating	0.88 ± 0.1	3.95 ± 0.1	22.4 ± 3.3
	25%	High pitch	1.48 ± 0.2	4.13 ± 0.2	35.8 ± 4.3
	(1.0 mm/4.0 mm)	Gating	1.40 ± 0.2	4.00 ± 0.1	34.9 ± 4.6
	50%	High pitch	1.98 ± 0.2	4.08 ± 0.2	48.6 ± 4.3
	(2.0 mm/4.0 mm)	Gating	1.98 ± 0.2	4.00 ± 0.1	49.6 ± 4.6
796	12,5%	High pitch	1.27 ± 0.1	4.35 ± 0.4	29.2 ± 2.4
	(0.5 mm/4.0 mm)	Gating	1.18 ± 0.1	4.52 ± 0.4	26.2 ± 2.6
	25%	High pitch	1.80 ± 0.4	4.52 ± 0.4	39.7 ± 5.9
	(1.0 mm/4.0 mm)	Gating	1.71 ± 0.4	4.70 ± 0.5	36.1 ± 5.0
	50%	High pitch	2.39 ± 0.4	3.99 ± 0.3	59.6 ± 7.1
	(2.0 mm/4.0 mm)	Gating	2.22 ± 0.3	3.93 ± 0.2	56.3 ± 5.9

The lowest density plaque phantoms (197 mmHA/cm^3) were not measurable as no sufficient contrast could be established between the lumen and the plaque mimic.

performed resulting in a total of 2,880 data points. The repeated measurements were averaged and used for statistical analyses.

Statistical analyses

Statistical analysis was performed using SPSS 19 (SPSS Inc., Chicago, Illinois, USA) and MedCalc (MedCalc Software, Mariakerke, Belgium). Tests performed were Analysis of Variances with post-hoc testing and Bland-Altman as well as Mountain plot method comparisons. P-values of 0.05 or lower were considered statistically significant, multiple testing correction (Bonferroni) was performed where applicable. Additional tests were performed using non-parametric Mann–Whitney-U analyses.

Results

The plaque phantom featuring the lowest calcification level (197 mmHA/cm^3) was not measureable with the applied methods due to low contrast between plaque and vessel lumen (Figure 3). The following data result from the measurements of the intermediately (401 mmHA/cm^3) and heavily (796 mmHA/cm^3) calcified plaque phantoms.

Comparison to phantom dimensions

In comparison to the phantom vessel dimensions retrospectively ECG-gated and prospectively ECG-triggered high pitch scanning provided vessel diameters of between 3.93 ± 0.2 mm and 4.70 ± 0.5 mm with a tendency to a slight overestimation (Table 1). The plaque thickness was measured at between 0.88 ± 0.1 mm and 1.27 ± 0.1 mm (0.5 mm/12.5%), 1.40 ± 0.2 mm and 1.80 ± 0.4 mm (1 mm/25%) and 1.98 ± 0.2 mm and 2.39 ± 0.4 mm (2 mm/50%) again showing an overestimation for both cardiac CT techniques which was more pronounced for high-pitch scanning. These findings led to the following degrees of stenoses: 22.4 ± 3.3% and 29.2 ± 2.4% (12.5% stenoses), 34.9 ± 4.6% and 39.7 ± 5.9% (25% stenoses) and 48.6 ± 4.3% and 59.6 ± 7.1% (50% stenoses) for retrospectively gated and prospectively triggered high pitch, respectively.

Separated by heart rate of the phantom, both examination protocols showed an overestimation of vessel diameter, plaque diameter and degree of stenosis which was more pronounced for the 12.5% in comparison to the 50% stenosis and for the high pitch protocol in comparison to ECG-gated scanning. Diameter measurements for the same degree of stenosis at different heart rates did not show relevant differences (Table 2).

Table 3 Average difference in degree of stenosis (Δ percentage) and measured plaque diameter (Δ diameter) between the two cardiac CT methods and tube voltages (first vs. second mentioned)

Comparison	Δ Percentage	Δ Diameter
Gated/high pitch	2 ± 8 PP	0.09 ± 0.31 mm
100 kV/120 kV	3 ± 8 PP	0.14 ± 0.32 mm

(PP: percent points).

Table 2 Absolute plaque/stenosis diameters (true diameters: 12.5%: 0.5 mm, 25%: 1.0 mm, 50%: 2.0 mm), measured vessel diameters (true diameter 4.0 mm) per heart rate and cardiac CT method

True stenosis [%]	Heart rate [bpm]	Method	Plaque diameter [mm]	Vessel diameter [mm]	Stenosis [%]	Deviation [PP]
12.5%	50	High pitch	1.13 ± 0.19	4.17 ± 0.35	27.0 ± 3.5	14.5
		Gating	1.03 ± 0.19	4.23 ± 0.45	24.4 ± 3.7	11.9
	70	High pitch	1.12 ± 0.18	4.14 ± 0.35	27.1 ± 3.4	14.6
		Gating	1.03 ± 0.19	4.26 ± 0.41	24.1 ± 3.6	11.6
	90	High pitch	1.11 ± 0.19	4.15 ± 0.30	26.7 ± 3.5	14.2
		Gating	1.03 ± 0.19	4.22 ± 0.40	24.4 ± 3.4	11.9
25%	50	High pitch	1.63 ± 0.34	4.35 ± 0.38	37.2 ± 5.7	12.2
		Gating	1.53 ± 0.33	4.35 ± 0.49	35.0 ± 4.6	10.0
	70	High pitch	1.65 ± 0.33	4.33 ± 0.36	37.8 ± 5.1	12.8
		Gating	1.53 ± 0.34	4.35 ± 0.51	34.8 ± 4.6	9.8
	90	High pitch	1.66 ± 0.35	4.29 ± 0.39	38.4 ± 5.8	13.4
		Gating	1.61 ± 0.36	4.36 ± 0.51	36.7 ± 5.2	11.7
50%	50	High pitch	2.19 ± 0.37	4.06 ± 0.20	53.9 ± 8.0	3.9
		Gating	2.08 ± 0.28	3.95 ± 0.18	52.7 ± 6.2	2.7
	70	High pitch	2.16 ± 0.36	4.00 ± 0.23	54.0 ± 7.9	4.0
		Gating	2.11 ± 0.27	3.99 ± 0.14	52.9 ± 6.1	2.9
	90	High pitch	2.20 ± 0.38	4.05 ± 0.21	54.4 ± 8.4	4.4
		Gating	2.11 ± 0.32	3.96 ± 0.19	53.1 ± 6.7	3.1

Deviations are given in percentage difference to the true diameters as specified by the phantom manufacturer. (PP: percent points).

Comparison of trigger types

High pitch scanning resulted in a larger depiction of the plaques in comparison to the ECG-gated scan method (0.09 ± 0.31 mm). This difference accounted for an additional overestimation of the stenoses by 2 ± 8 percent points (PP) (Table 3). Bland-Altman plotting (Figure 4) revealed this systematic difference, while mountain plotting additionally revealed no outliers and a narrow distribution profile.

Table 4 Average difference in degree of stenosis (Δ percentage) and measured plaque diameter (Δ diameter) per heart rate between the two cardiac CT examination protocols (PP: percent points)

Heart rate	Δ Percentage (gating vs. high pitch)	Δ Diameter
50 bpm	2 ± 7 PP	0.10 ± 0.28 mm
70 bpm	2 ± 8 PP	0.09 ± 0.31 mm
90 bpm	2 ± 8 PP	0.07 ± 0.35 mm

Trigger type and heart rate

Comparing the two CT imaging methods with respect to their plaque depiction depending on heart rate, a descending difference of the measured plaque diameter was found with increasing heart rate (50 bpm: 0.1 ± 0.28 mm, 70 bpm: 0.09 ± 0.31 mm and 90 bpm: 0.07 ± 0.35 mm, Table 4). However, the difference was so small at all heart rates that no clinically relevant effect on the degree of stenosis (2 ± 7–8 PP) was observed (Table 4).

Tube voltage

In comparison to 120 kV tube voltage 100 kV CT imaging resulted in a difference of 0.14 ± 0.32 mm regarding plaque diameters. This led to a 3 ± 8 PP overestimation of the stenosis diameter using 100 kV scan protocols (Figure 5, Table 4).

Reconstruction kernels

Smooth reconstruction kernels (B26f, I26f) showed a higher deviation from the true plaque diameters in comparison to the sharp kernels (B70f, I70f). This result was even more pronounced for the heavily calcified plaques which were significantly overestimated regarding their diameter when smooth kernels were used for image reconstruction. The B46f kernel exhibited a intermediate performance, with the least deviation in the less calcified plaque and a deviation between the standard and iterative kernels in the heavily calcified setting. The comparison between corresponding standard and iterative reconstruction kernels (B26f vs. I26f; B70f vs. I70f) did not reveal any relevant difference (Table 5, Figure 6).

Radiation dose comparison

Radiation doses were significantly lower for high pitch CT in comparison to ECG gated scanning (258.0 mGy vs. 2829.8 mGy for CTDIvol, 36.3 mGycm vs. 341.2 mGycm for the dose-length-product, DLP), and lower for 100 kV vs. 120 kV scan protocols (962.6 mGy vs. 2125.2 mGy CTDIvol and 115.1 mGycm vs 262.4 mGycm DLP). All these differences were statistically significant ($p \leq 0.0001$ for trigger type and $p \leq 0.0005$ for tube voltage, Tables 6, 7).

Motion artifacts

Coronal reconstruction revealed motion artifacts, present at the proximal end of the coronal phantom for the 90 bpm high pitch prospectively gated scans (Figure 7), which were not present in retrospectively gated scanning or the 50 or 70 bpm high pitch experiments. No other occurrences of motion artifacts were observed.

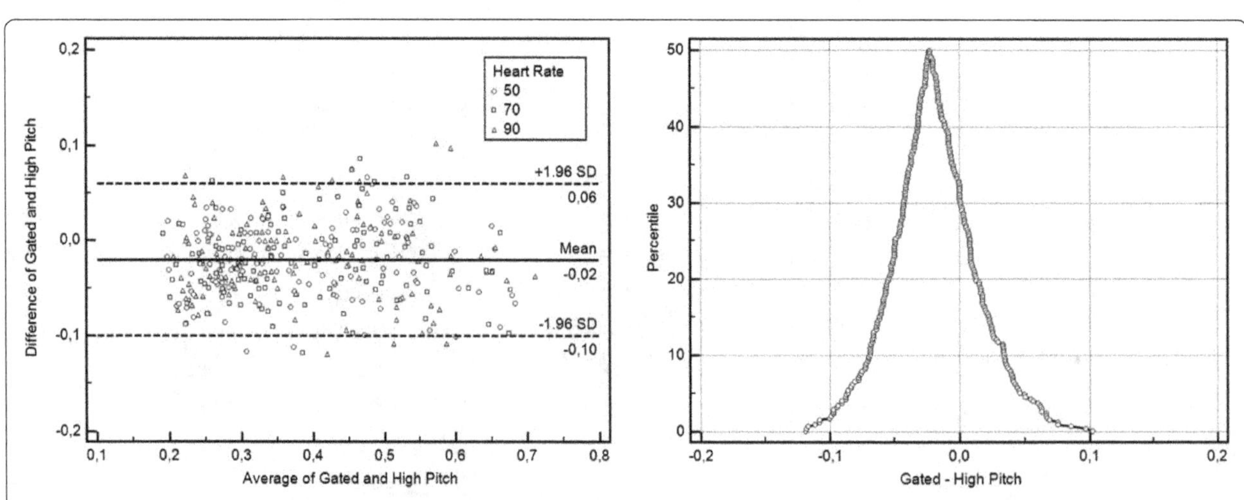

Figure 4 Method comparisons for the two trigger types under investigation. Bland-Altman-Plotting reveals a slight overestimation of stenosis percentage (2 ± 8%). Mountain plotting shows no relevant outliers.

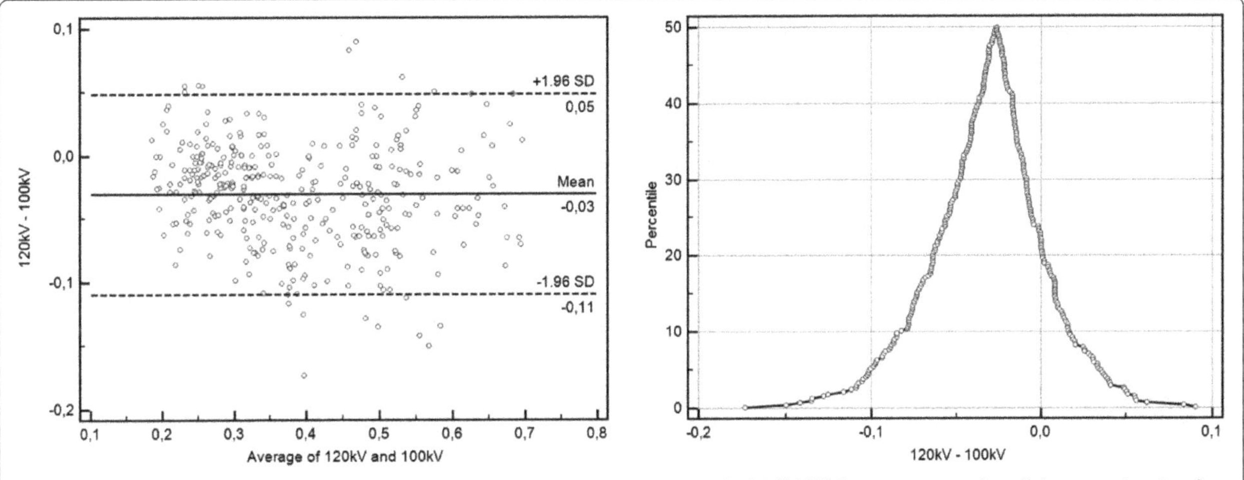

Figure 5 Method comparison plots for the tube voltage comparison at 100 and 120 kV. While on average only a slight overestimation for 100 kV is shown, some outliers are present in mountain plotting.

Discussion

Despite the fact that coronary CTA has found its way into the clinical workup of patients with suspected coronary artery disease, there are still major concerns regarding the applied radiation dose, which was determined to be in the typically order of 12 mSv (8–18 mSv) [10]. In comparison the effective radiation doses applied during invasive coronary angiography are reported to be approximately 5 mSv [11] with ranges from 2.3 to 22.7 mSv [3]. Because of its ability to rule out hemodynamically relevant coronary stenoses with a high negative predictive value, coronary CTA is especially suited for patients presenting with typical symptoms but having a low pre-test likelihood for coronary artery disease [12]. During the last few years different technical developments have been introduced in clinical routine practice in order to significantly reduce radiation dose of coronary CTA. These techniques include the use of lower tube voltage (e.g. 100 instead of 120 kV) [13] and the application of ECG-dependent tube current modulation. The latter bases upon the reduction of tube current of up to 80% during systolic phase and full dose is only applied during diastolic phase. This approach allows for dose reduction of up to 50% [14]. Another technique resulting in substantial reduction of radiation dose is realized by the use of prospective ECG-triggered transverse data acquisition (also known as "step and shot acquisition") instead of retrospective gated spiral scanning [15].

With the introduction of a modern dual-source CT scanner with simultaneous acquisition of 64 slices and a gantry rotation time of 330 ms a temporal resolution of 83 ms became technically feasible [16]. Latest generation of dual-source scanners reduced the rotation time to 0.28 s. Furthermore, due to the ca. 95° offset of both x-ray tubes within the gantry of dual source CT in combination with fast and precise table movement the use of high-pitch (>3.0) scan protocols for coronary CTA could be performed. The result was the ability to cover the whole heart within a single cardiac cycle [17]. Since then, different studies showed the diagnostic value of prospectively ECG-triggered high-pitch spiral coronary CTA [18,19].

The aim of the presented study was to investigate influence of scan protocol in combination with ECG-synchronization (prospective triggered high-pitch vs. retrospective ECG-gated spiral CT), tube voltage (100

Table 5 Pairwise comparisons of the average difference in degree of stenosis (Δ percentage) and measured plaque diameter for all used kernels

	796 mmHA/cm^3		401 mmHA/cm^3	
	Δ Diameter	Δ Percentage	Δ Diameter	Δ Percentage
B26f	0.88 ± 0.26 mm	15.9 ± 4.2%	0.39 ± 0.27 mm	8.6 ± 6.8%
I26f	0.86 ± 0.25 mm	10.8 ± 5.0%	0.38 ± 0.26 mm	4.3 ± 6.5%
B46f	0.53 ± 0.27 mm	9.2 ± 6.6%	0.18 ± 0.26 mm	6.9 ± 6.9%
B70f	0.36 ± 0.33 mm	15.3 ± 4.0%	0.26 ± 0.27 mm	8.5 ± 6.6%
I70f	0.34 ± 0.33 mm	8.9 ± 6.7%	0.21 ± 0.26 mm	5.8 ± 6.6%

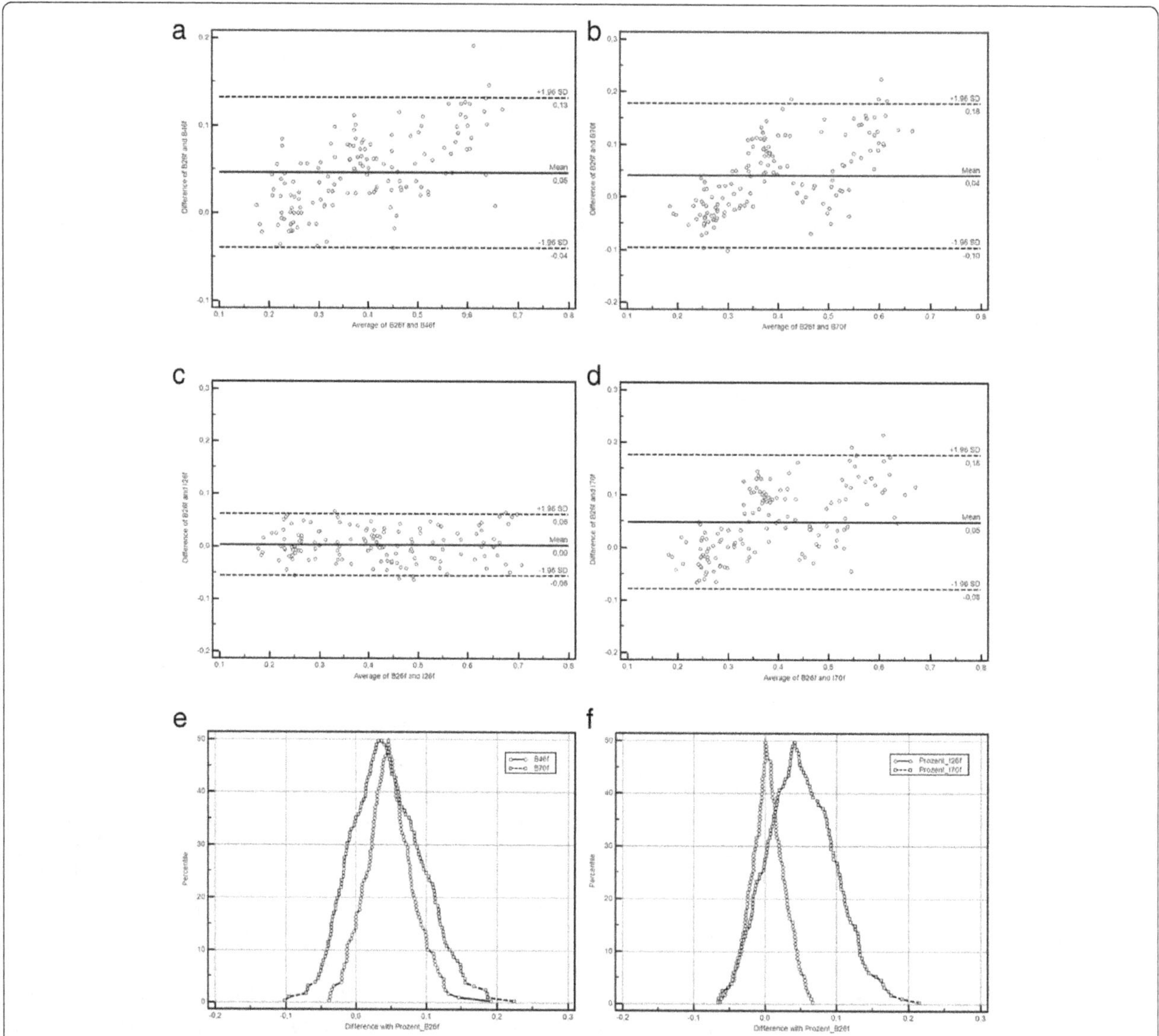

Figure 6 Method comparison plots for kernel comparisons (a-d Bland-Altman plots, e-f mountain plots). Shown are the differences between the standard B26f and the other kernels under investigation (**a**, **e**: B46f, **b**, **e**: B70f, **c**, **f**: I26f, **d**, **f**: I70f). While for B26f and I26f align perfectly, skewed distributions with outliers are visible for all other comparisons.

vs. 120 kV) and heart rate (50, 70, 90 bpm) on quantification of coronary artery stenosis due to plaques with different calcification levels. In general, all used CT examination protocols resulted in an overestimation of stenoses which increased with increasing calcium content and decreased with increasing grade of stenoses. This overestimation was slightly higher for the high pitch examination protocols in comparison to the retrospective ECG-gated technique. Both observations (overestimation of small lesions, which are highly calcified) are mainly due to blooming artifacts which occur when sharp edges with high attenuation differences are encountered in the scan volume [20,21]. A reason for the slight worsening of this phenomenon, when high pitch examination protocols are used, may be the fact that attenuation data of two separate detectors are used for image reconstruction. However, in the clinical situation this finding may be of little relevance due to a maximum difference of 3 percent points regarding grade of stenosis (small, highly calcified plaque).

In most of the recently published clinical studies on prospective ECG-triggered high pitch cardiac CT a heart rate more than 60 bpm was defined as an exclusion criterion [4,18]. In our experimental setup there were no significant differences regarding vessel diameter, plaque diameter and grade of stenoses between the different heart rates (50, 70, 90) although we found a slight trend to larger deviations of the measured parameters comparing the 50 and the 90 bpm data (Table 2). The motion artifacts observed at

Table 6 Dose comparison between the two used cardiac CT methods

Trigger	Gated	High pitch	Statistics
CTDIvol [mGy]	2829.8 ± 1539.4	258.0 ± 66.3	$p < 0.0001$
DLP [mGycm]	341.2 ± 150.7	36.3 ± 9.6	$p < 0.0001$

Both DLP and CTDIvol are significantly lower for high pitch cardiac CT protocols in comparison to gating.

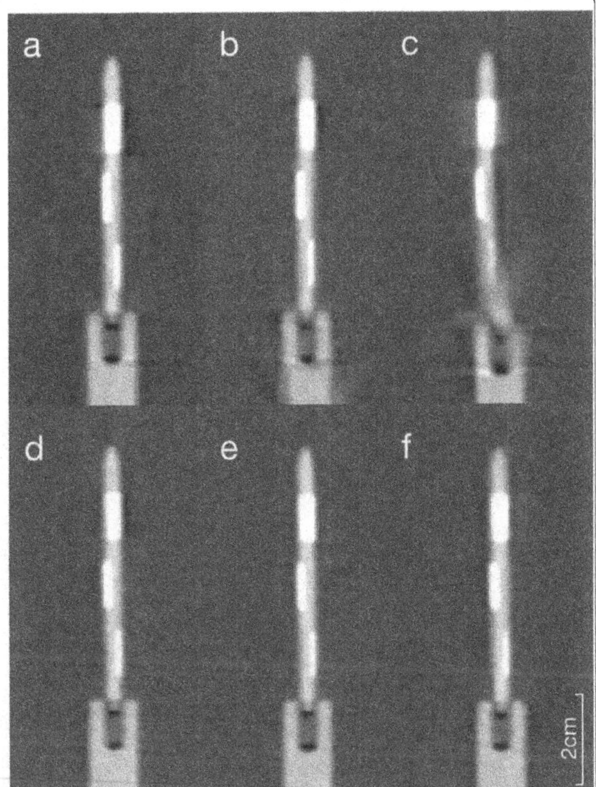

Figure 7 Coronary reformation of the phantom scans (a-c prospectively triggered high-pitch, d-f: retrospective gating) at different heart rate settings (a/d: 50 bpm, b/e: 70 bpm, c/f: 90 bpm).

90 bpm high pitch scanning should however raise concerns about the applicability of the technique at such heart rates (Figure 8). This finding is at least to some degree in contrast to clinical findings which were recently published [22]. Scharf et al. reported about a cohort of 111 consecutive patients who underwent prospectively ECG-triggered high-pitch spiral CT of the chest for non-cardiac reason. The evaluation of image quality showed a significant difference of mean heart rate and mean heart rate variability between patients with diagnostic and non-diagnostic images of the coronary arteries. The optimal values were calculated with a heart rates lower than 64 bpm and heart rate variabilities of less than 13 bpm. With respect to this result it needs to be discussed that we used an extremely reliable experimental setup providing an absolutely stable heart rate. Nevertheless, our results may be a hint that prospectively ECG-triggered high-pitch cardiac CT may also be suited for patients presenting stable heart rates > 60 bpm and a low heart rate variability. This hypothesis is supported by the results of Feuchtner et al. who found significantly higher diagnostic image quality in patients with stable sinus rhythm but without premedication for heart rate control in comparison to patients with arrhythmia using a prospective triggered "step and shoot" CT-examination mode [23]. In this study a mean heart rate of 66.2 ± 8 bpm in patient group with stable sinus rhythm was associated with only 0.5% non-diagnostic coronary segments whereas 4% of coronary segments were scored non-diagnostic in the arrhythmia group with a mean heart rate of 70 ± 15 bpm.

In our experimental setting the use of a prospectively ECG-triggered high-pitch spiral examination protocol resulted in a reduction of radiation exposure of approximately 90% in comparison to a retrospective ECG-gated cardiac CT-examination (Table 6). This finding is mainly due to the significant oversampling using a pitch of 0.19 for retrospective ECG-gating in order to acquire enough data in all cardiac phases. On the other hand this allows quantification of cardiac function in addition to the evaluation of coronary arteries. Comparing the measured diameters for the 100 and 120 kV examination modes we found a slight overestimation for the 100 kV CT-protocol (Table 3). However, we consider the differences (3 ± 8%) clinically not relevant whereas reduction of tube voltage results in further reduction of radiation dose applied to the patient. Due to the fact that lower tube voltage leads to increased image noise some authors used 100 kV scan protocols in patients < 100 kg body weight and 120 kV for > 100 kg, respectively [24].

Table 7 Dose comparison between the two used tube voltages

kV	100	120	Statistics
CTDIvol [mGy]	962.6 ± 862.9	2125.2 ± 2082.3	$p = 0.0005$
DLP [mGycm]	115.1 ± 93.4	262.4 ± 225.2	$p = 0.0002$

Both DLP and CTDIvol are significantly lower for 100 kV in comparison to 120 kV.

Due to the experimental design of the study our results cannot be directly transferred into the clinical situation. The employed phantom provides a stable sinus rhythm without any variability due to arrhythmia or respiration. Furthermore, motion of the patient is not an issue in this setup. Another limitation that needs to be discussed is the fact that we did not really measure the applied radiation dose but simply compared the dose indices derived from the CT-scanner's software. Moreover, regarding the different tube voltages (100 vs. 120 kV) we cannot make conclusion regarding image quality in obese patients due to

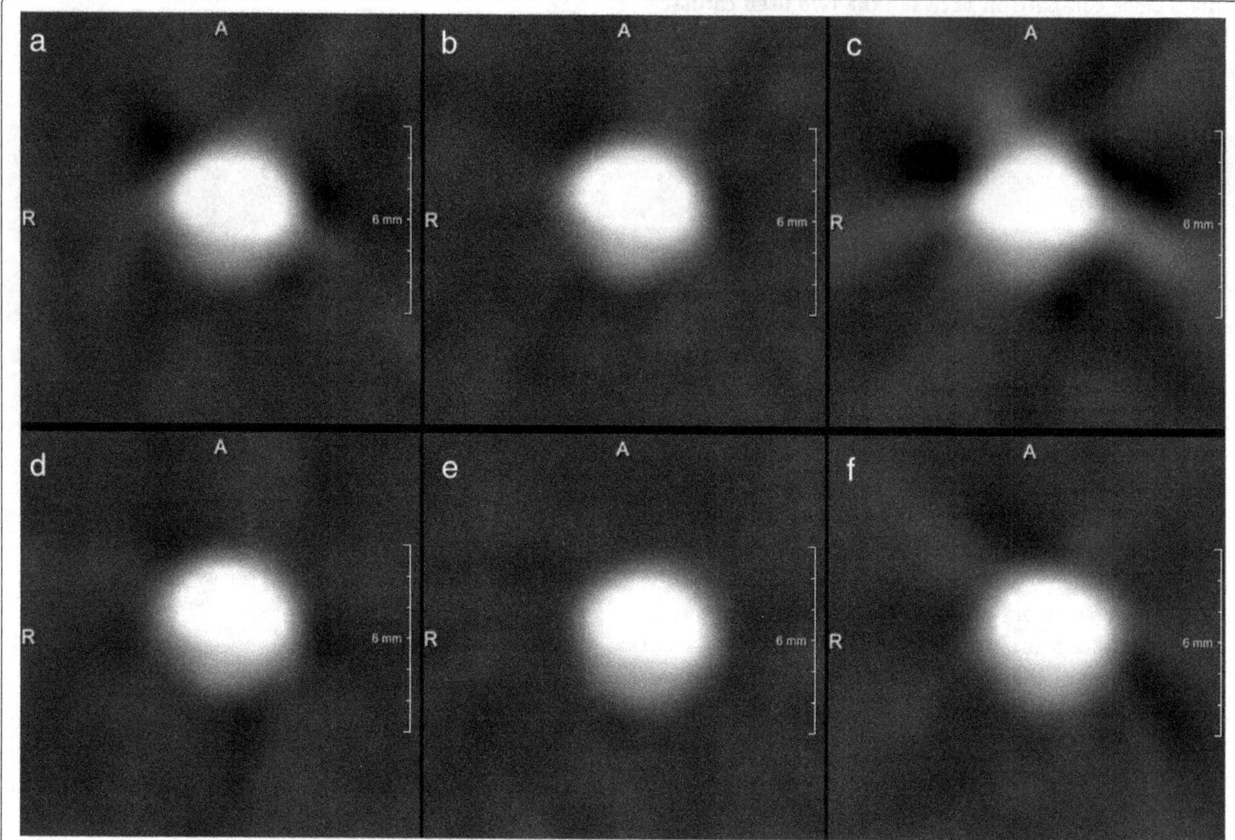

Figure 8 Image data reconstructed in different heart rate settings (a/d: 50 bpm; b/e: 70 bpm; c/f: 90 bpm, B26f) using either prospectively ECG-triggered high-pitch scanning (a – c) or retrospectively ECG-gated cardiac CT (d – f).

the fact that the phantom does not account for different subject weight. Further experiments should include these factors, for instance by applying different attenuation phantoms in the setup.

Conclusion

In conclusion, the presented results do not reveal any relevant differences in vessel diameter, plaque diameter and grade of stenoses between prospectively ECG-triggered high-pitch spiral CT in comparison to retrospectively ECG-gated spiral data acquisition in differently calcified plaques using a motion phantom. While there was reasonable agreement even at higher heart rates (90 bpm) between both examination modes, the presence of motion artifacts at 90 bpm questions the full applicability of the high pitch technique under these circumstances.

Competing interests

The study was carried out as part of a research agreement with Siemens Healthcare – CT Division -, Forchheim, Germany. TA is an employee of Siemens Healthcare, Forchheim, Germany.

Authors' contributions

Study design: TP, ED, PI, TA, CKK, AHM, PB, experiments, measurements: TP, ED, PI, TA, PB, manuscript draft: TP, PI, TA, CKK, AHM, PB. All authors read and approved the final manuscript.

Author details

[1]Department of Diagnostic and Interventional Radiology, Aachen University Hospital, RWTH Aachen University, Pauwelsstr. 30, 52074 Aachen, Germany. [2]Surgical Planning Laboratory, Department of Radiology, Brigham and Women's Hospital, 75 Francis Street, 02115 Boston, USA. [3]Applied Medical Engineering, Helmholtz-Institute Aachen, RWTH Aachen University, Pauwelsstr. 20, 52074 Aachen, Germany. [4]Siemens Healthcare, CT Division, Forchheim, Germany. [5]Department of Diagnostic and Interventional Radiology, University Hospital Marburg, Philipps University of Marburg, Marburg, Germany.

References

1. Vorobiof G, Achenbach S, Narula J: **Minimizing radiation dose for coronary CT angiography.** *Cardiol Clin* 2012, **30**(1):9–17.
2. Alkadhi H: **Radiation dose of cardiac CT–what is the evidence?** *Eur Radiol* 2009, **19**(6):1311–1315.
3. Einstein AJ, Moser KW, Thompson RC, Cerqueira MD, Henzlova MJ: **Radiation dose to patients from cardiac diagnostic imaging.** *Circulation* 2007, **116**(11):1290–1305.
4. Achenbach S, Marwan M, Ropers D, Schepis T, Pflederer T, Anders K, Kuettner A, Daniel WG, Uder M, Lell MM: **Coronary computed tomography angiography with a consistent dose below 1 mSv using prospectively electrocardiogram-triggered high-pitch spiral acquisition.** *Eur Heart J* 2010, **31**(3):340–346.
5. Flohr TG, Leng S, Yu L, Allmendinger T, Bruder H, Petersilka M, Eusemann CD, Stierstorfer K, Schmidt B, McCollough CH: **Dual-source spiral CT with pitch up to 3.2 and 75 ms temporal resolution: image reconstruction and assessment of image quality.** *Med Phys* 2009, **36**(12):5641–5653.
6. Flohr TG, McCollough CH, Bruder H, Petersilka M, Gruber K, Suss C, Grasruck M, Stierstorfer K, Krauss B, Raupach R, Primak AN, Kuttner A, Achenbach S, Becker C, Kopp A, Ohnesorge BM: **First performance evaluation of a dual-source CT (DSCT) system.** *Eur Radiol* 2006, **16**(2):256–268.

7. Morsbach F, Gordic S, Desbiolles L, Husarik D, Frauenfelder T, Schmidt B, Allmendinger T, Wildermuth S, Alkadhi H, Leschka S: **Performance of turbo high-pitch dual-source CT for coronary CT angiography: first *ex vivo* and patient experience.** *Eur Radiol* 2014, **24**(8):1889–1895.
8. Gordic S, Husarik DB, Desbiolles L, Leschka S, Frauenfelder T, Alkadhi H: **High-pitch coronary CT angiography with third generation dual-source CT: limits of heart rate.** *Int J Cardiovasc Imaging* 2014, **30**(6):1173–1179.
9. Ulzheimer S, Kalender WA: **Assessment of calcium scoring performance in cardiac computed tomography.** *Eur Radiol* 2003, **13**(3):484–497.
10. Hausleiter J, Meyer T, Hermann F, Hadamitzky M, Krebs M, Gerber TC, McCollough C, Martinoff S, Kastrati A, Schomig A, Achenbach S: **Estimated radiation dose associated with cardiac CT angiography.** *JAMA* 2009, **301**(5):500–507.
11. Coles DR, Smail MA, Negus IS, Wilde P, Oberhoff M, Karsch KR, Baumbach A: **Comparison of radiation doses from multislice computed tomography coronary angiography and conventional diagnostic angiography.** *J Am Coll Cardiol* 2006, **47**(9):1840–1845.
12. Hoffman U, Venkatesh V, White RD, Woodard PK, Carr JJ, Dorbala S, Earls JP, Jacobs JE, Mammen L, Martin ET, Ryan T, White CS: *ACR Appropriateness Criteria: Acute Nonspecific Chest Pain - low Probability of Coronary Artery Disease.* Reston, VA, USA: American College of Radiology; 2011. ACR Appropriateness Criteria.
13. Pflederer T, Rudofsky L, Ropers D, Bachmann S, Marwan M, Daniel WG, Achenbach S: **Image quality in a low radiation exposure protocol for retrospectively ECG-gated coronary CT angiography.** *AJR Am J Roentgenol* 2009, **192**(4):1045–1050.
14. Paul JF, Abada HT: **Strategies for reduction of radiation dose in cardiac multislice CT.** *Eur Radiol* 2007, **17**(8):2028–2037.
15. Maruyama T, Takada M, Hasuike T, Yoshikawa A, Namimatsu E, Yoshizumi T: **Radiation dose reduction and coronary assessability of prospective electrocardiogram-gated computed tomography coronary angiography: comparison with retrospective electrocardiogram-gated helical scan.** *J Am Coll Cardiol* 2008, **52**(18):1450–1455.
16. Flohr TG, Bruder H, Stierstorfer K, Petersilka M, Schmidt B, McCollough CH: **Image reconstruction and image quality evaluation for a dual source CT scanner.** *Med Phys* 2008, **35**(12):5882–5897.
17. Achenbach S, Marwan M, Schepis T, Pflederer T, Bruder H, Allmendinger T, Petersilka M, Anders K, Lell M, Kuettner A, Ropers D, Daniel WG, Flohr T: **High-pitch spiral acquisition: a new scan mode for coronary CT angiography.** *J Cardiovasc Comput Tomogr* 2009, **3**(2):117–121.
18. Achenbach S, Goroll T, Seltmann M, Pflederer T, Anders K, Ropers D, Daniel WG, Uder M, Lell M, Marwan M: **Detection of coronary artery stenoses by low-dose, prospectively ECG-triggered, high-pitch spiral coronary CT angiography.** *JACC Cardiovasc Imaging* 2011, **4**(4):328–337.
19. Kropil P, Rojas CA, Ghoshhajra B, Lanzman RS, Miese FR, Scherer A, Kalra M, Abbara S: **Prospectively ECG-triggered high-pitch spiral acquisition for cardiac CT angiography in routine clinical practice: initial results.** *J Thorac Imaging* 2012, **27**(3):194–201.
20. Dey D, Slomka P, Chien D, Fieno D, Abidov A, Saouaf R, Thomson L, Friedman JD, Berman DS: **Direct quantitative *in vivo* comparison of calcified atherosclerotic plaque on vascular MRI and CT by multimodality image registration.** *J Magn Reson Imaging* 2006, **23**(3):345–354.
21. Joseph PM, Spital RD: **The exponential edge-gradient effect in x-ray computed tomography.** *Phys Med Biol* 1981, **26**(3):473–487.
22. Scharf M, Bink R, May MS, Hentschke C, Achenbach S, Uder M, Lell MM: **High-pitch thoracic CT with simultaneous assessment of coronary arteries: effect of heart rate and heart rate variability on image quality and diagnostic accuracy.** *JACC Cardiovasc Imaging* 2011, **4**(6):602–609.
23. Feuchtner G, Goetti R, Plass A, Baumueller S, Stolzmann P, Scheffel H, Wieser M, Marincek B, Alkadhi H, Leschka S: **Dual-step prospective ECG-triggered 128-slice dual-source CT for evaluation of coronary arteries and cardiac function without heart rate control: a technical note.** *Eur Radiol* 2010, **20**(9):2092–2099.
24. Lell M, Marwan M, Schepis T, Pflederer T, Anders K, Flohr T, Allmendinger T, Kalender W, Ertel D, Thierfelder C, Kuettner A, Ropers D, Daniel WG, Achenbach S: **Prospectively ECG-triggered high-pitch spiral acquisition for coronary CT angiography using dual source CT: technique and initial experience.** *Eur Radiol* 2009, **19**(11):2576–2583.

Permissions

All chapters in this book were first published in MI, by BioMed Central; hereby published with permission under the Creative Commons Attribution License or equivalent. Every chapter published in this book has been scrutinized by our experts. Their significance has been extensively debated. The topics covered herein carry significant findings which will fuel the growth of the discipline. They may even be implemented as practical applications or may be referred to as a beginning point for another development.

The contributors of this book come from diverse backgrounds, making this book a truly international effort. This book will bring forth new frontiers with its revolutionizing research information and detailed analysis of the nascent developments around the world.

We would like to thank all the contributing authors for lending their expertise to make the book truly unique. They have played a crucial role in the development of this book. Without their invaluable contributions this book wouldn't have been possible. They have made vital efforts to compile up to date information on the varied aspects of this subject to make this book a valuable addition to the collection of many professionals and students.

This book was conceptualized with the vision of imparting up-to-date information and advanced data in this field. To ensure the same, a matchless editorial board was set up. Every individual on the board went through rigorous rounds of assessment to prove their worth. After which they invested a large part of their time researching and compiling the most relevant data for our readers.

The editorial board has been involved in producing this book since its inception. They have spent rigorous hours researching and exploring the diverse topics which have resulted in the successful publishing of this book. They have passed on their knowledge of decades through this book. To expedite this challenging task, the publisher supported the team at every step. A small team of assistant editors was also appointed to further simplify the editing procedure and attain best results for the readers.

Apart from the editorial board, the designing team has also invested a significant amount of their time in understanding the subject and creating the most relevant covers. They scrutinized every image to scout for the most suitable representation of the subject and create an appropriate cover for the book.

The publishing team has been an ardent support to the editorial, designing and production team. Their endless efforts to recruit the best for this project, has resulted in the accomplishment of this book. They are a veteran in the field of academics and their pool of knowledge is as vast as their experience in printing. Their expertise and guidance has proved useful at every step. Their uncompromising quality standards have made this book an exceptional effort. Their encouragement from time to time has been an inspiration for everyone.

The publisher and the editorial board hope that this book will prove to be a valuable piece of knowledge for researchers, students, practitioners and scholars across the globe.

List of Contributors

Robert Rusina
Department of Neurology, Thomayer Teaching Hospital and Institute for Postgraduate Education in Medicine, Prague, Czech Republic

Jaromír Kukal and Tomáš Bělíček
Department of Software Engineering in Economy, Faculty of Nuclear Science and Physical Engineering, Czech Technical University, Prague, Czech Republic

Marie Buncová
Department of Nuclear Medicine, Institute for Clinical and Experimental Medicine, Prague, Czech Republic

Radoslav Matěj
Department of Pathology and Molecular Medicine, Thomayer Teaching Hospital, Prague, Czech Republic

Ilse M Purmer, Erik P van Iperen, Jan M Binnekade Marcus J Schultz and Janneke Horn
Department of Intensive Care Medicine, Academic Medical Center Amsterdam, The Netherlands

Ludo F M Beenen
Department of Radiology, Academic Medical Center, Amsterdam, The Netherlands

Michael J Kuiper
Department of Intensive Care, Medicine, Medical Center LeeuwardenLeeuwarden, The Netherlands

Peter W Vandertop
Neurosurgical Center Amsterdam, Academic Medical Center, Amsterdam, The Netherlands

Azusa Tokue and Yoshito Tsushima
Department of Diagnostic and Interventional Radiology, Gunma University Hospital, 3-39-22 Showa-machi, Maebashi, Gunma 371-8511, Japan

Hiroyuki Tokue
Department of Radiology, Maebashi Red Cross Hospital, Maebashi, Gunma, Japan
Department of Diagnostic and Interventional Radiology, Gunma University Hospital, 3-39-22 Showa-machi, Maebashi, Gunma 371-8511, Japan

Chung-yao Yu and Neville Sammel
Cardiology Department, St Vincent's Hospital, Darlinghurst, Sydney 2010, Australia

James M Otton, Justin Phan, Michael Feneley and Jane McCrohon
University of New South Wales, Sydney, NSW, Austra
Cardiology Department, St Vincent's Hospital, Darlinghurst, Sydney 2010, Australia

Richard E Jacob and James P Carson
Biological Sciences Division, Pacific Northwest National Laboratory, 902 Battelle Blvd., Richland, WA 99352, USA

Dominik Vollherbst, Miguel F Wachter, Ulrike Stampfl, Daniel Gnutzmann, Nadine Bellemann, Anne Schmitz, Hans U Kauczor, Boris A Radeleff and Christof M Sommer
Department of Diagnostic and Interventional Radiology, University Hospital Heidelberg, Heidelberg, Germany

Jens Werner and Stefan Fritz
Department of General, Abdominal and Transplantation Surgery, University Hospital Heidelberg, Heidelberg, Germany

Sascha Zelzer
Medical and Biological Informatics, German Cancer Research Center, Heidelberg, Germany

Maya B Wolf
Department of Radiology, German Cancer Research Center (dkfz) Heidelberg, INF 280, Heidelberg, Germany

Jürgen Knapp
Department of Anesthesiology, University Hospital Heidelberg, Heidelberg, Germany

Philippe L Pereira
Clinic for Radiology, Minimally-invasive Therapies and Nuclear Medicine, SLK Kliniken Heilbronn GmbH, Heilbronn, Germany

Hennie Verburg, Laurens C van de Ridder and Peter Pilot
Department of Orthopaedics, Reinier de Graaf Groep, Reinier de Graafweg 3, 2625 AD Delft, The Netherlands

Vincent WJ Verhoeven
Department of Nuclear Medicine, Reinier de Graaf Groep, Reinier de Graafweg 3, 2625 AD Delft, The Netherlands

Makoto Ishii, Kazuma Yagi, Mizuha Haraguchi, Masako Matsusaka, Shoji Suzuki, Takanori Asakura, Takahiro Asami, Fumitake Saito, Koichi Fukunaga, Sadatomo Tasakan and Tomoko Betsuyaku
Division of Pulmonary Medicine, Department of Medicine, Keio University School of Medicine, 35 Shinanomachi, Shinjuku-ku, Tokyo 160-8582, Japan

Ho Namkoong
Japan Society for the Promotion of Science, Tokyo, Japan
Division of Pulmonary Medicine, Department of Medicine, Keio University School of Medicine, 35 Shinanomachi, Shinjuku-ku, Tokyo 160-8582, Japan

Naoki Hasegawa and Hiroshi Fujiwara
Center for Infectious Diseases and Infection Control, Keio University School of Medicine, Tokyo, Japan

Thomas Baum, Eduardo Grande Garcia, Olga Gordijenko, Hans Liebl, Pia M. Jungmann, Tina Zahel, Ernst J. Rummeny and Simone Waldt
Institut für Radiologie, Klinikum rechts der Isar, Technische Universität München, Ismaninger Str. 22, 81675 München, Germany

Rainer Burgkart and Eduardo Grande Garcia
Klinik für Orthopädie, Abteilung für Biomechanik, Klinikum rechts der Isar, Technische Universität München, Ismaninger Str. 22, 81675 München, Germany

Michael Gruber
Universitätsklinik für Radiologie und Nuklearmedizin, Abteilung für Neuroradiologie und Muskuloskeletale Radiologie, Medizinischen Universität Wien, Währinger Gürtel 18-20, 1090 Wien, Austria

Jan S. Bauer
Abteilung für Neuroradiologie, Klinikum rechts der Isar, Technische Universität München, Ismaninger Str. 22, 81675 München, Germany

An De Crop, Tom Van Hoof, Katharina D'Herde, Hubert Thierens and Klaus Bacher
Department of Basic Medical Sciences, Ghent University, Proeftuinstraat 86, B-9000 Ghent, Belgium

Merel Vergauwen, Tom Dewaele, Eric Achten, Koenraad Verstraete, Mathias Van Borsel and Peter Smeets
Department of Radiology, Ghent University Hospital, De Pintelaan 185, B-9000 Ghent, Belgium

Hideyuki Suenaga, Kazuto Hoshi and Tsuyoshi Takato
Department of Oral-Maxillofacial Surgery, Dentistry and Orthodontics, The University of Tokyo Hospital, 7-3-1 Hongo, Bunkyo ku, Tokyo 113 8656, Japan

Huy Hoang Tran and Ken Masamune
Department of Mechano-Informatics, Graduate School of Information Science and Technology, The University of Tokyo, Tokyo, Japan

Hongen Liao
Department of Bioengineering, Graduate School of Engineering, The University of Tokyo, Tokyo, Japan
Department of Biomedical Engineering, School of Medicine, Tsinghua University, Beijing, China

Ken Masamune
Faculty of Advanced Technology and Surgery, Institute of Advanced Biomedical Engineering and Science, Tokyo Women's Medical University, Tokyo, Japan

Takeyoshi Dohi
Department of Mechanical Engineering, School of Engineering, Tokyo Denki University, Tokyo, Japan

Alexandra Platon, Minerva Becker, Christoph D. Becker and Pierre-Alexandre Poletti
Department of Radiology, University Hospital of Geneva, 4, rue Gabrielle-Perret-Gentil, 1211, Geneva, Switzerland

Eric Lock
Scientific Police, Geneva State Police, Geneva, Switzerland

Hans Wolff
Division of Correctional Medicine and Psychiatry, University Hospital of Geneva, ch. du Petit-Bel-Air 2, 1225, Chêne-Bourg, Switzerland

Thomas Perneger
Division of Clinical Epidemiology, University Hospital of Geneva, 4, rue Gabrielle-Perret-Gentil, Geneva, Switzerland

Vipula R. Bataduwaarachchi
Department of Pharmacology and Pharmacy, Faculty of Medicine University of Colombo, Colombo 8, Sri Lanka

Nirmali Tissera
Department of Medicine, National Hospital, Ward Place, Colombo, Sri Lanka

Krisztián Szigeti, Ildikó Horváth, Dániel S. Veres and Domokos Máthé
Department of Biophysics and Radiation Biology, Semmelweis University, Tűzoltó utca, Budapest H-1094, Hungary

Ilona Czibak, Tibor Szabó, Márta Pócsik and Domokos Máthé
CROmed Translational Research Centers Ltd., Baross utca 91-95, Budapest H-1047, Hungary

Kinga Karlinger and Csaba Korom
Department of Radiology and Oncotherapy, Semmelweis University, Üllői út 78/A, Budapest H-1082, Hungary

Zoltán Gyöngyi and Ferenc Budán
Department of Public Health Medicine, University of Pécs, Szigeti út 12, Pécs H-7624, Hungary

Ralf Bergmann
Institute of Radiopharmaceutical Cancer Research, Helmholtz-Zentrum Dresden-Rossendorf, Dresden D-01314, Germany

Ferenc Budán
MedProDevelop Kft, Irgalmasok utcája 16, Pécs H-7621, Hungary

Hsu-Chao Chang
Department of Radiology, Taipei Tzu-Chi Hospital, Buddhist Tzu-Chi Medical Foundation, No. 289, Jianguo Rd, Xindian Dist, New Taipei City 23143, Taiwan

Mei-Chen Yang
School of Medicine, Tzu Chi University, Hualien, Taiwan
Division of Pulmonary Medicine, Department of Internal Medicine, Taipei Tzu-Chi Hospital, Buddhist Tzu-Chi Medical Foundation, No. 289, Jianguo Rd, Xindian Dist, New Taipei City 23143, Taiwan

Yu-Ying Lin, Yi-Shuan Hwang and Kar-Wai Lui
Department of Medical Imaging and Intervention, Chang Gung Memorial Hospital at Linkou, 5 Fushing Street, Kweishan, Taoyuan 333, Taiwan, Republic of China
Department of Medical Imaging and Radiological Sciences, College of Medicine, Chang Gung University, Taoyuan, Taiwan

Hui-Yu Tsai
Institute of Nuclear Engineering and Science, National Tsing Hua University, Hsinchu 300, Taiwan

M. Peters
Department of Internal Medicine, Division of Rheumatology, Maastricht University Medical Centre, NL-6202 Maastricht, AZ, the Netherlands
NUTRIM School for Nutrition and Translational Research in Metabolism, Maastricht University, Maastricht, the Netherlands

P. Geusens, A. van Tubergen, A. Scharmga and M. Peters
CAPHRI, Care and Public Health Research Institute, Maastricht University, Maastricht, the Netherlands
Department of Internal Medicine, Division of Rheumatology, Maastricht University Medical Centre, NL-6202 Maastricht, AZ, the Netherlands
NUTRIM School for Nutrition and Translational Research in Metabolism, Maastricht University, Maastricht, the Netherlands

D. Loeffen and R. Weijers
Department of Radiology, Maastricht University Medical Centre, Maastricht, the Netherlands

J. de Jong
Department of Radiology, Maastricht University Medical Centre, Maastricht, the Netherlands
Department of Internal Medicine, Division of Rheumatology, Maastricht University Medical Centre, NL-6202 Maastricht, AZ, the Netherlands
NUTRIM School for Nutrition and Translational Research in Metabolism, Maastricht University, Maastricht, the Netherlands

S. K. Boyd and C. Barnabe
Cumming School of Medicine, McCaig Institute for Bone and Joint Health, University of Calgary, Calgary, Canada

K. S. Stok
Department of Biomedical Engineering, the University of Melbourne, Melbourne, Australia

B. van Rietbergen
Faculty of Biomedical Engineering, Eindhoven University of Technology, Eindhoven, the Netherlands
Department of Orthopaedic Surgery, Maastricht University Medical Centre, Maastricht, the Netherlands

J. van den Bergh
Department of Internal Medicine, VieCuri Medical Centre, Venlo, the Netherlands
Department of Internal Medicine, Division of Rheumatology, Maastricht University Medical Centre, NL-6202 Maastricht, AZ, the Netherlands
NUTRIM School for Nutrition and Translational Research in Metabolism, Maastricht University, Maastricht, the Netherlands

Hui Yu, Haijun Wang, Yao Shi and Yuzhen Cao
Department of Biomedical Engineering, Tianjin University, Tianjin, China

Ke Xu
Department of Orthopedic, Tianjin Medical University General Hospital, Tianjin, China

Xuyao Yu
Department of Radiation Oncology, Tianjin Medical University Cancer Institute & Hospital, Tianjin, China

Jamshid Sadiqi and Hidayatullah Hamidi
Department of Radiology, French Medical Institute for Mothers & Children (FMIC), behind Kabul Medical University, Jamal mina, Kabul, Afghanistan

C Jason Liang, Richard A Kronmal and Elizabeth R Brown
Department of Biostatistics, University of Washington, Seattle, WA, USA

Matthew J Budoff
Division of Cardiology, Los Angeles Biomedical Research Institute at Harbor- UCLA Medical Center, Torrance, CA, USA

Joel D Kaufman
Environmental & Occupational Health Sciences, Medicine, and Epidemiology, University of Washington, Seattle, WA, USA

Elizabeth R Brown
Vaccine and Infectious Disease and Public Health Sciences Divisions, Fred Hutchinson Cancer Research Center, Seattle, WA, USA

Gianni Frisardi and Flavio Frisardi
"Epochè" Orofacial Pain Center, Nettuno (Rome), Italy
Department of Prosthetic Rehabilitation, University of Sassari, Italy

Giacomo Chessa
Department of Prosthetic Rehabilitation, University of Sassari, Italy

Sandro Barone, Alessandro Paoli and Armando Razionale
Department of Mechanical, Nuclear and Production Engineering, University of Pisa, Italy

Ke-Zeng Li, Yuan Gao, Ru Zhang and Tao Hu
State Key Laboratory of Oral Diseases, West China College of Stomatology, Sichuan University, Chengdu, P.R. China

Bin Guo
Institute of Stomatology, Chinese PLA General Hospital, Beijing, P.R. China

Andrew L Chan, Maya M Juarez and Timothy E Albertson
Division of Pulmonary/Critical Care and Sleep Medicine, University of California, Davis Medical Center, Sacramento, CA and VA Northern California Health Care System, USA

David K Shelton and Taylor MacDonald
Department of Radiology, University of California, Davis Medical Center, Sacramento, CA, USA

Chin-Shang Li
Department of Public Health Sciences, Division of Biostatistics, University of California, Davis, CA, USA

Tzu-Chun Lin
Department of Statistics, University of California, Davis, CA, USA

Alijavad Moosavi
Department of pulmonary diseases, Rasoul-e-Akram Hospital, Tehran University of Medical Sciences, Sattakhan street, Tehran(1445613131), Iran

Hanieh Raji
Department of pulmonary diseases, Jundishopur University of Medical Sciences, Golestan boulevard, Ahvaz, Iran

Mojtaba Teimoori
Nephrology and Urology Research Center, Medical Faculty, Baqyatallah University of Medical Sciences, Mollasadra street, Tehran, Iran

Shadi Ghourchian
Medical student, Scientific students' research center of Tehran University of Medical Sciences, DDRI of Rasoul hospital, Sattakhan street, Tehran (1445613131), Iran

Eva Donandt and Christiane K Kuhl
Department of Diagnostic and Interventional Radiology, Aachen University Hospital, RWTH Aachen University, Pauwelsstr. 30, 52074 Aachen, Germany

Thomas Allmendinger
Siemens Healthcare, CT Division, Forchheim, Germany

Index

www.ingramcontent.com/pod-product-compliance
Lightning Source LLC
Chambersburg PA
CBHW082022190326
41458CB00010B/3246

* 9 7 8 1 6 3 9 2 7 0 6 8 2 *